Sergio Starkstein

A Conceptual and Therapeutic Analysis of Fear

palgrave
macmillan

Sergio Starkstein
University of Western Australia
Fremantle, WA, Australia

ISBN 978-3-030-08683-1 ISBN 978-3-319-78349-9 (eBook)
https://doi.org/10.1007/978-3-319-78349-9

Softcover re-print of the Hardcover 1st edition 2018

Cover credit: Ian Dagnall/Alamy Stock Photo

Printed on acid-free paper

This Palgrave Macmillan imprint is published by the registered company Springer International Publishing AG part of Springer Nature
The registered company address is: Gewerbestrasse 11, 6330 Cham, Switzerland

A Conceptual and Therapeutic Analysis of Fear

"Surprising though it may seem, fear has a history, and in this elegant and wide-ranging study Sergio Starkstein, with his combined experience as linguist, philosopher, and psychotherapist, shows clearly how the concept has varied from classical antiquity to today. With a judicious selection of texts, Starkstein provides a kaleidoscopic image of fear, at the same time revealing the weakness, evasions, and arbitrary generalisations of theories old and new. It is a masterful achievement."

—David Konstan, *Professor of Classics, New York University, USA*

"With his monumental work about how fear and related apprehensive emotions have been understood and remedied in Western philosophical and psychological traditions, Starkstein completes a notable gap in the literature on affective states and their treatment that is particularly welcome in today's era, dominated by reductive biomedical and neuroscientific models. Writing with a profound clinical appreciation of the devastating effects of such negative emotions, Dr Starkstein shows himself equally adept as a scholar of ancient, as well as modern, and contemporary, philosophy."

—Jennifer Radden, *Professor emerita of Philosophy, University of Massachusetts, Boston, USA*

"This book on the concept of Fear shows the same precision, originality and scholarship shown by Professor Starkstein's neuropsychiatric publications. As it only happens to few researchers, he has come to realize that in the field of psychiatry 'explanation' is but an incomplete conceptual device. Consequently, he has started his long pilgrimage towards the more satisfactory but elusive 'understanding'. Whether expert or neophyte, the reader will find something valuable in this book. It could not be otherwise as it vividly maps the cultural and clinical biography of fear, a concept that remains central to the understanding of human behaviour."

—German E Berrios, *Emeritus Professor of Psychiatry, University of Cambridge, UK*

For Peta

Preface

Fear is a critical emotion in everyday life as it permeates many of our minor and major decisions. Explicitly or implicitly, fear is one of the emotions that most strongly shape human life. In this book, fear and its philosophical remedies will be analysed through the work of western philosophers and thinkers selected on the basis of their overall contributions in conceptualizing fear and suggesting therapies for reducing its more damaging effects.

This book describes how Epicurus, Cicero and Seneca considered fear as the main obstacle to achieving peace of mind and that their ethical systems were primarily focused on dealing with this emotion by proposing eclectic philosophical therapies. In a similar vein, Montaigne presented a humanist therapy of fear instrumented as a critical self-analysis.

In contrast, a reductionist trend in thinking about fear emerged during the seventeenth century with the growth of materialistic philosophy. Thomas Hobbes reduced fear into a necessary tool for social control, whereas René Descartes demoted fear to a secondary emotion enacted by a dualist mechanism. This trend continued with William James's conception of fear as a sensory-somatic reflex and with Sigmund Freud's hypothesis of a neurotic fear resulting from universal unconscious laws.

The book also discusses how current neuroscience has reduced fear to decontextualized neural changes and how the dominant trend in psychiatry has reified anxiety into arbitrary nomenclatures of unclear validity. On a completely different tack, Ludwig Wittgenstein provided a broad 'perspicuous presentation' of fear, but his nuanced analysis has been largely ignored in philosophical studies.

Overall, it can be seen that, in keeping with the scientific revolution, the influential perspectives throughout the philosophical history of fear change from understandings that philosophy itself and reason are the best therapies for fear towards the medicalization of fear that is dominant today. By following these specific and diverse historical convergences, however, their criss-crossing insights and oversights, this work aims to enhance the conceptual understanding of fear and the variety of perspectives and therapies available for accommodating its enduring influence in our lives.

Fremantle, Australia | Sergio Starkstein

Acknowledgements

After several decades of doing empirical research in the field of neurosciences, I began my degree of philosophy at the Universidad del Salvador, in Buenos Aires. After migrating to Australia, I finished my Honours degree in philosophy at the University of Western Australia. Wanting to pursue a Ph.D. in the philosophy of emotions, I had the fortune of meeting Dr. Peta Bowden at Murdoch University. Her friendliness and enthusiasm convinced me that Peta would be an ideal supervisor, and we embarked together into investigating the philosophical aspects of fear from different perspectives. My first drafts came back with the 'red sea' of Peta's corrections, and I will always cherish our monthly meetings in the cafeteria of Fremantle Prison (of all places!). After having published several hundred papers and three books in neuroscience, I realized that I had to learn how to write meaningfully in a very different field all over again. It was Peta who, with utmost patience, taught me how to write in a clear style, without leaving loose ends, and always conveying a hopefully original view. I will always thank her for having shown me the way to write philosophy in a professional way. Besides, Peta made the famous motto of 'philosophy as a way of life' a true reality, as we both had to go through troublesome times during the ten years we worked together. Peta, you are a true model of a philosopher in the full sense of the term.

I also want to thank Emeritus Professor German Berrios (University of Cambridge) who for the past five years educated me in the intricacies of writing philosophy from historical and conceptual perspectives. German is, in my opinion, the most accomplished psychiatrist and philosopher in the western hemisphere, and what I have learnt from him opened new perspectives in my professional life.

Finally, I want to thank my wife, Corina, and my children Lucila, Guillermo and Cecilia (in chronological order), for their understanding through the many long hours I had to devote to writing this book, secluded in my 'garret'. I love them all.

Contents

List of Figures

1
Introduction

> Empty is the argument of the philosopher by which no human disease is healed; for just as there is no benefit in medicine if it does not drive out bodily diseases, so there is no benefit in philosophy if it does not drive out the disease of the soul.
>
> Porphyry, *To Marcella* (Inwood and Gerson 1994, p. 82)

Fear is one of the most significant emotions in shaping human life. Fear permeates many of our minor and major decisions, and explicitly or implicitly influences our choices and behaviour. We fear events, such as making mistakes at work, and we fear real objects, such as snakes and spiders, fictional objects, such as running into ghosts in the dark, or non-material objects, such as the uncertainty of the future. Fear sometimes protects us from short- and long-term dangers, but it may also be a source of severe distress. We may appreciate this distinction in the life of Pyrrho of Ellis (c.360 BCE–c.270 BCE), one of the most fearless philosophers of Antiquity. His ethics of suspension of judgment included a remarkable impassivity in daily life events. Diogenes Laertius describes Pyrrho as "taking no precaution, but facing all risks as they came, whether carts, precipices, dogs or what not…he was kept out of harm's way by his friends who…used to follow close after him"

S. Starkstein, *A Conceptual and Therapeutic Analysis of Fear*,
https://doi.org/10.1007/978-3-319-78349-9_1

(Laertius 1925: 9.61).[1] Pyrrho lived in a state of extraordinary tranquillity and emotional indifference. It was his friends who suffered the fear Pyrrho seems to have lacked.

Fear has been relatively neglected as an object for philosophical study in proportion to its importance. In its more detrimental severity, fear has been addressed by sociologists writing on the concept of 'risk society' (Adam et al. 2004, p. 88),[2] as well as historians and psychologists conceptualising the twentieth Century as the 'age of anxiety' (Dunant and Porter 1996).[3] During the twentieth century severe manifestations of fear, such as anxiety, panic and phobias have been increasingly managed by psychiatrists and psychologists. A personal anecdote related to this trend may help to illustrate the interest of anxious individuals about philosophical therapies.

While working as a practicing psychiatrist in an anxiety clinic, I began studies on Epicurean and Stoic philosophy and became markedly impressed by the relevance of fear in Hellenistic texts, and especially by the variety of remedies recommended by these philosophical schools. I then assembled a short pamphlet that included brief remarks from Epicurus, Cicero and Seneca with advice on managing fear, for patients to read in the waiting area. To my surprise, that little pamphlet was strongly demanded and ran through several reprints including expansions and revisions. Furthermore, a sizeable number of patients reported feeling better after reading the short text. This personal experience kindled my interest in providing a conceptual analysis of fear and its therapies as proposed by philosophers and major thinkers.

---

[1]Reference to Diogenes Laertius is provided as year of publication, followed by volume and section numbers.

[2]'Risk society' (Adam et al. 2004, p. 5) is conceptualised as a social condition produced by specific economic, political and cultural variables, and is characterised by a pervasive increase in uncertainty influencing social structures.

[3]In their text entitled *The Age of Anxiety* Dinant and Porter (p. xvi) describe the twentieth century as an age of expanding choices but limited by a decrease in the sense of social control and an increase of fear of the future. In a comic vein, they consider that the new millennia placed humans at a crossroad, where "one path leads to despair and utter hopelessness, the other to total extinction. Let us pray that we have the wisdom to choose correctly" (p. xviii).

It is necessary at this stage to provide more clarification of the object of this work. I shall examine the concept and therapies of fear, where I take fear to include several semantically-related emotional conditions, such as anxiety, phobias, dread, panic, and anguish. The reason for this broad take on fear is justified by a brief lexical analysis presented below which shows that these terms have crisscrossing uses and intertwined histories that do not allow for exhaustive distinctions between them and the phenomena they denote.

1.1 A Lexical Introduction to the Concept of Fear

In the secular Old Greek lexicon, *phobos* had the meaning of "someone or something that is to be feared," of terror (usually when referring to a single individual), or panic (when referring to a group) (Liddell and Scott 1996, p. 1947).[4] In Homer, *phobos* was used to denote panic or flight (Konstan 2006a); Herodotus used it as generic fear or terror; Hippocrates used *phobos* in the milder sense of doubt or scruple; and it also had the theological connotation of awe and reverence for a divine being, as well as meaning dread and the act of, or the object for, striking terror into someone (Liddell and Scott 1996, p. 1947). The Old Greek also included the noun *alusmos* to denote the somatic aspects of fear (e.g. restlessness, palpitations, sweating, tremor) (Liddell and Scott 1996, p. 74). The root *aluo* had the meaning of wandering restlessly and being uneasy, whereas *alusmos* meant "anguish, inquietude, uneasiness, being troubled," as well as "tossing about" in the specific case of the sick. The derivation *alusis* had the meaning of distress and anguish, and in the colloquial Greek, the adjective *lusiteles* meant "unprofitable", whereas in medicine it was used to mean "unfavourable prognosis" (Liddell and Scott 1996, p. 74). Other derivatives of *alusmos* were

[4]In this section I am drawing heavily on Liddell and Scott's lexical work on Greek-English, along with Konstan's thorough discussion of fear in his book *The Emotions of the Ancient Greeks* (Konstan 2006a).

used as medical terms only. For instance, in the Hippocratic corpus the adjective *allusmotes* was used to denote states of feeling uneasy or troubled (Liddell and Scott 1996, p. 74).[5]

Despite these relevant semantic differences, recent texts on the philosophy of emotions define 'fear' and 'anxiety' in rather idiosyncratic ways, and a few words on the current technical use of these terms is in order. In her translation of Cicero's *Tusculan Disputations* Graver (2002) takes the Latin noun *aegritudo* to denote mental pain at present and *metus* for mental pain in the future. However, this categorical distinction is rendered more equivocal by the fact that *aegritudo* derives from *aeger*, an adjective denoting sickness from both body and mind. In the latter case ("*aeger animus*"), this term not only has the connotation of pain but also of "any agitation of the passions or feelings, of love, hope, *fear, anxiety*, sorrow" as well as being "troubled, *anxious*, dejected, sad, sorrowful" (Lewis and Short 1891, p. 53) (my italics). Moreover, the early use of *aegritudo* only had the connotation of illnesses of the body ("of men and brutes"), and it was Cicero who began using *aegritudo* in the psychological sense of mental grief and sorrow (Lewis and Short 1891, p. 84). Another important difference in translation is Graver's rendering of the Latin *passio* as 'emotion'. Graver acknowledges the different etymologies of these terms, but based on an analysis of Stoic fragments and current use, she considers it is more reasonable to use 'emotion' rather than the old 'passion' (Graver 2002, pp. 2–3). While this is a debatable decision, these lexical dilemmas show the difficulty of rendering, psychological terms used many centuries ago in a non-anachronistic way. In this book, I have also used 'emotion' to render the Latin *passio*, except when the text being analysed requires using the original term, for example when addressing Descartes's *The Passions of the Soul*,

[5]Konstan has drawn attention to the important work of Robert Zaborowski, who catalogued all the words related to the concept of fear in the Homeric epics. Zaborowski considers that the emotions of fear and courage are indispensable for the description of the human condition (Zaborowski 2002). According to this author, his lexicographical description is based on a contextual analysis of the texts, as well as on analyses of metaphors and specific behaviours. Zaborowski remarks on the importance of analysing the cause of the emotion, its object, its results, and its relation with other psychological forces for a deeper semantic understanding (Zaborowski 2002, p. 325).

where he uses the terms passion and emotion with different technical connotations (see Chapter 6).

This brief lexical description of Old Greek and Latin terms demonstrates that even in antiquity the noun 'fear' had a rich semantic network and its meanings acquired specificity when analysed in their proper contexts. As argued by Dixon, coining new words or endowing old ones with new meanings "can create new concepts, and even new worldviews, which may strongly influence people's capacity to understand the world and themselves" (Dixon 2012, p. 338). Some philosophers addressed in this book used the noun 'passion', a term largely replaced around the middle of the nineteenth century in both the philosophical and medical literature by 'emotion' (Dixon 2003). However, whereas 'passion' has the connotation of passivity and disease, 'emotion' has been used since the early nineteenth century with the connotation of a vivid feeling, usually detached from pathological considerations (Dixon 2003). It is also the case that the same word may remain in use in different historical times, but gain different connotations with each successive period. An example of such a lexical rejuvenation is provided by the noun 'anxiety', which was rarely used in its current psychological meaning in the psychiatric or philosophical literature before the late nineteenth century (Berrios 1999), but became of common technical and vernacular use after Freud described the syndrome of 'anxiety neurosis' in 1895 (see Chapter 8). Other terms conceptually related to fear such as 'phobia' and 'panic' acquired a strong medical connotation during the twentieth century, and have acted as a linchpin for the medicalization of fear (see Chapter 9). In contemporary colloquial use the sense of fear is implicit whenever using semantically related words such as 'fright', 'dread', 'terror', 'horror', 'panic', 'alarm', 'dismay', 'consternation', 'trepidation', 'apprehension', 'anxiety' and 'timidity', and the selection of which term is used is influenced by a host of variables, such as the acuteness and severity of the event producing the emotion, the presence of people, the age and social status of the agent, the possibility of escape, and other contextual factors (Hollander 2004).

Finally, it is important to remark that there is no single concept of fear, given that this emotion may be analysed from the different perspectives of philosophy, theology, psychology, sociology, psychiatry, the neurosciences, the history of emotions and lexical uses. Nevertheless, some philosophers consider it is possible to provide categorical definitions to fear-related terms. For instance, the philosopher Jesse Prinz suggests that the "folk" category of fear consists of two different states, which he termed *panic* and *anxiety* (Prinz 2004, p. 152). 'Panic' is defined as a response to an immediate physical threat which is behaviourally related to a flight response, whereas 'anxiety' is defined as a response to impending danger which is behaviourally related to freezing (p. 153). The main problem with this classification is the attempted reduction of these terms to concepts defined in purely behavioural terms (e.g. flight or freezing responses), which may allow for ease in studying fear in laboratory settings, but may not reflect other technical or colloquial uses. For instance, Prinz's concept of anxiety is no more than one among many alternative definitions. He could have referred to Boissier du Sauvage's use of the term in the early medical nosologies when 'anxiety' had both psychological and somatic connotations (Boissier de Sauvages 1772), or to Freud's concept of anxiety which has a purely psychological connotation (see Chapter 8), or the complex spiritual connotation of anxiety in Kierkegaard's *Concept of Anxiety* (see Chapter 9), or the current psychiatric conceptualisation of anxiety as a mental disorder (see Chapter 9), where anxiety is defined as including restlessness rather than Prinz's freezing.[6]

To conclude, the object of this work is the emotion of fear, with the important clarifications that first, the term 'fear' includes a variety of semantically-related terms united by 'family resemblances' but with fuzzy boundaries, and second, that fear-related terms have not 'crystallised' in time, but have evolved with changes in their colloquial and technical meanings. After this necessary discussion and clarification of the object of this text, I shall now address the meaning of 'conceptual analysis' of emotions.

---

[6]Other philosophers who wrote extensively on the philosophy emotions provide very different classifications of fear. Solomon, for instance, divides fears into the categories of "rational and reasonable" and "irrational and unreasonable" depending on the response (adequate or exaggerated) to a given object (Solomon 2007, p. 36). Against Prinz's theory, Solomon considers that physical symptoms should not be confused with the emotion of fear which, in his opinion, is the act of recognizing a danger (p. 37).

1.2 The Conceptual Analysis of Fear

In his well-known text *Emotions: An Essay in Aid of Moral Psychology*, the philosopher Robert Roberts has defined the conceptual analysis of emotions as "an approach to the investigation of emotions that takes major clues about them from the ways people talk about the emotions in the contexts of their life," and from examining examples of a given emotion as it occurs in specific narrative contexts (Roberts 2003, p. 4). Roberts proposes a "common-sense realism" type of conceptual analysis given that, in his opinion, people from any historical period are able to be roused by fear and provide reasons for this emotional state (Roberts 2003, p. 11).[7] Roberts also considers that observation of emotional features is more relevant for conceptual analysis than philosophical theories, given that, in his view, the emotional display used for conceptual analysis has remained relatively stable in the history of humanity. For example, the progression from Aristotelian *pathe* to Stoic passions deals with the same "old familiar facts of anger, fear, joy and hope" (Roberts 2003, p. 13). Roberts wants to avoid the extremes of conceptualising emotions as the exclusive result of neurophysiological or sociocultural processes. In his own words "an imperialistically social constructivist account of emotions is as far from the truth about [the concept of emotions] as a purely neurological account" (Roberts 2003, p. 13). Finally, Roberts considers that for a conceptual analysis of emotions a lexical-historical approach is "*useful but not necessary*" (italics in the original) (Roberts 2003, p. 10).

For this work, I have selected the philosophical strategy of conceptual analysis given that, as I shall discuss, this is a powerful technique not only for clarifying the concept of fear, but also to help in understanding

[7] As Roberts acknowledges, this 'folk' or 'common-sense' approach to the concept of emotions was criticised by Amelié Rorty (1984), who suggested that an adequate concept of emotions requires consideration of the philosophical background from which the concept originated, as well as a historical and lexical approach.

the best therapeutic approaches.[8] The selection of different Western philosophers and thinkers from different periods is relevant for providing perspicuous views and didactic differences that would not be otherwise obtained by analysing a single philosopher or period. In other words, rather than trying to arrive at a synthesis, I will follow the Wittgenstenian tradition of enriching and illuminating differences on the concept and therapy of fear that only an eclectic selection of thinkers can provide.[9] This is the reason I have not only included perspectives from different Western philosophical traditions, but I have also drawn on concepts of fear from psychoanalysis, psychiatry, sociology and the neurosciences.

Some differences between the conceptual investigation in this work and Roberts's conceptual analysis technique should be mentioned. A solely philosophical form of argumentation may be sufficient for Roberts's analytical purposes, but for the present work, which spans several millennia, a historical approach, with consideration of biographical aspects and important idiosyncrasies in lexical use should be employed. I am not arguing that a conceptual analysis of fear should follow a strict chronological trajectory, or that a detailed lexical analysis is sufficient in illuminating the concept of fear of the ancients, but I consider that historical and lexical aspects cannot be ignored. As I shall discuss, historical factors are important for understanding the Hellenistic search for therapies of fear (Konstan 2006a), as well as for understanding Hobbes's political concept of fear. The brief lexical analysis above is an important

[8]Daniel Hutto has argued against the type of conceptual analysis that defines its object in terms of 'necessary and sufficient' conditions (Hutto 2009, p. 196). Hutto remarks that the "correctness" of conceptual analysis requires a standard against which this activity is evaluated, but given the lack of such standards of general agreement, concepts are idiosyncratic rather than "stable and unambiguous" constructs (p. 201). Concepts are not only unstable, but their existence depends on current uses. Therefore, any conceptual analysis is restricted to the time at which it is carried out. Given that no philosophical conclusions can be assessed as final, concepts have no immutable "essences," and as Hutto proposes, concepts can be refined or replaced with alternative ones (p. 202). I agree with Hutto's criticism of the futility of searching for "essential" concepts, and I explicitly reject pursuing a 'definite' concept of fear. In fact, one of the main aims of this work is addressing the major differences in the concept of fear among philosophers from different traditions and other thinkers and scientists selected for analysis.

[9]I will justify below the reasons behind the selection of particular thinkers.

reminder that a generic concept of fear will only result in limited concepts and therapies if lexical richness and the historical background are ignored. The philosopher Sellars rightly remarks that biographies were regarded by the ancients as relevant for the understanding of philosophical texts, as philosophy was considered a practice rather than an activity limited to textual analysis (Sellars 2003). According to Sellars, biographical information may clarify the congruency (or lack thereof) between the philosophers' doctrines and their way of life. In this work, biographical information will be provided whenever necessary for a better understanding of the argument under discussion. I shall examine several examples where biographical aspects and the context in which philosophers lived are relevant for understanding their conceptualization of fear. Such is the case of Cicero and Seneca (discussed in Chapter 2), Montaigne (Chapter 3), Hobbes (Chapter 4), and Descartes (Chapter 5).

1.3 The Philosophical Therapy of Fear

Fear is an emotion with a wide spectrum of intensities, ranging from everyday fears of minor relevance, to severe fears expressed in marked psychomotor reactions. Fear is also an emotional disposition, with some individuals having the habit of constantly worrying about any minor foreseeable danger, and on occasions, even feeling paralysed and unable to engage in their daily activities. For these individuals, fears may become a mental torment, which may motivate the affected person to seek professional help. It is this understanding of fear as constitutively requiring some sort of therapeutic treatment that is the other principal focus of this work, and investigating the therapy of fear in these terms has required drawing from philosophical, psychological, neuroscientific, psychoanalytic, psychiatric and sociological sources. Roberts has made the interesting comment that in the past 25 years "the crop" of philosophers interested in the field of emotions have preferred to focus on understanding ethical rather than functional underpinnings, such as the subtlety and unpredictability of emotions, aspects that are strongly related to language and best understood by conceptual analysis (Roberts 2003, p. 37). Martha Nussbaum is one of the few contemporary philosophers with an interest in the philosophical therapy of emotions.[10] To my knowledge, the concept of fear and its therapies has never been the exclusive focus of philosophical analysis.[11]

The roots of philosophical therapy have been thoroughly examined by the philosopher and psychiatrist Pedro Laín Entralgo, who stressed the early split between physicians, using the healing power of herbs by the *mutas artes* (mute arts), and Cicero's philosophical *medicina mentis* (medicine of the mind) (Laín Entralgo 1970, p. 71). According to Laín Entralgo, in the Athens of the fifth century BCE an important philosophical dilemma arose concerning the question as to whether the passions might be diseases sensu stricto (in a strict sense), and whether the use of words could be developed into a therapeutical technique.[12] This important question is addressed in Chapters 2 and 3, which discuss the Epicurean and Stoic remedies for healing the distress caused by fear. Focusing on these Hellenistic schools, the philosopher Pierre Hadot stressed the role of philosophy, not only as providing a therapy for the passions, but also as bestowing ethical principles for pursuing a philosophical way of life, such as concern for one's destiny and spiritual progress, assessing moral needs, and seeking peace of mind (Hadot 1995, p. 88). This way of life included a corpus of techniques that were used as remedies for the passions (see Chapters 2 and 3), such as living in the present and ceasing to worry, the Cyrenaic *premeditatio malorum* (meditation about potential misfortunes), and the Epicurean detachment

---

[10]See principally her *The Therapy of Desire: Theory and Practice in Hellenistic Ethics* (Nussbaum 1994).

[11]I should nevertheless point to important chapters on fear by Konstan (2006b), Tappolet (2010), and Canfield (2007, 2009).

[12]Already the Greek sophist Gorgias (c.485–c.380 BCE) remarked on the power of words as remedies for the soul. In his *Encomium of Helen*, Gorgias writes that "Speech is a powerful ruler. Its substance is minute and invisible, but its achievements are superhuman; for it is able to stop fear and to remove sorrow and to create joy and to augment pity" (Gorgias 2005, p. 23). He also compares words with drugs ("*pharmakon*"), stating that "the power of speech bears the same relation to the ordering of the mind as the ordering of drugs bears to the constitution of bodies. Just as different drugs expel different humours from the body, and some stop it from being ill but others stop it from living, so too some speeches cause sorrow, some cause pleasure, some cause fear, some give the hearers confidence, some drug and bewitch the mind with an evil persuasion" (Gorgias 2005, p. 25).

from the future in the search for relaxation and serenity (Hadot 1995, p. 88). Hadot also remarks on the relevance of the philosopher as a therapist adapting the use of words or *logotherapy* to the listener's needs with the aim of bringing a cure for the passions. The legacy of the Ancients, Hadot considers, "has never been surpassed" (Hadot 1995, p. 69),[13] and this legacy constitutes the starting point for the analysis of the therapies of fear in this work.

1.4 Aims and Methodological Challenges

To sum up, I believe there is an important gap in the philosophical literature concerning the concept of fear and its remedies, and this book has been designed to examine different concepts of fear that inform its therapy. This aim has guided the selection of the philosophers and thinkers included for discussion, allowing for a comparison of concepts and therapies. As discussed above, while the book is structured as a historical-philosophical investigation of the concept of fear, it is not a purely historical rendition of fear, nor does it present an 'anatomy of fear' which includes all philosophical writings on this subject. Instead it provides a broad brushwork rendition of the main concepts of fear as presented by selected philosophers and thinkers, and how they have approached its therapy.

Any work that takes a historical approach to its subject manner must be selective. The history of thinking about fear is no exception as the large number of philosophers and scholars who have discussed this emotion reflects its pervasive influence in human life. This work aims at providing the benefits of a conceptual overview, deciding which philosophers and thinkers to include, and what works of those thinkers will best represent their views is a complex and fraught task. The philosophers and thinkers discussed in the following chapters were selected

[13]Hadot contrasts the therapeutic preoccupations of the Ancients with those of contemporary philosophy, stating that "philosophical discourse now tends to have as its object nothing but more philosophical discourse" (Hadot 1995, p. 76).

based on their overall contribution to the conceptualisation of fear and their suggestion of therapies for reducing its more damaging effects. While many scholars have discussed fear in different ways my focus here is specifically on works that are concerned with the type of problems that fear presents in our lives and the ways in which those difficulties might be alleviated. Some examples may help to clarify this important issue.[14]

It might be asked why, for example, Epicurus's concept of fear and the Epicurean therapies have been selected over the work of Aristotle. The principal reason here is that, in my opinion, Epicurus's concept of anxiety is closer to human daily concerns and it lends to a readier translation into therapy compared with that of Aristotle. While there is room for debate over this, of course, Konstan's chapter on fear in Aristotle's work provides a useful lead (Konstan 2006a). Konstan discusses Aristotle's concept of fear, which in the *Rhetoric* is defined as a pain in relation to a future evil, with the qualification that the pain has to be "great" and its object relatively close in time (Konstan 2006a, p. 130). Konstan concludes that for Aristotle the fear of death does not exist because it is far in the future. I want to argue that this definition of fear limits the concept of this emotion to rather exceptional events, and denies one of the main fears of humankind. Moreover, this concept does not render fear of death amenable to therapy, let alone a discussion of fear of death as one of the main human emotional concerns. On the other hand, for Epicurus an essential step for achieving *ataraxia* was that death should not be feared, tacitly admitting that fear of death is a strong human emotion in need of treatment. Furthermore, as argued by

[14]I will argue that that the concept of fear has evolved in divergent directions. Whereas Hellenistic and Roman philosophers used a wide scope for fear, and this trend continued with thinkers of the Renaissance humanism such as Michel de Montaigne, this conceptual approach changed with the rise of materialism and the desire for social control in the eighteenth century. This is manifested by the political and dualist reductionism of Hobbes and Descartes, respectively, continued with the psychobiological perspective of William James, and brought into contemporary times with the medicalization of fear by Sigmund Freud and the current neurobiological trend in psychiatry. Against the latter context of a narrow concept of fear due to multiple reductions, the philosophies of Soren Kierkegaard and Ludwig Wittgenstein generated an important challenge, although their conceptual efforts are rarely discussed in current philosophical texts (see for instance Goldie's recent *Handbook on the Philosophy of Emotions* (Goldie 2010)).

Konstan, it was Epicurus who stressed that the fear of death underlies many human irrational fears and desires (Konstan 2006a, b, p. 149), and it was the Epicurean school that accepted fears with and without concrete objects as relevant emotions, a concept rejected by Aristotle for whom fear always requires an object.[15]

A similar question may arise as to why Descartes's concept of fear has been given preference over Spinoza's. I want to argue that Descartes's *Passions of the Soul* (Descartes 2015) provides a concept of fear that opens a new perspective by using a mechanistic approach that has witnessed several iterations until current times (see the mechanism proposed by Damasio as discussed in Chapter 7). Furthermore, Descartes's text was born from an epistolary exchange between the philosopher and Princess Elizabeth of Bohemia, who at the time was suffering from fears and distress. These letters present Descartes not only as a philosopher and mathematician, but also as a physician of the soul, advising on various philosophical remedies to heal Elizabeth's emotional ailments. This material provides an illuminating and didactic counterpoint between theory and practice which is missing in Spinoza.

For some readers, too, it may be surprising that no chapter is devoted to existentialist philosophers, although specific reference is made to Kierkegaard's *Concept of Anxiety* in Chapter 9. Instead, I have prioritised a discussion of Freud's concept of anxiety, given that it is the father of psychoanalysis who began the process of medicalization of fear, turning anxiety into a specific psychological pathology. While the concept of *Angst* developed by Heidegger provides a significant but complex perspective (Mulhall 2005), in practical terms during the twentieth century it has been the field of neurosciences and psychiatry that have elaborated the main conceptual material that translated into specific therapies.

The question may be raised as to whether Chapter 7, which focuses on a critical analysis of dualism and reductionism, may have little relevance for the therapy of fear. I discuss in this chapter how the strong reductionist approach to the empirical study of fear in the field of

---

[15]See Konstan (2006a, p. 150).

current neurosciences ignores the richness and complexity of this emotion and its diffuse connections with, rather than definite demarcation from, other emotions with which it shares a 'family resemblance.' As I discuss in the next two chapters, this narrow approach has strongly influenced clinical practice for more than a century, with a potentially negative impact upon therapeutic progress.

1.5 A Summary of the Chapters

Epicurus was among the first philosophers to recognise the negative impact of fear and anxiety upon peace of mind.[16] I will argue in Chapter 2 that the Epicurean *telos of ataraxia* was only to be achieved after a systematic therapy of fear, and above all by fighting the fear of death. Whereas Epicureanism had a strong social acceptance, it was the Greek Stoic school which provided the first systematic conceptualisation of emotions. In Chapter 3, I shall first discuss Cicero's concept and therapy of fear and distress. While not a Stoic, his *Tusculan Disputations* are strongly influenced by Stoicism. Chapter 3 also examines Seneca's concept of fear and his therapeutic recommendations. While belonging to the Stoic school, Seneca used an eclectic approach to conceptualise and treat fear. An original aspect of his therapy is that his recommendations were delivered in an epistolary style, but related to the reader in the shape of a therapeutic manual. The connection with the reader is even stronger in Montaigne's *Essays*, which also provide a broad narrative of fears (Chapter 4). These are conveyed by describing a full palette of fear-related emotions, from individual doubts and avoidance, to terror and generalised panic.

[16]The noun *anxiety* has been used to translate fragments from the Epicurean school (see Long and Sedley's *The Hellenistic Philosophers*, volume 2, pages 116, 128, 144 and 158 (1987), and the Preface in Inwood and Hutchinson (Inwood and Gerson 1994)). Striker (1990) uses *anxiety* to translate the Greek noun *tarache* present in Epicurean texts. Fear and anxiety are semantically related terms, but providing an in-depth philological and historical analysis of this relation exceeds the aims of this book. As Everts and Jackson have discussed, semantic similarities and differences between these terms have been the focus of lengthy debates (Jackson and Everts 2010).

The search for therapies of fear, from Hellenistic times onwards, and the significance of this emotion for human life underwent a major change with the reductionist stance that began with the philosophical materialism of the seventeenth century. Thomas Hobbes conceptualised fear as a powerful tool for social control. He used the biblical figure of Leviathan as a symbol of a powerful sovereign capable of enforcing a strong political system by using the fear of punishment. Hobbes's important insight is that fear underlies human curiosity, prudence and foresight, an idea which is addressed by recounting the myth of Prometheus, as I discuss in Chapter 5. René Descartes performed a different reduction, by conceiving of emotions as based on a hydraulic mechanism. In *The Passions of the Soul*, his main treatise on the passions, Descartes investigates the passions from the perspective of a physiologist rather than a philosopher. Conceptually, Descartes's approach is a strong departure from the humanist concept of emotions, employing as it does a physiological strategy consisting of the separation of soul and body as different ontological entities in constant interaction.

By the end of the nineteenth century, the philosopher and physician William James suggested that the emotions result from the perception of somatic changes, thus implying that fear does not depend on an appraisal of danger, being instead the result of a complex neural reflex. As discussed in Chapter 7, James's theory was the departing point for the neurobiological paradigm of fear, which flourished in the second half of the twentieth century. I shall also discuss how Ludwig Wittgenstein warned against the dangers of reductionism and provided thoughtful remarks towards a broad concept of fear, stating that emotions are nuanced feelings and behaviours evolving in a specific context. Wittgenstein conceptualised emotions in terms of his metaphor of 'language games', where 'language' refers to both verbal and non-verbal behaviours. Thus, in the case of fear, mastering its language game implies using the appropriate verbal expression or non-verbal behaviours interpreted against a distinct backdrop. Wittgenstein also provided arguments to support his contention that the complex human manifestations of fear cannot be exclusively construed as activity in putative neural circuits. However, these warnings have largely been ignored and the reduction of fear to specific neural mechanisms, as extensively described by the neurologist Antonio Damasio, is the current dominant scientific paradigm.[17]

Another major shift in the concept of fear occurred in 1895 when Sigmund Freud separated out from the syndrome of 'neurasthenia'[18] a specific entity he termed 'Neurosis Anxiety.'[19] This conceptual demarcation had major consequences for the nosology of fear and anxiety, and most importantly, Freud's delimitation of pathological anxiety resulted in the description of a specific pathogenesis and the creation of a therapy, both instrumental in medicalising fear. Chapter 8 thus provides a critical analysis of Freud's construction of normal and pathological fear and anxiety, and the conceptual problems arising from this psychophysical reductionism.

Both, Freudian theories and treatment of anxiety were replaced during the second half of the twentieth century with theories based on empirical findings in the field of biological psychiatry along with the revolutionary discovery of medications able to provide dramatic relief to anxious people. The twenty-first century is rich in nosological systems and phenomenological descriptions of anxiety. However, as I argue in Chapter 9, the problem of what counts as abnormal is not empirical but conceptual, and has not yet been satisfactorily addressed, let alone resolved.

To conclude, this work will provide a historical-conceptual analysis of fear based on the writings of Western philosophers and thinkers who have examined this emotion in innovative ways, and who have also extended their interest into the care for unhealthy fears. Conceptual problems still plague the wide topic of fear and related emotions, and it is my hope that this book will help by illuminating conceptual riddles and by providing philosophical leads to help with future studies in the field.

---

[17]This is the reason for having included Damasio, rather anachronistically, in this chapter.

[18]Neurasthenia is a medical syndrome, coined in 1869 by the American neurologist George Miller Beard, that includes a variety of somatic and psychological symptoms such as headaches, dizziness, fatigue after mental effort, muscle tension, poor concentration, anxiety and depressed mood, among others (Beard 1881). This nosological construct is still extant in the International Classification of Diseases (10th version) of the World Health Organization (1993).

[19]The original German term is *Angstneurose*, and translating the German *Angst* with the English *anxiety* is considered by some authors as inadequate (Berrios 1999).

References

Adam, B., Beck, U., & Van Loon, J. (2004). *The risk society and beyond*. London: Sage.

Beard, G. M. (1881). *American nervousness, its causes and consequences*. New York: G. P. Putnam's Sons.

Berrios, G. (1999). Anxiety disorders: A conceptual history. *Journal of Affective Disorders, 56*(2–3), 83–94.

Boissier de Sauvages, F. (1772). *Nosologie Méthodique, ou distribution des maladies en classes, en genres et en especes, suivant l'esprit de Sydenham, et la méthode des botanistes* (M. Gouvion, Trans., Vol. 1). Lyon: Jean-Marie Bruyset.

Canfield, J. V. (2007). Wittgenstein on fear. In D. Moyal-Sharrock (Ed.), *Perspicuous presentations: Essays on Wittgenstein's philosophy of psychology*. London: Palgrave Macmillan.

Canfield, J. V. (2009). The self and the emotions. In Y. Gustafsson, C. Kronqvist, & M. McEachrane (Eds.), *Emotions and understanding: Wittgenstenian perspectives*. London: Palgrave Macmillan.

Descartes, R. (2015). *The passions of the soul and other late philosophical writings* (M. Moriarty, Trans.). Oxford: Oxford University Press.

Dixon, T. (2003). *From passions to emotions*. Cambridge: Cambridge University Press.

Dixon, T. (2012). "Emotion": The history of a keyword in crisis. *Emotion Review, 4*(4), 338–344.

Dunant, S., & Porter, R. (1996). *The age of anxiety*. London: Virago Press.

Goldie, P. (2010). *The Oxford handbook of philosophy of emotion*. Oxford: Oxford University Press.

Gorgias. (2005). *Encomium of Helen*. London: Bristol Classic Press.

Graver, M. R. (2002). *Cicero on the emotions* (M. R. Graver, Trans.). Chicago: The University of Chicago Press.

Hadot, P. (1995). *Philosophy as a way of life: Spiritual exercises from Socrates to Foucault* (A. I. Davidson, Trans.). Malden, MA: Blackwell Publishing.

Hollander, J. (2004). Fear itself. *Social Research, 71*(4), 865–886.

Hutto, D. D. (2009). Lessons from Wittgenstein: Elucidating folk psychology. *New Ideas in Psychology, 27*, 197–212.

Inwood, B., & Gerson, L. P. (1994). *The Epicurus reader: Selected works and testimonia*. Indianapolis: Hackett Publishing Company.

Jackson, P., & Everts, J. (2010). Anxiety as social practice. *Environment and Planning, 42*, 2791–2806.

Konstan, D. (2006a). *The emotions of the ancient greeks: Studies in Aristotle and classical literature*. Toronto: University of Toronto Press.

Konstan, D. (2006b). Fear. In *The emotions of the ancient Greeks: Studies in Aristotle and classical literature* (pp. 129–155). Toronto: University of Toronto Press.

Laertius, D. (1925). *Lives of eminent philosophers* (R. D. Hicks, Trans., Vol. 185). Cambridge, MA: Harvard University Press.

Laín Entralgo, P. (1970). *The therapy of the word in classical antiquity* (L. J. Rather & J. M. Sharp, Trans.). New Haven: Yale University Press.

Lewis, C. T., & Short, C. (1891). *A new Latin dictionary*. Oxford: Clarendon Press.

Liddell, H. G., & Scott, R. (1996). *Greek-English Lexicon*. Oxford: Clarendon Press.

Long, A. A., & Sedley, D. N. (1987). *The Hellenistic philosophers. Vol. 2: Greek and Latin texts with notes and bibliography*. Cambridge: Cambridge University Press.

Mulhall, S. (2005). *Routledge philosophy guidebook to Heidegger and being and time* (T. Crane & J. Wolff, Eds.). London: Routledge.

Nussbaum, M. C. (1994). *The therapy of desire: Theory and practice in Hellenistic ethics*. Princeton, NJ: Princeton University Press.

Prinz, J. J. (2004). *Gut reactions: A perceptual theory of emotion*. Oxford: Oxford University Press.

Roberts, R. C. (2003). *Emotions: An essay in aid of moral psychology*. Cambridge: Cambridge University Press.

Rorty, A. (1984). Aristotle on the metaphysical status of "Pathe". *The Review of Metaphysics, 37*(3), 521–546.

Sellars, J. (2003). *The art of living: The Stoics on the nature and function of philosophy*. London: Bloomsbury Academic.

Solomon, R. C. (2007). *True to our feelings: What our emotions are really telling us*. Oxford: Oxford University Press.

Striker, G. (1990). Ataraxia, happiness as tranquillity. *Monist, 73*(1), 97–110.

Tappolet, C. (2010). Emotion, motivation, and action: The case of fear. In P. Goldie (Ed.), *The Oxford handbook of philosophy of emotion*. Oxford: Oxford University Press.

World Health Organization. (1993). *The ICD-10 classification of mental and behavioural disorders*. Geneva: WHO.

Zaborowski, R. (2002). *La crainte el le courage dans l'Illiade et l'Odysée*. Varsaw: Stakroos.

2
The Epicurean Concept of Fear and the Road to *Ataraxia*

> What produces unsurpassed jubilation is the contrast of the great evil escaped: and this is the nature of good, if you apply your mind rightly and then stand firm and do not stroll about.
>
> Saying of Epicurus in Plutarch's *Moralia, A Pleasant Life Impossible* (1086) (Plutarch 1927)

> The fool's life is empty of gratitude and full of fears; its course lies wholly toward the future.
>
> Saying of Epicurus in Seneca's *Epistles XV, 9* (Seneca 2015)

2.1 Introduction

Fear of death, fear of the gods, fear of poverty, and fear of pain have been the most relevant fears of humankind. These fears figure prominently already in the Book of Job as well as in the Homeric texts, and it is appropriate for this work to begin by analysing these fears, considered

S. Starkstein, *A Conceptual and Therapeutic Analysis of Fear*,
https://doi.org/10.1007/978-3-319-78349-9_2

by the Hellenistic philosopher Epicurus as the main obstacle to achieving peace of mind, or *ataraxia.*[1]

Epicurus, born in the Greek island of Samos in 341 BCE, was one of the most influential Hellenistic philosophers, and Epicureanism remained an active school of philosophy for centuries. Epicurus began teaching philosophy at the Greek city of Mytilene and a few years later at Lampsacus, and finally set up his school in Athens in 306 BCE. He bought a house named *Ho Kepos* ('The Garden'), where he established his school, at a time when Athenian philosophy was dominated by Plato's Academy and Aristotle's Lyceum (Grant 1990, pp. 239–244). At the Garden, Epicurus provided philosophical teachings aimed towards helping his students in achieving *ataraxia.* Life at the Garden was frugal, with water and barley bread as the main staple, and simple shelter for men and women alike (Clay 2009, pp. 9–28). Epicurus was a prolific writer, but little of this material was preserved, and extant writings are found mostly in letters to his friends and the maxims produced for his students to memorise. For Epicurus, pleasure was the state of mind that resulted from removing pain in the body (*aponia*) and fear in the soul (*ataraxia*) (Warren 2002, p. 166), and, as I shall argue, removing fear was the principal goal of Epicurean ethics.

---

[1]Like many Greek philosophical terms, *ataraxia* has several connotations. Epicurus used ataraxia as a noun to denote "impassiveness" and "calmness;" as a verbal derivative to denote "to keep calm" and "to act with perfect composure;" and as the adverbial form "calmly" (Liddell and Scott 1996, p. 268). *Atarbes* is a lexically-related adjective meaning "fearless" and "not dreaded," and has a verbal derivative meaning "causing no fear" (Liddell and Scott 1996, p. 268). Diogenes Laertius conveyed *ataraxia* as "neither suffering pain nor anxious fear" (Diogenes Laertius 1925; 10.128). It is important to note that the concept of *ataraxia* had precursors in Greek philosophy, and was not an Epicurean creation. Democritus used the term *athambia* (defined by Cicero as "id est animum terrore liberum" ("freedom from alarm") (Cicero 1914; 5.87–8) to refer to the state of human happiness in which the soul is "disturbed by no fear" (Sedley 2009, p. 39). Anaxarchus, a follower of Democritus, left a few fragments that are mostly related to the influence of fear upon human behaviour. For Anaxarchus much learning can cause "distress and misfortune" (Warren 2002, p. 83). Nausiphanes of Teos, Epicurus' teacher, described the aim of life as *akataplexia,* "a correct attitude to things which normally cause fear or astonishment" (Warren 2002, p. 165). Nevertheless, *akataplexia* is not synonymous with *ataraxia,* since the latter not only includes the indifference to fearful events, but also the rejection of unnatural and unnecessary desires (Warren 2002, p. 166). The terms "happiness," "ataraxia" and "peace of mind" are used interchangeably by Inwood and Gerson (1994, pp. 32–36).

In this chapter, I shall examine the Epicurean concept and philosophical treatment of fear. After a short discussion on the historical context of Epicureanism, I shall examine the relevance of fear for Epicurus's ethical system by describing the main objects of fear, their relevance for the Epicurean way of life, and the different 'remedies' proposed by Epicurus and his followers to manage fear.[2]

2.2 The Historical Context of Hellenistic Philosophical Schools

A notable introspective turn in the human condition started with the fall of Athens under Alexander the Great (Grant 1990, p. 214). For several centuries before the Macedonian invasion, the city-state of Athens enjoyed a democracy in which Athenian citizens participated actively. The mind-set of the Athenians was mostly focused 'outwards', that is, on participating in political, cultural or other civic events. With Alexander's invasion, the golden times of the city-state were gone, as Athens became part of the Macedonian empire. According to Michael Grant this period is considered the origin of Hellenistic "individuality" (Grant 1990, p. 214). With the demise of Athens as a city-state, the busy political life came to an end and Athenians no longer participated in the decision-making process of the city. This was a dramatic change in the political system since the future of Athens was no longer in their hands, and it also generated great uncertainty about citizens' personal futures, leading to fear and anxiety (Grant 1990, p. 214). Accordingly, this community shift resulted in a personal shift, since the Athenians become more introspective, increasingly concerned about their present and future condition. In other words, with the collapse of the city-state emerged the fear of what the new political system would bring. This mixture of increasing uncertainty and distrust generated a need for a

[2]All the references to Epicurus extant remains correspond to the translation by Inwood and Gerson unless explicitly stated (1994). The numeral next to the text reference corresponds to Usener's notation system.

better understanding of fear and effective management of it. According to Gordon and Suits (2004, pp. 5–16) there were three main ways of addressing the uncertainties of fortune: first, astrology, as this practice could provide advice relevant to how to control and plan one's life; second, the mystery cults of Greek religion to seek protection from the Olympian gods; and third, Epicurean philosophy. Tarn and Griffith (1952, pp. 327–328) suggest that the political changes in Athens influenced some individuals in such a way that their feelings of social belonging drove them into Stoic philosophy, whereas others, affected by the oppression of fear and a wish to escape, selected Epicureanism.[3]

Epicurus' philosophy is considered 'hedonistic' given that its main goal is achieving a state of physical and mental pleasure. As I shall now discuss, the state of mental pleasure or *ataraxia* could only be achieved after major fears were removed. In fact, many of the extant Epicurean fragments are orientated towards discussing the objects of fear, providing advice on how to obtain protection from social danger.

2.3 The Epicurean Concept of Fear

The most recent translation of Epicurus' extant works starts its Introduction with a bold statement: "The fundamental obstacle to happiness says Epicurus, is anxiety" (Inwood and Gerson 1994, p. i).[4] Epicurean fragments are rife with references to fear and anxiety, although they do not include a conceptual analysis of these emotions. Rather, Epicurus provided numerous examples of fear and worries from everyday life, discussed in a didactic fashion. An Epicurean follower,

[3]Other historians and philosophers of the Hellenistic period offer a more nuanced view of the religious and social changes. Graham Shipley considers that the cult of *Tyche* should not be elevated into "a paradigm of Hellenistic religion" (Shipley 2014, p. 175), and that interpreting the fear of Hellenistic Greeks as due to social changes may be anachronistic (Shipley 2014, p. 190).

[4]A paragraph in the *Letter to Menoeceus* (128) is translated by Warren as "For it is for the sake of ataraxia that we do everything—so that we may feel neither pain nor anxiety" (Warren 2002, p. 3), whereas Inwood and Gerson translate this paragraph as follows: "For we do everything for the sake of being neither in pain nor in terror" (p. 29) (my italics). This discrepancy shows the difficulty of translating ancient into current emotional terms.

Diogenes of Oenoanda, distinguished two types of fear. The first corresponds to the ordinary concept of fear, such as avoiding dangerous objects (Konstan 2008, p. 48). The second belongs to a more indefinite category of fear, which Konstan considers corresponds to the current concept of anxiety: "the fear lies hidden within us, and we cannot simply escape the danger" (Konstan 2008, p. 48). It is the second type of fear that most often impedes achieving *ataraxia* given that it is difficult to track down.[5]

The goal of Epicurean ethics, as already noted, was achieving *ataraxia*, "for we do everything for the sake of being neither in pain nor in terror" (*Letter to Menoeceus*, 128).[6] Pleasure is nothing more than having no pain in the body and no fear in the soul (*Letter to Menoeceus*, 131), and this will become the main Epicurean mantra, one of those maxims to be memorised and rehearsed by his followers.[7] This modest concept of pleasure led to a frugal lifestyle, avoiding any excess that could result in bodily pain through sickness. Epicurus was also concerned about the anxiety of losing those pleasures to which many people were habituated, given that the impact of this anxiety could be greater than the potential pleasure. Therefore, although the Epicurean philosophy is considered "hedonistic" we may agree with Marcuse that it is a "negative hedonism" since pleasure is achieved by avoiding the ordinary fears of life rather than actively seeking pleasure (Marcuse 1967).

[5]Warren (2004, p. 11) provides a different explanation for the two types of fear described by Diogenes of Oenoanda. He considers that the fear that is manifest and clear is the fear of death, whereas the fear 'creeping into our nature' is the fear of pain.

[6]One major influence in Epicurean ethics and physics was Democritus of Abdera (Warren 2002, p. 36). Diogenes Laertius wrote, "[Democritus] says that *euthymia* is the goal of life—which is not identical with pleasure as some have mistakenly understood, but is the state in which the soul proceeds peacefully and well settled, disturbed by no fear or superstition…" (Laertius 1925; 9.61). Warren suggests that Democritus' concept of *euthymia* (the precursor of Epicurus' *ataraxia*) as the removal of fear influenced the Epicurean *tetrapharmakos* (see below) (Warren 2002, p. 36).

[7]"Practise these and the related precepts day and night, by yourself and with a like-minded friend, and you will never be disturbed either when awake or in sleep, and you will live as a god among men" (*Letter to Menoeceus*, 135).

Epicurus placed great importance on obtaining assurance about preserving *ataraxia* in the future.[8] While Epicurus stated that the satisfaction of simple desires such as food and shelter is sufficient for a happy life, he also claimed that happiness depends on the confidence that what is necessary will be always available.[9] There is here a subtle tension between the concept of *ataraxia* as a state of mind based on the present condition, and *ataraxia* as a mental state greatly dependent on the potential outcome of future events. As Plutarch rightly pointed out in his criticism of Epicurus, the body will sooner or later become sick or injured, and consequently, humans "cannot but suffer constant dismay and anguish for the body in facing the future."[10] Thus, *ataraxia* is a delicate state of mind, feeding in the present moment, but greatly dependent on the future. This dependency on future events is expressed in the Epicurean recommendation to enjoy the present without delay for fear of future misfortunes,[11] and explains the central role of safety (*asphaleia*) in the Epicurean ethical system, as I describe below.

2.4 The Role of Fear and Safety in Epicurean Ethics

An analysis of extant Epicurean maxims and fragments shows that avoiding fear and anxiety is critical to achieving *ataraxia*. The relevance of fear for Epicurean ethics is manifested by the fact that 20 of the 40

[8]The relevance of a safe future was also stressed by Epicurus' followers such as Porphyry, who stated that "It is better for you to have confidence [about the future] while lying on a cheap bed than to be disturbed while possessing a golden couch and extravagant table" (Inwood and Gerson 1994, p. 81).

[9]"The cry of the flesh: not to be hungry, not to be thirsty, not to be cold. For if someone has these things *and is confident of having them in the future*, he might contend even with Zeus for happiness" (my italics) (*Vatican Sayings*, 31).

[10]Plutarch, *A pleasant life* (Plutarch 1927; 1090b).

[11]"Life is ruined by delay and each and every one of us dies without enjoying leisure" (*Vatican Sayings*, 14) (see also footnote 19).

aphorisms in the *Kuriai Doxai* (or 'Key Doctrines')[12] are directly related to fear. The words *fear, terror* and *alarm* (as translated by Inwood and Gerson from the original Greek) appear in seven of them,[13] fear-related themes are addressed in another eight aphorisms,[14] and five are related to security and safety.[15,16]

The *Kuriai Doxai* also addresses other frequent topics of Hellenistic ethics, such as virtue, prudence, and the role of knowledge, justice and friendship for a happy life. For ease of explanation, I have divided the aphorisms into the following categories[17]: (i) principal causes of fear,[18] (ii) pain and fear,[19] (iii) safety,[20] (iv) knowledge and fear,[21] (v) friendship and safety,[22] and (vi) ethics and fear.[23] A conceptual analysis of these groupings is provided below.

---

[12]The *Kuriai Doxai* is a collection of brief quotes preserved by Diogenes Laertius (1925) which present a very abridged version of the main tenets of Epicurean ethics, for quick consultation or memorization.

[13]#10–12, 18, 20, 34, and 39.

[14]#2, 16, 22, 28, 31–33, and 35.

[15]#6–7, 13–14, and 40.

[16]Another collection of Epicurean maxims, the *Vatican Sayings*, includes many aphorisms dealing with fear and related themes, such as safety, fortune, danger, procrastination about the future, confidence, hope and distrust.

[17]The aphorisms in the *Kuriai Doxai* have been divided into subgroups based on various criteria by different authors. The Spanish philosopher Garcia Gual (2001, p. 134) divided the *Kuriai Doxai* into fragments dealing with the "*tetrapharmakos*" (1–4), followed by the conditions for a happy life and the relationship between pleasures and virtues (5–21), the criteria for knowledge and moral action (22–26), the relevance of friendship, a classification of desires (27–30), and social justice and its relationship to the life of the wise man (31–40). Long and Sedley (1987, pp. 102–157) classified the fragments into aphorisms about fear and virtue, aphorisms about fear and science, and aphorisms about fear and social life.

[18]#1, 2, 1 5, 21 and 26.

[19]#3, 4, 8, 9, 19, and 30.

[20]#6, 7, 10, 14, 16 and 17.

[21]#11, 12, 13, 18, 20, 22, 23, 24, 29 and 38.

[22]#27, 28 and 39.

[23]#31, 32, 33, 34, 35, 36, 37, 40.

2.4.1 The Principal Causes of Fear

The main causes of human fear, which are described in the first four aphorisms of the *Kuriai Doxai*, were briefly summarised by Epicurus' follower Philodemus in the famous *tetrapharmakos* or the four-fold remedy (Erler and Schofield 1999)[24]: "Don't fear god, Don't worry about death; What is good is easy to get, and What is terrible is easy to endure." The *tetrapharmakos* is structured in a hierarchy that facilitates a philosophical treatment of fears. The first step is to eliminate the fear of the afterlife, which should allow an easier removal of the fear of death. Once this step is achieved, the remaining fears can be diminished or removed by following the Epicurean ethics of a frugal life and Epicurus' maxims regarding fear and safety (see below). I shall now analyse the *tetrapharmakos* in its four individual components.

2.4.2 Don't Fear God

During the Hellenistic period, as already noted, there was a widespread belief that human life was in the control of *Tyche*, the goddess of fortune. Religion became one alternative to escape from the grasp of an uncertain destiny, although imparting its own fears. For example, individuals could ask the gods for protection, but at the same time had to seek protection from the gods' anger. Gordon (Gordon and Suits 2004, pp. 5–16) considers this ambivalent status of the Hellenistic gods as the origin of the human fear of the divine. Dickinson (1911, p. 8) suggested that in the Hellenistic era the Greeks were terrified by the powers of nature, which became impersonated in spiritual beings. Later, these beliefs crystallised in a religious system that made the gods more familiar and natural phenomena less frightening. The Greek gods acquired a human form and could interfere with human affairs in both positive and negative ways. According to Epicurus, fear of the gods is

---

[24]Philodemus *Ad Contubernales* (To His Companions) (PHerc 1005, col. 4.9–14) (Erler and Schofield 1999). Long considers that the *tetrapharmakos* encapsulates "Epicurus' entire philosophy" (Long 2006, p. 178).

readily dispatched once it is recognised that the gods are disinterested in human affairs. The first aphorism in the *Kuriai Doxai* states that the gods cause no trouble, given that they are devoid of passions in their "blessed and immortal nature" (*Kuriai Doxai*, 1). Epicurus' gods live in their own Garden, aloof from human life. Because the gods have no passions and therefore no anger towards humans, they do not represent a danger. Once this is understood, humans are released from fears of the supernatural and the afterlife.

2.4.3 Don't Worry About Death

The second aphorism of the *Kuriai Doxai* states that "death is nothing to us" given that, for the materialistic Epicurean ontology, death is no more than the dissolution of the human being (body and soul) into its constituent atoms.[25] According to Epicurus, whatever is good or bad is provided by sense-experience, and given that death is the privation of sensation, nothing good or bad is lost. The understanding that death is not to be feared also removes the quest for immortality. These arguments suggest (as Martha Nussbaum argues in *Therapy of Desire*) (Nussbaum 1994, p. 124) that for Epicurus whether one is alive or dead was a matter of indifference.[26] However, Epicurus explicitly considered life desirable even for an "old man" (*Letter to Menoeceus*, 126), and the desire to die foolish. Epicurus' main argument for appreciating life is the variety of pleasures available to the Epicurean, such as the '*katastematic*' or passive pleasure of being in the state of *ataraxia* and *aponia*, and the 'kinetic' or active pleasures of enjoying friendship (Diogenes Laertius 10.136–138, in Inwood and Gerson 1994).

[25]"Death is nothing to us. For what has been dissolved has no sense-experience, and what has no sense-experience is nothing to us" This concept of death is also alluded to in another fragment: "So death, the most frightening of bad things, is nothing to us; since when we exist, death is not yet present, and when death is present, then we do not exist. Therefore, it is relevant neither to the living nor to the dead, since it does not affect the former, and the latter do not exist" (*Letter to Menoeceus*, 125).

[26]Warren has addressed relevant inconsistencies in the Epicurean account of death, but discussing his provocative arguments are beyond the scope of this work (Warren 2009).

One conceptual limitation of the Epicurean maxim on not fearing death is that it does not consider the instinct of self-preservation, the well-established phenomenon that a living entity will remove itself from any situation that may pose a danger to its life. Thus, Nussbaum considers this Epicurean maxim as "inhuman," given that this goal is beyond human emotional capacity. This instinctive fear, usually expressed by typical physiological changes and automatic behavioural responses such as flight will occur regardless of any rational argument about the relevance of death. On the other hand, humans have the capacity of creating habits from strong beliefs, which may reduce or even remove the fear of death. This is the case for Buddhists believing in reincarnation, and Christians and Muslims believing in the possibility of a heavenly life. In other words, some individuals with strong religious faith are not afraid of death, and some may even seek it intentionally.

Epicurus was well aware that for most individuals removing the fear of death is a difficult achievement. As he acknowledged, "One can attain security against other things, but when it comes to death all men live in a city without walls" (*Vatican Sayings*, 31). Humans are constantly exposed to the fear of death, and therefore, to tame or remove this fear, they have to continually remind themselves that death is not to be feared. Thus, Epicurus urges Menoeceus to "*become accustomed* to the belief that death is nothing to us" (my italics). Epicurus strongly advocated for the need to remove the fear of death since this fear is the foundation and origin of most human fears (Warren 2004, p. 12). For the Epicureans, fear of death was the main underlying cause of violence and greed, in so far as power and wealth are means of avoiding death (Segal 1990, p. 15). The Epicurean poet Lucretius described how fear of death feeds "avarice and the blind lust of distinction," sometimes "transgressing the bounds of law" (Lucretius 1924; 3.59–70). Rather than enjoying a stable life, Lucretius considered that humans live in a chronic state of fear, and in their quest for escaping death they "amass wealth by civil bloodshed…piling murder upon murder; cruelly they rejoice at the mournful death of a brother, they hate and they fear a kinsman's hospitality" (Lucretius 1924; 3.59–74). In other words, fear of death not only explains many human vices but also social phenomena such as war, the end of friendships, and the lack of trust.

In conclusion, the fear of death has a central role in Epicurean ethics, as it shapes the mental conditions of the human way of life. It is only after removing this fear that people can attain a tranquil life and achieve *ataraxia*.

2.4.4 What Is Good Is Easy to Get

After dealing with the two most important human fears, namely the gods' anger and death, Epicurus addressed the third main source of fear, which is poverty. Epicurus considered this fear to be strongly related to the quality and quantity of desires. Thus, in *Kuriai Doxai-29* Epicurus articulated his well-known aphorism: "Of desires, some are natural and necessary, some natural and not necessary, and some neither natural nor necessary but occurring as a result of a groundless opinion." Desires that are both natural and necessary are those for food, clothing and shelter. These are natural because seeking nourishment and protection against inclement weather and wild animals are basic behaviours shared with non-human animals. These desires are also necessary because without them life is short. Examples of natural but *unnecessary* desires are those for sophisticated foods and clothing, which Epicurus urged should be avoided. He suggested that unnecessary desires are recognised by the fact that not satisfying them does not result in pain (*Kuriai Doxai*, 30). Most often, Epicurus argued, pursuing these desires may result in harm (*Kuriai Doxai*, 26). Finally, desires that are neither natural nor necessary are wealth and honours, and these should also be avoided since "groundless opinions extend without limit,"[27] and the continuous search for wealth and glory makes human life miserable. Konstan suggests that there is a vicious circle between fear and desires, where fear of death brings about limitless desires, and in turn, excessive desires result in anxiety (Konstan 2008). He also argues that for Epicurus, excessive desire is the cause of irrational fear, and the deep insight and

[27]"The stomach is not insatiable, as the many say, but rather the opinion that the stomach requires an unlimited amount of filling is false" (*Vatican Sayings*, 59).

sophistication of Epicurean ethical philosophy is the discovery of the strong bond between fear and desire.

An important aspect of Epicurean ethics, namely its almost systematic ambiguity, needs discussion. In the extant material, Epicurus provides strong advice in some maxims, and in others, he provides divergent suggestions on the same subject. For instance, in *Kuriai Doxai-2* Epicurus suggests that we should procure only what is natural and necessary for a tranquil life, whereas in *Kuriai Doxai-7* he remarks that there is nothing intrinsically bad in achieving wealth and fame, as long as their acquisition produces no fear or anxiety. Epicurus also speculated about the use of an algebraic equation to make decisions, for instance, accepting some pain in the present when this could result in a future pleasure. These inconsistencies may suggest a lack of coherence of Epicurean ethics, but the explanation I will defend is that these maxims were devised for use by Epicurean followers as a guide in life, but not to be applied in a dogmatic fashion. We shall see similarly ambiguous remarks when discussing the Epicurean concept of justice, safety and friendship.

2.4.5 What Is Terrible Is Easy to Endure

This section brings the analysis of the *tetrapharmakos* to its conclusion. The previous three components addressed fears produced by mistaken beliefs (e.g. that the gods mingle with human affairs, that death is terrible, that many objects of desire are overvalued). The final aphorism of the *tetrapharmakos* is the only one not dealing with false beliefs, as it refers to physical pain. For Epicurus, bodily pain is a great evil, since it invariably results in mental pain. His therapeutic advice was rather simplistic, suggesting that pain should not be feared since a pain that is acute and severe indicates that the end is close, whereas a chronic pain is mild and even pleasurable (*Kuriai Doxai*, 4). The weakness of this argument is that severe pains may not be necessarily short-lasting (as Epicurus would know himself, after suffering from kidney stones for several years). Nor is it true that chronic pains, even mild ones, are not burdensome. Epicurus considered that it was the role of the philosopher to teach how to overcome the most severe pains by increasing mental pleasure. For this purpose, he used the strategy of recalling sweet memories, such as conversations with friends, to appease the severity of bodily pain (Tsouna 2009, p. 251). This was an important training for Epicureans, since pleasant memories were frequently available to those living in the Garden (O'Keefe 2001, p. 133). This technique was used by Epicurus himself while he was dying with kidney stones. Another Epicurean strategy to minimise the impact of bodily pain was to argue that physical pain is felt in the present only, whereas mental pain is felt in the present but has roots in the past and projects into the future (Laertius 1925; 10.137). This argument is also weak, since suffering pain almost always raises the question of its duration, about how one's future will be affected by pain, and it may even raise the fear of oncoming death. This argument further illustrates the difficulty of separating bodily from mental pain, thus challenging Epicurus' categorical separation of *aponia* and *ataraxia*. In other words, bodily pain often results in mental suffering, whereas the latter usually has somatic concomitants. The Roman Epicurean poet Lucretius argued that in the case of "vehement fear" we should be able to see the spirit through the perspicuous bodily changes: "sweatings and pallor hence arise over the whole body, the speech falters, the voice dies away, blackness comes before the eyes, a sounding is in the ears, the limbs give way beneath..." (Lucretius 1924; 3.155–158).

In conclusion, the *tetrapharmakos* is not only considered "the basis of the Epicurean moral system" (Bailey 1970, p. 347), but it also provides, in a condensed manner, the first specific philosophical medicine against fear and anxiety. The four maxims may be considered as harsh therapy, since the beliefs to be modified are part of entrenched instinctive and cultural behaviours that are very difficult to modify using the technique of changing beliefs. A less radical reading may consider the *tetrapharmakos* as a compass, guiding the student towards a life with less fear but without necessarily meeting the stringent criteria of the fourfold remedy. Epicurus himself recognised that against death we live in a city without walls, meaning that fear of death is difficult to remove. He also accepted that humans will always pursue empty (that is, unnecessary) desires, with the fear of not obtaining the desired object or of being unable to keep it. The *tetrapharmakos* is a medicine to be swallowed slowly. The benefits will only appear after arduous practice, and it is not suited to everybody.

The remaining aphorisms about fear in *Kuriai Doxai* and in the *Vatican Sayings* provide gentler advice than the *tetrapharmakos*, and constitute the backbone of the Epicurean ethical system which is discussed below.

2.5 Epicurean Ethics and the Road to *Ataraxia*

Most Epicurean followers lived in the Garden, and this living arrangement was replicated in other Greek cities (Grant 1990, p. 236). The Garden provided shelter to Epicurean followers by securing them with food and a place to live, but there also were Epicurean followers living in cities who were unable to enjoy the 'safety net' provided by the Garden. Nevertheless, these individuals could always benefit from the Epicurean ethical doctrine that could be studied and practiced outside the Garden.

2.5.1 Living Unnoticed

One example of Epicurean ethical advice is the famous *lathe biosas*, or 'live unnoticed' (Roskam 2007). The concept of living unnoticed meant to refrain from occupying prominent positions in the political or social system. Epicurean followers living in the city were supposed to carry out their professions with a low social profile, looking at city life as from a balcony, without mingling with those pursuing empty desires (Konstan 1973, p. 8). Nevertheless, this ethical advice should not be considered as promoting a 'monastic rule', since Epicurus approved of political participation as long as this activity is practiced safely. Furthermore, he encouraged participating in politics whenever the individual feels that not participating is more painful than potential suffering in the future (Plutarch, *On Tranquillity of Mind*, 337: 173) (Plutarch 1927). This not only demonstrates the eclecticism of the Epicurean ethical system, but also suggests that the accusation, discussed below, that Epicureanism fostered an egotistic lifestyle should be strongly moderated (Nussbaum 1994, p. 139). The concept of 'living unnoticed' also implied living a frugal life, without extravagances that could place the Epicurean at the mercy of financial misfortunes. Thus, the Epicurean follower was guided towards self-sufficiency to minimise dependency on others and reduce the concomitant anxieties that this dependency could bring (*Vatican Sayings*, 81). For Epicurus living wisely was living prudently, and making the right choices after careful analysis of risks and benefits.[28] Another essential element for a life free of fears was *asphaleia* or safety, which I discuss in the next section.

2.5.2 Living Safely

Epicurus considers that obtaining security from natural disasters and from fellow humans is an "instinct from nature,"[29] and this is the central theme of six aphorisms in the *Kuriai Doxai*. For Epicurus, obtaining safety from being harmed by others is so relevant that any means to remove this fear was considered a "natural good" (*Kuriai Doxai*, 6). In other words, if the individual is in danger, the Epicurean maxim that empty desires should be avoided is revoked. Thus, Epicurus tolerates the pursuit of wealth and fame as long as these non-essential elements provide safety to the individual. In a radically pragmatic fashion, Epicurus conceded that even a dissolute life ("the pleasures of profligates") is acceptable if it helps to remove fear and anxiety.[30]

[28] Long (2006, p. 9) considers that Epicurean prudence is a "mental disposition" and a "rational outlook on life" which examines the cause of choices and removes confusing opinions.

[29] "Some men want to become famous and respected, believing that this is the way to acquire security against [other] men. Thus, if the life of such men is secure, they acquire the natural good; but if it is not secure, they do not have that for the sake of which they strove from the beginning according to what is naturally congenial" (*Kuriai Doxai*, 7).

[30] "If the things which produce the pleasures of profligate men dissolved the intellect's fears about the phenomena of the heavens and about death and pains and, moreover, if they taught us the limit of our desires, then we would not have reason to criticize them, since they would be filled with pleasures from every source and would contain no feeling of pain or distress from any source" (*Kuriai Doxai*, 10).

In conclusion, the Epicurean ethical system was pragmatic and flexible, adapting to specific situations. Epicurean ethical advice ranges from a rigid practice of frugality and self-effacement to the engagement in an antithetical behaviour whenever personal safety is at stake. This malleability of Epicurean ethics is strongly related to minimising the anxiety produced by living in a community with limited capacity to provide the necessary safety to achieve tranquillity of mind. The strong association between safety and *ataraxia* also underlines the relevance of retributive justice for Epicurean ethics. According to Epicurus, justice originated from a natural pact between people not to harm each another (*Kuriai Doxai*, 31), and from the fear of retaliation.[31] In other words, for Epicurus the concept of justice was not dogmatic but relative. A human act is considered 'unjust' only when the agent is afraid of being punished. But the wrongful act comes at a price, since Epicurus considered that fear will always follow the offender, even if "he escapes detection ten thousand times." In conclusion, the Epicurean ethical system was in large part based on defensive practices generated by fear.[32]

An important caveat to the Epicurean system of justice, however, is his view that pacts forged out of fear do not last indefinitely. Life circumstances frequently change, and the usefulness of pacts depends on the safety they provide to both parties at a given time in a given context. Another problem is that the concept of justice and vice based on fear of punishment and the struggle for security creates significant tensions within the Epicurean ethical system. On the one hand, Epicurus considered that a virtuous life was generally better than a life with vices, as the wise and virtuous person, that is, the one that follows the Epicurean precepts, will obtain continuous safety against adverse fortune, whereas the "unjust" will live in the greatest disquietude.[33] On the other hand,

[31]"Injustice is not a bad thing in its own right, but [only] because of the fear produced by the suspicion that one will not escape the notice of those assigned to punish such actions" (*Kuriai Doxai*, 34).

[32]"Let nothing be done in your life, which will cause you to fear if it is discovered by your neighbour" (*Vatican Sayings*, 70).

[33]"The just life is most free from disturbance, but the unjust life is full of the greatest disturbance" (*Kuriai Doxai*, 17). In *Kuriai Doxai-14* Epicurus remarks that whereas fame and wealth may provide security against other men, a quiet and secluded life brings greater safety ("The purest

like a Machiavelli *avant la lettre*, Epicurus considered that any means of procuring safety is a natural end, thus ethically justified (*Kuriai Doxai*, 37). This ethical conflict may lead to untoward consequences, since individuals are entitled to defend themselves against others, which may end in a state of war.[34] Thrasher (2013, pp. 423–436) has recently commented on the incompatibility of pursuing *ataraxia* while simultaneously complying with the requirements of justice.[35] He observes a similar inconsistency in the Epicurean concept of friendship, especially with Epicurus' remark that "Every friendship is worth choosing for its own sake, though it takes its origin from the benefits [it confers on us]" (*Vatican Sayings*, 23). This remark suggests that friendship is a good in itself, but that its origin is instrumental. I shall now analyse the Epicurean concept of friendship in more detail, given its relevance for the concept of fear.

2.5.3 The Benefits of Friendship

In keeping with other ancient Greek philosophers such as Aristotle, Epicurus regarded friendship as one of the greatest assets of social life and highly significant for a life without fear.[36] Nevertheless, Epicurean

---

security is that which comes from a quiet life and withdrawal from the many, although a certain degree of security from other men does come by means of the power to repel [attacks] and by means of prosperity").

[34]Vander Waerdt (1987, p. 402) has a different view, and considers that wise individuals will not commit injustice given that this is against their self-interest. Their aim is *ataraxia* and they will therefore avoid any wrong-doing because of fear of punishment. In this case, the fear is instrumental to achieving *ataraxia*. Therefore, Epicurus states that the wise person has to live justly in order to live pleasantly ("It is impossible to live pleasantly without living prudently, honourably, and justly and impossible to live prudently, honourably, and justly without living pleasantly. And whoever lacks this cannot live pleasantly" (*Kuriai Doxai*, 5). See Julia Annas (1987) for a similar account of instrumental virtue.

[35]Thrasher (2013, p. 424) concludes that the Epicurean concept of justice is both possible and necessary once the Epicurean social arrangement is understood to reconcile justice and pleasure. Discussion of this suggestion is beyond this work.

[36]"For since a solitary life without friends is full of dangerous traps and fear, reason herself advises us to get some friends; and when we do so our mind is reassured and becomes indissolubly linked to the expectation that pleasures will thereby be acquired" (Cicero, *On Goals*; 1.66) (Inwood and Gerson 1994).

friendship is not of the type idealised by Aristotle in the *Nichomachean Ethics*; rather Epicurus' conception was mainly instrumental, that is, based on the security that friendship may provide. Thus, immediately after an aphorism stating that friendship is the most blessed human possession (*Kuriai Doxai*, 27), friendship is considered valuable for the protection it brings against life's adversities, present and future (*Kuriai Doxai*, 28). The concept of friendship is another example of Epicurean ethical ambivalence. Friendship has instrumental value, for the protection it provides to those in the relationship, while simultaneously being a source of happiness unmixed with fears (Laertius 1925; 10.120). Thus, not everything is instrumental in Epicurean friendship. The Epicurean Philodemus (1998; fr. 28), while discussing friendship, considered that "there is nothing so grand as having one to whom one will say what is in one's heart and who will listen when one speaks." Furthermore, Epicurus felt unselfish gratitude towards friends (Laertius 1925; 10.120), and suggests that we should run risks or even die for the sake of a friendship (*Vatican Sayings*, 28). Eventually, Epicurus seemed to prefer friends with a moderate self-interest, rejecting those that mostly expect benefits from the relation as well as those who are indifferent to gains and unhelpful in case of future need (*Vatican Sayings*, 39).

The answer to these ethical ambiguities regarding justice and friendship may lie in a dual concept of happiness, briefly mentioned by Diogenes Laertius and rarely discussed in philosophical texts. Whereas the pinnacle of Epicurean happiness is *ataraxia*, a mental state that cannot be increased by any pleasure, this is not the only state of happiness accessible to humans. Diogenes Laertius cites this comment from Epicurus, "Two sorts of happiness can be conceived, the one the highest possible [*ataraxia*]", but there is another "admitting addition and subtraction of pleasures," (Laertius 1925; 10.121) which is much closer to the common concept of happiness. This duality is also present in the Epicurean concept of friendship, which oscillates between moments of instrumental speculation and moments of mutual enjoyment.

In conclusion, friendship was for Epicurus, an oscillating relationship, originating in the fear of future misfortunes and the need of protection, evolving into a relation of disinterested pleasure, and ending in a solid bond where fear no longer had a relevant role. We shall now examine the impact of fear on learning and knowledge, where the instrumental role of these activities is also evident.

2.5.4 The Benefits of Qualified Knowledge

Epicurus despised all knowledge that was not instrumental for achieving *ataraxia*, and his theory of nature was shaped in a way that justified and promoted a tranquil way of life.[37] Thus, if fear of gods was an obstacle to *ataraxia*, the gods were conceptualised as beings that are disinterested in human affairs. Another example is the false belief that the gods cause frightening natural phenomena.[38] In this context, the study of atmospheric phenomena is relevant to dispel false beliefs.[39] For instance, geological phenomena such as earthquakes may create great fears, but once they are properly understood as the expression of physical forces and not due to the wrath of the gods, natural events no longer become a source of mental unrest. Similarly, if the fear of death destroys peace of mind, death becomes a mere physical event characterised by the dissolution of atoms.[40] It is for the purpose of tranquillity that Epicureans

[37]"Natural philosophy does not create boastful men nor chatterboxes nor men who show off the 'culture' which the many quarrel over, but rather strong and self-sufficient men, who pride themselves on their own personal goods, not those of external circumstances;" (*Vatican Sayings*, 45) and "In the first place, remember that, like everything else, knowledge of celestial phenomena, whether taken along with other things or in isolation, has no other end in view than peace of mind and firm conviction" (Laertius 1925; 10.85). There was a philosophical tradition, starting with Democritus of Abdera, of rejecting any learning not necessary for a tranquil life. Warren (2002, p. 83) cites fragments by Anaxarchus stating, for instance that "much learning can especially benefit, and especially harm him who has it."

[38]"The greatest anxiety of the human mind arises through the belief that the heavenly bodies are blessed and indestructible, and that at the same time they have volitions and actions and causality inconsistent with this belief" (Laertius 1925; 10.81).

[39]"I recommend constant activity in the study of nature, and with this sort of activity more than any other I bring calm to my life" (*Letter to Herodotus*, 37).

[40]"Hence, we must attend to present feelings and sense perceptions, whether those of mankind in general or those peculiar to the individual, and also attend to all the clear evidence available, as given by each of the standards of truth. For by studying them we shall rightly trace to its cause and banish the source of disturbance and dread, accounting for celestial phenomena and for all other things which from time to time befall us and cause the utmost alarm to the rest of mankind" (Laertius 1925; 10.82). It is interesting to note the use of different words in Sections 81

require the study of natural phenomena, since without "the study of nature there is no enjoyment of unmixed pleasures."[41] Thus, in the *Letter to Pythocles* (87) Epicurus remarks that the benefit of studying physics lies entirely in obtaining "freedom from disturbance" and avoiding "irrationally and groundless opinion" (*Letter to Pythocles*, 87).

For Epicurus, the study of philosophy only had instrumental value, and his own philosophy was the only one that he considered able to provide the necessary and sufficient knowledge to achieve *ataraxia* (Pascual 2011, p. 54). Epicurus is proposing a philosophical system that is not to be defended by argument but, rather, one to be memorised and practised.[42] As already mentioned, the most important task of Epicurean philosophy was to bring reason to bear on the passions as they relate to vain desires and bodily pleasures, to stress that fear is based on false beliefs, and to highlight the relevance of setting a limit to seeking pleasures and gain.[43] According to Epicurus, the value of his philosophy was in providing the rationale for *ataraxia* as the best mental state, as well as teaching how to reach it. In his view, any other philosophical system providing much knowledge about the world but ignoring both the importance of, and the road to, *ataraxia* could result in even more fear.[44] Therefore, Epicurus recommended moderation in learning and qualified knowledge, sufficient to dispel fears and

---

and 82 pertaining to the 'language game' of fear. Thus, Epicurus' translators use 'anxiety', 'evil', 'dread', 'terror', and 'alarm' to denote the same emotional state.

[41]As I shall discuss in Chapter 4, Montaigne was in agreement with the subordination of knowledge to maintaining peace of mind, stating that "some sects have rather followed truth, others utility, whereby the latter have gained credit" (Montaigne 1991, p. 380).

[42]"Do and practise what I constantly told you to do, believing these to be the elements of living well" (*Letter to Pythocles*, 123).

[43]"Poverty, if measured by the goal of nature, is great wealth; and wealth, if limits are not set for it, is great poverty" (*Vatican Sayings*, 25).

[44]"People who know about these things, if they are ignorant of what the natures [in question] are and what the most important causes are, have fears just the same as if they did not have this special knowledge—and perhaps even more fears, since the wonderment which comes from the prior consideration of these phenomena cannot discover a resolution or the orderly management of the most important factors" (*Letter to Herodotus*, 79).

anxieties.[45] His advice is not without contemporary interest, since we live in an age where an excess of information may increase fear and anxiety at individual and social levels. The relevant question as to how to fight fear using Epicurean remedies is examined in the next section.

2.6 The Epicurean Therapy of Fear

Epicurean therapy was strongly influenced by Democritus, whom Warren considers to be the pioneer on the therapeutic arguments employed by Hellenistic schools (Warren 2002, p. 47). Democritus suggested examining the lives of those in pain and assessing one's own situation "…so that you will not suffer psychic distress through desire for more" (Warren 2002, p. 47). This self-examination should allow taming our desires, and realising that wealth and fame are unnecessary, if not damaging. Excessive desire leads to an unstable an anxious life, the antithesis of Democritus' *euthymia*. According to Democritus, *euthymia* was not mere mental tranquillity, but also included pleasant experiences in the context of *symmetria*, or a balance between excessive and deficient states (Warren 2002, p. 55). Democritus also suggested valuing the present moment and whatever is sufficient for a tranquil life, rather than relying on an uncertain future, since "the desire for more destroys what is present" (Warren 2002, p. 55). He further considered that "only fools disregard the security of the present" (p. 55), striving for uncertain goods while making themselves vulnerable to external contingencies.

Epicurus continued the therapeutic work of Democritus' by stressing the relevance of fighting fear by increasing one's own safety and by taming empty desires.[46] The strong therapeutic attribute of the

[45]"…if men do not set bounds to their terror, they endure as much or even more intense anxiety than the man whose views on these matters are quite vague. But mental tranquillity means being released from all these troubles and cherishing a continual remembrance of the highest and most important truths" (Laertius 1925; 10.81).

[46]Segal (1990, p. 19) has suggested that the Epicurean therapy may be relevant to our times, since in his opinion Hellenistic therapy is similar to modern psychotherapy (for instance, in its focus on false beliefs), and also because "the needs of the soul have changed relatively little over the last two millennia". This is a questionable remark, but discussing the risks of anachronism is beyond the possibilities of this work.

Epicurean philosophy is forcefully conveyed by the Epicurean Porphyry, who claimed: "Empty is the argument of the philosopher by which no human disease is healed; for just as there is no benefit in medicine if it does not drive out bodily diseases, so there is no benefit in philosophy if it does not drive out the disease of the soul" (Inwood and Gerson 1994) (Porphyry, *To Marcella*, 31). Thus, Epicurean therapy was to the soul what medicine was to the body, and this philosophical therapy followed a medical model. Given the complexity and the difficulty of healing emotional problems, the Epicurean treatment included a variety of therapeutic methods, such as the already discussed *tetrapharmakos* (Tsouna 2009, pp. 263–265). Epicurean therapy catered for all ages, young or old. The old may benefit from practised gratitude for the good things received, whereas the young will benefit from "lack of fear of what is to come" (*Letter to Menoeceus*, 122).

Porphyry warned against the hazards of living with fear, as this type of life may itself result in dangers that were meant to be avoided.[47] This is an important concept that requires further discussion. Fear is usually conceptualised as a 'protective' emotion,[48] as it preserves humans from danger. However, excessive fear may be paralysing, preventing the affected person from making rational decisions. Long (2006, p. 187) considers that irrational fears and empty desires are the two main internal (that is, context-independent) impediments to *ataraxia*, and that both can be removed by using Epicurean prudence.[49] To protect oneself from excessive fear, Epicurus advised living prudently, a way of life that he considered "a more valuable thing than philosophy" (*Letter to Menoeceus*, 132) (Bergsma et al. 2008, p. 404).

The Epicurean treatment of fear of death deserves specific attention, given that treating this fear is an essential step towards *ataraxia* (Warren 2004, pp. 154–159). For the Epicureans, fear included cognitive and

---

[47]"Most men are afraid of parsimony in their life-style and because of this fear, proceed to actions which are most likely to produce it" (Inwood and Gerson 1994) (Porphyry, *To Marcella*, 28).

[48]See discussion in the next section on Nussbaum's interpretation of Epicurean therapy.

[49]Inwood and Gerson (1994) (Porphyry *To Marcella*, 29) "For a man is unhappy either because of fear or because of unlimited and groundless desire; and by reining these in, he can produce for himself the reasoning [which leads to] blessedness."

non-cognitive components,[50] and the therapeutic approach has to cater for both. For Epicurus, a sort of 'cognitive' therapy was the most relevant method, consisting in the removal of false beliefs. Thus, fear of death is eliminated by purging the desire for immortality and by being mindful of the present, keeping away the distress caused by anticipation. This therapy also included techniques of persuasion and intellectual advice (Tsouna 2009, p. 263). For instance, Epicurean students had to be convinced that life is valuable for the pleasure it brings and not for its duration, and they had to understand that philosophical practice "produces a good life and a good death" (*Letter to Menoeceus*, 126). This is a slow therapy, as Epicurus advised to "accustom ourselves" (*Letter to Menoeceus*, 124) to putting his precepts into practice. As Warren suggests (2009, p. 235), this idea cannot be rapidly incorporated into our belief system, as it requires consideration of personal attitudes towards life and the context in which we live, as well as generating new habits. Warren (2004, p. 15) is also sceptical about the power of persuasion or similar psychological techniques in convincing an individual that death is not to be feared, and suggests that "fearing death is simply part of what it is to be human, like the feelings of hunger or thirst". Warren considers fear of death to be a deep-rooted instinct, a type of fear not amenable to removal by psychological intervention. It could be argued, however, that Epicurus was pointing to a type of fear of death that is conscious and feels oppressive, generating greed for power and wealth. This type of fear of death could be amenable to Epicurean cognitive therapy. This view is in line with Warren's suggestion (2004, p. 16) that there is no single concept of fear of death, but a family of related concepts more or less amenable to Epicurean treatment. It is the conscious fear of death that, as Warren suggests, has a strong influence on how we conduct ourselves in life, especially in terms of having excessive desires and greed. For Epicurus, an important cause of "the anxious dread of fear of death" was attaining safety (Konstan 2008, p. 54). Konstan argues that material safety is unable to provide the necessary security to

[50]The cognitive component of fear is the value judgment of impending harm, whereas the non-cognitive components are the physiological concomitants, as described by Lucretius (1924).

remove the fear of death, and as a result people who fear death tend to engage in building "ever higher bastions of wealth and power," regardless of justice and with the selfish intention of protecting oneself "from an anxiety that dwells within" (p. 54). This anxiety was to be treated by removing the fear of death and the quest for unnecessary objects.

Epicurean therapy also included behavioural techniques, such as getting used to a frugal life; drawing on memory, such as reflecting on good past moments when in mental pain; and the use of imagination, such as thinking about what Epicurus would say and do in a fearful situation. The most famous Epicurean behavioural technique was the *lathe biosas* or 'living unnoticed' (Roskam 2007), already discussed. This way of life allows individuals freedom from chasing fame or seeking unnecessary goods, allowing them to enjoy the present moment. On the other hand, the Epicurean concept of *asphaleia* implied that a political position could be pursued if such activity would increase one's level of security. This illustrates what Roskam (2007, p. 35) terms the Epicurean philosophy of "conditional qualifications," which considered power and fame as having a neutral value, intrinsically, which could change depending on whether obtaining political power may increase one's security or not. I believe it is more accurate to state that for Epicurus fame and power have an a priori negative value, although his ethical system provided enough latitude to change this value for the positive in exceptional circumstances (*Vatican Sayings*, 14).

Parrhesia, or frank speech, was another Epicurean therapeutic method (Tsouna 2009, p. 252). In the introduction to Philodemus' *On Frank Criticism*, David Konstan considers that the technique of conversation and reasoning was essential to Epicurean therapy, with the aim of forming character and mitigating the fears "that destroy human happiness" (Philodemus 1998, p. 8). This technique was a form of confession during which Epicurean friends had the opportunity to express their fears for open criticism, and for correction and emotional improvement. *Parrhesia* also consists in providing therapeutic advice on moral aspects of life to Epicurean students, advice which was adapted to the interlocutor's state of mind and personality. Teachers were also scrutinized for their moral and intellectual attributes, and were advised to recognise the different needs of the students, as well as when they should refrain from using this technique. Philodemus recommended a gentle and empathic approach, avoiding the use of harsh speech. Thus, depending on the student's personality the cure could use 'drugs' (mild words) for those that adapted well to treatment, or use the 'scalpel' for those recalcitrant students in need of a 'surgical approach' consisting of sharp speech.[51] The Epicurean admonishment could be "caring" or it could be "an irony that pleases but pretty much stings everyone" (Philodemus 1998, p. 43).

Another method of Epicurean therapy is self-reflection, which included reading Epicurean texts (a Hellenistic version of 'self-help' literature). Reading was considered by the Epicureans to be a powerful remedy (Tsouna 2009, p. 254), as it was accessible to anybody at any time. As mentioned before, repetition and memorization of Epicurean maxims was another therapeutic method, aiming at creating a habit of "moral reflexes" (Tsouna 2009, p. 255), as well as being mindful of the present, since fear is removed when we switch our attention from future dangers into the present time. This therapy can be modified whenever anticipated pleasures are significant and properly considered. Importantly, for all these therapies, the active participation of the student is necessary. Epicurean therapy was not a mere 'recipe' for removing fears but it provided comprehensive methods for a way of life conducive to *ataraxia* (Striker 1990, pp. 97–110).[52]

The Epicurean therapy has been thoughtfully analysed and criticised by Martha Nussbaum in her book, *Therapy of Desire* (1994, pp. 102–139).[53] Given the influence of this work, I will discuss it at some length in what follows. Nussbaum begins her analysis by citing two fragments she considers of great relevance: "Empty is the philosopher's argument by which no human suffering is therapeutically treated"

[51]"...and having accomplished nothing he will again employ frankness toward the same man. If, although he has erred, he did not heed the frank criticism, the teacher will criticise frankly again. For although a doctor in the case of the same disease had accomplished nothing through a clyster, he would again purge..." (Philodemus 1998, p. 71).

[52]Tsuona mentions additional Epicurean techniques, such as developing an "impartial perspective", which enables individuals to separate themselves from the ordinary valuation of objects; and applying a right view about past and future events (Tsouna 2009, p. 259).

[53]This text includes an in-depth analysis of other relevant Epicurean sources, such as Lucretius and Philodemus, which are not fully addressed in my criticism below.

(from Porphyry, *To Marcella*, 116), and "what produces a jubilation unsurpassed is the contrast of the great evil escaped" (Plutarch 1927; 428: 47). The first remark stresses the importance that philosophical therapy had for Epicurus, whereas the second suggests that fear should be the main aim of philosophical therapy. Nussbaum highlights the Epicurean concept of the irrational society, where people fall victim to false beliefs and social manipulation, rushing "frenetically" to procure wealth, luxuries, and power. She agrees with Epicurus that anxiety is pervasive due to an ever-increasing desire for wealth and fame, and the consequent fear of losing them (p. 103). She also agrees that fear of death may be the cause of the social "frenetic activity" and of chasing material wealth. Once the irrational way of life is acknowledged, the Epicurean therapy begins by undoing empty desires. The desire for wealth is the product of believing that money will protect people from life's evils, and beliefs like this can be the origin of fear and anxiety. Uprooting false beliefs will allow people to achieve "the unimpeded functioning of the whole creature" (p. 109). Following the medical model, Nussbaum suggests that the therapy will consist of remedies of different intensity. The first step in Epicurean therapy consists in diagnosing false beliefs. A second step consists in modifying the false beliefs with the appropriate cognitive remedies to dissolve them. Finally, the third step consists in changing empty desires for those that are natural and necessary.

Finally, Nussbaum argues that the Epicurean therapy had "value-relativity," in other words, this therapy had the practical goal of achieving *ataraxia*. Given that desires are value laden; those based on false beliefs require treatment by the philosopher *cum* physician using different strategies according to the situation. These "medications" range from mild remedies for those already convinced of the need of removing false beliefs to strong "purgatives" providing a "devastating attack" to those living under the delusion of false beliefs (p. 125). The therapy is adjusted depending on whether students are able to find the road to *ataraxia* on their own, or whether they have to be guided or driven.

In summary, Nussbaum provides a faithful account of the main aspects of the Epicurean philosophical therapy for the removal of fear. She emphasises the importance that Epicurus placed on changing false beliefs and modifying the quality of desires, and provides a thorough account of the most frequent 'remedies' used by the Epicurean school. However, Nussbaum feels "unease" about the medical approach of Epicurean therapy, and wonders whether "digesting and memorizing maxims" should be called true philosophy (p. 129). She objects to the asymmetry between the commanding position of the philosopher/physician compared with that of the student. According to Nussbaum, this asymmetry is an impediment to dialectical discussion in the Aristotelian fashion. This 'medicalization of philosophy', she argues, not only forcefully indoctrinated Epicurus' followers, but also blunted their argumentative capacities.[54] Students at the Garden were supposed not only to memorise the Epicurean maxims and worship the head of the School, but also to "confess" to the School master their beliefs, actions, thoughts, and even their dreams. Nussbaum concludes that in the Garden reasoning was biased by a rigorous practice of maxims and precepts in a context of exhortations to follow the Epicurean ethical system without much arguing. She illustrates her conclusion by referring to Arcesilaus' response to the question as to why people were leaving philosophical schools for that of Epicurus, but never that of Epicurus for another (Laertius 1925; 4.43). Arcesilaus' answer was that "If one is a man, one can become a eunuch, but if one is a eunuch, one cannot become a man". Nussbaum considers that the Epicurean 'mental emasculation' resulted from providing students with 'ready-made' ethical conclusions without learning the process of reasoning leading to those conclusions. In other words, Nussbaum agrees with Arcesilaus that the 'brain-washing' methodology of the Epicurean school spoiled the philosophical capacities of those going to the Garden. Nussbaum (and Arcesilaus) makes fun of and underestimates those people flocking to the Garden, but without discussing why the Garden was such an attractive place.[55] And yet the answer may be very simple. The Garden was providing people with the peace of mind they were seeking and which they were unable to obtain in other philosophical schools.

---

[54]Limitations of Nussbaum's medical metaphor are discussed by Jordan (1990, pp. 142–143).

[55]"Aristotelians that we are, we would shrink back in distaste from giving one of our philosophy students such a summary of doctrine" (p. 129).

Another criticism of Epicurean therapy raised by Nussbaum is its instrumental quality. This applies, in her opinion, to the Epicurean concepts of friendship and justice, since for the Epicureans both human virtues only had the value of providing safety for the present and future. In contrast to the Epicurean school, Nussbaum considers the Aristotelian therapy of fear to be clearly superior.[56] In her view, Aristotle's philosophy is far more modest than Epicurus', given that the Aristotelian philosopher will accept the independent contribution and arguments of the students and foster independent reasoning. Nussbaum criticises Epicurus' "callous" and narrow approach to philosophy by comparison with the Aristotelian dialectics of emotions which may enable a broader approach to philosophical therapy (p. 138).[57]

Unlike Epicurus, Nussbaum considers fear of death as essential for self-preservation and for fostering, for the sake of self-protection, familial bonds and community values. Nussbaum argues that the search for immortality encourages having children and promoting better social policies. She disagrees with the relinquishing of non-essential goods required by the Epicurean way of life, since she considers pleasures to be important components of a fulfilling human life. Epicurean philosophy is for Nussbaum not only inhuman in despising death but also incoherent, since there is no rationality in seeking safety when death

[56]In support of the benefits of the Lyceum over the Garden, Nussbaum added "Had Nikidion [a fictional character] gone to Aristotle's school, she would have been exposed to a number of alternative positions and taught to examine their merits sympathetically, using her critical faculties" (p. 129). I find this statement both misleading and anachronistic. There is no way to know whether teachers at the Lyceum were more sympathetic than those at the Garden. Epicurus was a prolific writer but almost all his work is lost. Nevertheless, as Long suggests (2006, p. 185), the Garden may have given ample opportunity for the students to use their critical faculties.

[57]Nussbaum praises the Aristotelian dialectical philosophy as providing "a distinct sort of practical benefit" (p. 138), where public life is guided by social justice and informs the political system, which can use Aristotelian philosophy for improving social policies. She complains that "Epicurus should not have neglected this possibility…[as]…he seems to have sold both philosophy and society short, for the sake of saving *ataraxia* for a small group of individuals" (p. 138). She accepts that Epicurus' maxim of living unnoticed may have evolved from witnessing a corrupt political system and the fact that politicians may not have held philosophy as a heuristic tool in high regard, but she believes that Epicurus never demonstrated that philosophy had no impact on the political system and considers that the effort of trying to do so is worthwhile. This interesting point of view cannot be discussed further here, but it should be mentioned that Aristotle himself had to flee Athens to avoid being condemned to death.

is not to be feared. Further, she considers that the Epicurean strategy of removing fears will result in a less pleasurable and more selfish life, with little regard for participation in community affairs. Nussbaum's main criticism of Epicurean philosophy, however, is its treatment of "the human world and its accidents" (p. 237), accusing the Epicureans of being unconcerned with "alleviating the sufferings of others" (p. 237). This argument relates to the values and structures of desire. She claims that Epicureans fail to lead worthy lives given that their negative hedonism requires them to relinquish their pleasures and desires "in an anxious search for an end to fear" (p. 233), and concludes that the student's life is devalued by Epicurean philosophy. In essence, Nussbaum's main argument against Epicurean philosophy is aimed against the strong individualist strands of this therapy, focusing as it does on individual *ataraxia* rather than fostering communal bonds. Nussbaum claims that communal life should be an end in itself rather than simply instrumental to individual well-being. Moreover, there was, in fact, no benefit at the individual level, as the Epicurean philosophy lacked a structured system for teaching social virtues, and forced the student to despise what is valuable in human life.

There is an element of circularity in Nussbaum's argumentation, since without peace of mind at the individual level it may be difficult to achieve the fruitful social role that Nussbaum envisages. In other words, if individuals live in fear and anxiety, they will naturally enforce behaviours and laws to protect themselves, which, as Nussbaum acknowledges, will result in greed and frenetic activity. The Garden, in contrast, was a small community; the lifestyle was one of friendship, confidence, and exercise in frugal habits, providing a good example to the community at large of how to live a fulfilled life.[58] Long (2006, p. 184) argues against the notion that Epicurean ethics is socially irresponsible and suggests, instead, that Epicurean ethics fostered peaceful cooperation.[59]

[58]Nussbaum considers the Garden to be divorced from the community, but she does not develop her own concept of community. It is unclear whether she considers the city-state of Athens, the whole of Greece, or the whole of humankind to be the favoured model.

[59]Long (2006, p. 195) is critical about the lack of security in contemporary societies resulting from poverty, poor education, political ambitions, and religious fears, and stresses the philanthropic values of the Epicurean community to be used as a model of human culture.

It also seems that Nussbaum's remarks on the Epicurean asymmetry between master and student, and the blunting of students' dialectical capacities are exaggerated. I have already discussed the ways in which Epicurean therapy included a wide variety of techniques depending on the student's emotional and intellectual capacities, and the fact that the teacher was also scrutinized.[60] On the other hand, the Aristotelian concept of community which Nussbaum values excluded women and slaves, people who were openly received in the Garden (Hibler 1984, p. 47).

In conclusion, and against Nussbaum's reservations about Epicurean philosophical therapy, the Garden was not constituted by a small group of hedonistic and egotistic individuals. On the contrary, there were thousands of Epicureans living in communities in the main cities of the ancient world, sharing a cooperative lifestyle that lasted for centuries (Bergsma et al. 2008; Sedley 2009, pp. 29–45). In the Garden, Epicurus promoted cooperation with the legal system, a philanthropic cultivation of friendship, and a model of human culture (Long 2006, p. 185). This may explain why his therapeutic system remained essentially unchanged for centuries.[61]

What Epicurus brings to the world, despite the potential political and analytical shortcomings noted by Nussbaum, is a strong commitment to alleviating human fears and anxiety, his solidarity with any individual coming to the Garden for help or study, and a vivid example of how philosophy can be understood as a contented way of life. What is missing in Nussbaum's otherwise thorough analysis is the richness and engaged understanding of Epicurus' remarks on emotions in general and fear in particular. While Epicurus states that fear is based

[60]Philodemus remarked that when moved by a sad event "the man of understanding" will produce "a flow of tears" in front of his student, thus "admitting his own vulnerability" (Gordon and Suits 2004, p. 31).

[61]Roskam states that "the same irrational fears and vain desires always require the same healing method, a method which was as relevant in Athens 300 BC as in the late Roman republic." Roskam further suggests that the idea that the Epicureans lived a reclusive life in successive Gardens is erroneous, given the political involvement of many of the Epicurean leaders (Roskam 2007, p. 151).

on false beliefs, his interest is not epistemological but therapeutic. In other words, he is not interested in understanding the mechanism of fear per se, but on whether the false belief can be removed by using his therapy. Epicurus' take on fear may lack some of the finesse of Aristotle's treatment of this emotion,[62] but it is Epicurus who provides a philosophical therapy of fear, something not found in Aristotelian ethics. It is because of the negative impact of fear that humans live in an anxious state, pursuing empty desires, and forgetting to live in the present. It was Epicurus, and not Aristotle, who discussed the main causes of fear in humans, and whose epistemological endeavour was aimed at helping people to achieve peace of mind.

2.7 Conclusion

Epicurus emphasized in his philosophy the role of fear in shaping the human way of life: humans should not live with fear, but they cannot live without fear. Epicurus accepted this limitation and provided for the first time in the history of philosophy a systematic therapy of fear. His philosophical therapy was directed towards bringing humans to a peaceful end of life: "We should try to make the later stretch of the road more important than the earlier one, as long as we are on the road; and when we get to the end of the road, we should feel a smooth contentment" (*Vatican Sayings*, 48).

[62] As featured in Nussbaum's text, "there are some things that one must fear, that it is noble to fear, and not to do so is shameful" (Aristotle 1984; 1115a 12–13); the brave person fears death, but "in the appropriate way, and as reasoning instructs, he will stand his ground for the sake of the fine" (1115b 1–13); a person will be "more pained at the prospect of death the more he has complete virtue…for he will be aware that he is being deprived of the greatest goods, and this is painful" (1117b 10–13). It is of great interest to compare the concept of fear in Aristotle and Epicurus, but unfortunately, this is beyond the scope of this work.

References

Annas, J. (1987). Epicurus on pleasure and happiness. *Philosophical Topics, 15*(2), 5–28.

Aristotle. (1984). *The complete works of Aristotle* (J. Barnes, Ed.). Princeton: Princeton University Press.

Bailey, C. (1970). *Epicurus: The extant remains.* Hildesheim: Georg Olms Verlag.

Bergsma, A., Poot, G., & Liefbroer, A. C. (2008). Happiness in the garden of Epicurus. *Journal of Happiness Studies, 9*(3), 397–423. https://doi.org/10.1007/s10902-006-9036-z.

Cicero, M. T. (1914). *De Finibus Bonorum et Malorum* (H. Rackham, Ed., Vol. 40). Cambridge, MA: Harvard University Press.

Clay, D. (2009). The Athenian garden. In J. Warren (Ed.), *The Cambridge companion to Epicureanism* (pp. 9–28). Cambridge: Cambridge University Press.

Dickinson, G. L. (1911). *The Greek view of life* (23rd ed.). Chicago: University of Michigan.

Erler, M., & Schofield, M. (1999). Epicurean ethics. In A. Keimpe, J. Barnes, J. Maansfield, & M. Schofield (Eds.), *The Cambridge history of Hellenistic philosophy* (pp. 647–740). Cambridge: Cambridge University Press.

García Gual, C. (2001). *Sobre la Felicidad.* Barcelona: Debate Editorial.

Gordon, D. R., & Suits, D. B. (2004). *Epicurus: His continuing influence and contemporary relevance* (Rev. and Corrected ed.). Rochester, NY: RIT Gary Graphic Arts Press.

Grant, M. (1990). *The Hellenistic Greeks: From Alexander to Cleopatra* (New ed.). London: Weidenfeld & Nicolson.

Hibler, R. W. (1984). *Happiness through tranquillity: The school of Epicurus.* Lanham, MD: University Press of America.

Inwood, B., & Gerson, L. P. (1994). *The Epicurus reader: Selected works and testimonia.* Indianapolis: Hackett Publishing Company.

Jordan, R. W. (1990). Ancient concepts of philosophy. In *Issues in Ancient philosophy.* London: Routledge

Konstan, D. (1973). *Some aspects of Epicurean philosophy.* Amsterdam: Brill.

Konstan, D. (2008). *A life worthy of the gods: The materialist psychology of Epicurus* (Rev. and Expanded ed.). Las Vegas: Parmenides Publishing.

Laertius, D. (1925). *Lives of eminent philosophers* (R. D. Hicks, Trans., Vol. 185). Cambridge, MA: Harvard University Press.

Liddell, H. G., & Scott, R. (1996). *Greek-English lexicon*. Oxford: Clarendon Press.
Long, A. A. (2006). *From Epicurus to Epictetus*. Oxford: Clarendon Press.
Long, A. A., & Sedley, D. N. (1987). *The Hellenistic philosophers. Vol. 1: Translations of the principal sources with philosophical commentary*. Cambridge: Cambridge University Press.
Lucretius, T. C. (1924). *De Rerum Natura* (W. H. D. Rouse & M. F. Smith, Trans., Vol. 181). Cambridge, MA: Harvard University Press.
Marcuse, H. (1967). *Cultura y Sociedad: Acerca del Carácter Afirmativo de la Cultura* (E. Bulygin & E. Garzón Valdés, Trans.). Buenos Aires: Editorial Sur.
Montaigne, M. D. (1991). *The complete essays* (M. A. Screech, Trans.). London: Penguin.
Nussbaum, M. C. (1994). *The therapy of desire: Theory and practice in Hellenistic ethics*. Princeton, NJ: Princeton University Press.
O'Keefe, T. (2001). Would a community of wise Epicureans be just? *Ancient Philosophy, 21*(1), 133–146.
Pascual, J. (2011). Epicuro y Atenas: La creación de una comunidad identitaria distinta de la *pólis*. *Studia Historica. Historia Antigua, 29*, 39–63.
Philodemus, D. (1998). *On frank criticism* (D. Konstan, D. Clay, C. E. Glad, J. C. Thom, & J. E. Ware, Jr., Trans.). Atlanta: Scholars Press.
Plutarch. (1927). *Plutarch's Moralia*. Cambridge, MA: Harvard University Press.
Roskam, G. (2007). *Live unnoticed: On the vicissitudes of an Epicurean Doctrine*. Amsterdam: Brill.
Sedley, D. N. (2009). Epicureanism in the Roman Republic. In J. Warren (Ed.), *The Cambridge companion to Epicureanism*. New York: Cambridge University Press.
Segal, C. (1990). *Lucretius on death and anxiety: Poetry and philosophy in De rerum natura*. Princeton, NJ: Princeton University Press.
Seneca. (2015). *Letters on ethics: To Lucillius* (M. R. Graver & A. A. Long, Trans.). Chicago: The University of Chicago Press.
Shipley, G. (2014). *The Greek world after Alexander: 323–30 BC*. London: Routledge.
Striker, G. (1990). Ataraxia, happiness as tranquillity. *Monist, 73*(1), 97–110.
Tarn, W. W., & Griffith, G. T. (1952). *Hellenistic civilisation* (3rd ed.). London: E. Arnold.
Thrasher, J. J. (2013). Reconciling justice and pleasure in Epicurean contractarianism. *Ethical Theory and Moral Practice, 16*(2), 423–436. https://doi.org/10.1007/s10677-012-9348-5.

Tsouna, V. (2009). Epicurean therapeutic strategies. In J. Warren (Ed.), *The Cambridge companion to Epicureanism* (pp. 249–265). Cambridge: Cambridge University Press.

Vander Waerdt, P. A. (1987). The justice of the Epicurean wise man. *The Classical Quarterly, 37*(2), 402–422.

Warren, J. (2002). *Epicurus and Democritean ethics: An archaeology of ataraxia*. Cambridge and New York: Cambridge University Press.

Warren, J. (2004). *Facing death Epicurus and his critics*. Oxford: Clarendon Press.

Warren, J. (2009). Removing fear. In J. Warren (Ed.), *The Cambridge companion to Epicureanism*. Cambridge: Cambridge University Press.

3

Roman Fears: Cicero's and Seneca's Remedies

> Should I have died less cheerfully before having read the Tusculans?
> I think not. And now that I find myself closer to death,
> I feel that my tongue has grown richer,
> My courage not at all.
>
> Montaigne, *On Physiognomy* (Montaigne 1991)

3.1 Introduction

Montaigne's irony shows scepticism about his success in fighting the fear of death using Cicero's advice. Nevertheless, Montaigne's remark illustrates the widespread significance that the *Tusculan Disputations* (*Tusculans*)[1] acquired over the centuries not only as a philosophical treatise on the passions, but as a therapeutical 'manual' as well. In this

[1]The *Tusculans* was written in the year 45 BCE, and the name originates from Cicero's villa at Tusculum. The text is set in the form of dialogues intermixed with long expositions. The *Tusculans* brings together philosophical material from Epicurean, Cyrenaic and Stoic schools for use as 'remedies' against distress and fear (Cicero 1927, p. xi). I have used the recent translation

S. Starkstein, *A Conceptual and Therapeutic Analysis of Fear*,
https://doi.org/10.1007/978-3-319-78349-9_3

chapter I shall examine the concept and philosophical therapy of fear at the time of the Roman Empire, roughly the period from 27 BCE to 395 CE, as propounded by Marcus Tullius Cicero (106–43 BCE) and Lucius Annaeus Seneca (1–65 CE), two of the foremost Roman philosophers and followers of the "medical model" of treating passions (Nussbaum 1994). Both produced an abundance of texts, but Cicero's *Tusculans* and Seneca's *Letters on Ethics*[2] (*Letters*) have been selected for discussion because they provide in-depth discussion of the mechanism and philosophical therapy for distress, fear and anxiety.[3]

Before discussing the texts, I shall briefly provide their philosophical background. In Cicero's time, around 100 BCE, the Epicurean and Stoic schools had the highest number of followers in Rome (Cicero 1927, p. xxiv). For the Stoics, the main aim in life was to acquire virtue through reason; whereas, as we have seen in the previous chapter, for the Epicureans their *telos* was the frugal pleasure of *ataraxia*. The Stoics considered health, power and wealth as 'indifferent' for human life, that is, as objects that did not produce desire or aversion. This had a major impact on the Stoic system of the emotions, as I discuss below.

Cicero rejected both Epicureans and Stoics alike, as he considered that the former led to a dissipated life, whereas the latter showed contempt and a pedantic attitude towards ordinary human feelings. Cicero was a follower of Plato's Academy, which in Roman times had sceptical influences. This sceptical stance required the philosopher to study ethical concepts from other schools before arriving to the most plausible solution to a philosophical dilemma. Nevertheless, Cicero's main

---

of Books 3 and 4 by Margaret Graver (2002), which provides a modern translation with a focus on the emotional concomitants of the text. As noted in Chapter 1, Graver translates the Latin term *passio* as "emotion" rather than "passion" given that in her opinion, it would be anachronistic to label experiences such as fear, anxiety, anger and desire as "passions" since the latter currently have the connotation of extreme emotions (Graver, p. 3). For Books 1 and 2, I have used the Loeb translation (Cicero 1927).

[2]The *Letters* is a collection of 142 letters written by Seneca during his retirement. This text provides an eclectic collection of Stoic ethics, although Epicurean ethics are also addressed. Many of the letters focused on the cause and management of fear and anxiety. I have used the recent translation by Margaret Graver and A. A. Long (Seneca 2015).

[3]Unfortunately, there is not enough space for discussion of other seminal texts of Stoic ethical philosophy, such as those of the later Stoics Epictetus and Marcus Aurelius.

ethical work, the *Tusculans*, despite his explicit rejection of the Stoics was mostly influenced by this school.

During Seneca's time, about a century later, Stoicism was still a dominant school. Seneca studied philosophy with Attalus the Stoic, and while himself a Stoic, Seneca was also influenced by other schools such as Epicureanism and the Peripatetics. Since the immediate historical/political context also had a strong influence on both Cicero's and Seneca's ethical writings, I shall now provide a sketch of this aspect of their lives. Both philosophers were deeply involved in politics at a time when the Roman rulers were ruthless with anybody considered as an enemy, becoming almost paranoid about those close to them, such as Cicero and Seneca.

3.2 Fear in Roman Times

To understand Cicero and Seneca in their historical context, it is important to discuss the role of chance in the life of Romans, and its relevance for the emotions of fear and distress. The goddess *Fortuna* was one of the few deities who was extremely popular during the Roman Empire and survived well into the middle ages (Patch 1974, pp. 12–14). According to Patch, the goddess *Fortuna* grew in Roman times in parallel with the Greek goddess *Tyche* (mentioned in the previous chapter), and both symbolised the external forces that control human destiny. *Fortuna* was revered during the Roman Empire, being "enormously popular" (p. 12) and becoming the patron goddess of several emperors. This period was one of Roman expansion towards the unknown and its potential dangers. Patch views the Roman Empire as a period of social unfairness, when many people were at the mercy of chance. In this context, worship of the goddess *Fortuna* was an attempt to limit the unpredictability of life. Another way of reducing the power of chance is living the rational and virtuous life of the philosopher, which the goddess *Fortuna* cannot harm. Thus, the Stoics rejected the concept of fortune as they considered that humans are fully able to direct their lives successfully using their rational capacities. In other words, the Stoics considered that humans have the capacity to choose and direct their lives based on following moral rules. The Stoic concept of fate entailed that human life is pre-ordained by "Divine Reason" rather than chance, and therefore life has to be conducted following the program of nature (Grant 1990, p. 219). For instance, the Stoics thought it irrational to fear death given that dying is part of a natural process, and mortality is a necessary attribute of being human. The Stoic concept of humans, as by nature rational beings explains why their ethical system was directed against irrational emotions, such as the fear of death, and why the Stoic way to happiness was to follow reason, since it is a vigilant use of reason that will protect humans from external dangers. As clearly expressed by Veyne (2003, p. 73): "The Stoic is like a driver who must never take his eyes off the road for a single instant because at any moment a signal may appear or an accident may occur endangering his safety."

In summary, there were two main competing ways to confront the fear of human destiny and the frightening power of fortune in Roman times. One, adopted by the majority of Romans, consisted in a religious conviction that fortune was a fickle deity. The second was the philosophical way dominated by Epicureans and Stoics. These external factors, as well as personal calamities, explain why Cicero and Seneca were both concerned with the problem of fear and related emotions, such as distress and anxiety, for the achievement of a fulfilled life.

I begin with an analysis of Cicero's *Tusculans*, focusing on Cicero's discussion of human emotions, and on distress and fear in particular. The chapter continues with an examination of Seneca's *Letters*, a text that provides a variety of philosophical therapies for confronting fear and anxiety.

3.3 Distress, Fear and Anxiety in Cicero's *Tusculan Disputations*

Cicero was a Roman lawyer, orator and philosopher with a busy political career. He was strongly influenced by Greek culture, and was the first educated Roman known to have an interest in philosophy (Striker 1995). Cicero was a student of the Platonist, Antiochus, and the Sceptic, Philo. Antiochus endorsed both Platonic and Aristotelian ethics, proposing that the human good lay in the practice of virtue combined with moderate goods. These understandings, combined with Philo's anti-dogmatic philosophical ideas may explain Cicero's eclectic philosophical position (Striker 1995, pp. 53–61). Cicero had a strong interest in ethics and his detailed account of the classification, mechanism and treatment of the emotions is the earliest that is extant. His principal concern was to examine the emotion of distress,[4] and the main aim of the *Tusculans* was to advance recommendations as to how to assuage this emotion. Cicero also remarked on the conceptual link between distress and fear, suggesting that the therapy should be the same for both emotions. Striker observes that major tragedies in Cicero's private and public life provide the immediate context for his strong interest in analysing distress in the *Tusculans.* In the space of a few months, Cicero suffered serious misfortunes and these events influenced his philosophical interest in providing ethical advice on how to manage the emotions for daily life.[5]

Thus, Cicero was subjected to fear and distress for prolonged periods during his life. According to Sellars (2014, pp. 107–109), the way of life of a philosopher in later antiquity was critical in providing a tangible context for the ethical doctrines of their school, as well as serving as a paradigm for the implementation of ethical advice. The dialogues and arguments that constitute the *Tusculans* took place during Cicero's retirement to his villa at Tusculum and at this stage of his life, rather than developing new ethical theories, he was interested in providing "psychological guidance and moral education" (Striker 1995, p. 57).

The text is subdivided into five books: "On despising death" (Book I); "On enduring pain" (Book II), "On the alleviation of distress" (Book III), "On the remaining disorders of the soul" (Book IV); and

[4]Graver translates the Latin 'aegritudo' with the unavoidably anachronistic "distress," and the same translation is provided in the Loeb Collection.

[5]In the Introduction to the *Tusculan Disputations*, the translator J. E. King notes that "…The study of philosophy was, he found, his only comfort in distress. He had suffered cruelly in his family life. He had quarrelled with and divorced his wife Terentia, his second marriage was a failure, and in Feb. 45 BCE his beloved daughter Tullia had died. The public life in which he still longed to play his part was no longer open to a man of his convictions. The days were evil. There was nothing, he felt, for him to do in the Senate or the courts of law. Since the glories of his consulship in 63 BCE his political life had been one long disappointment" (Cicero 1927, pp. xii–xii).

"On virtue as sufficient for leading a fulfilled life" (Book V). A unifying theme running across all five books is how to relieve humans from fear and distress. Like Epicurus centuries before, Cicero considered fear of death to be the main obstacle for the achievement of peace of mind.[6] Therefore, several sections of the *Tusculans* are specifically aimed at providing therapeutic advice for this type of fear.

To facilitate understanding of Cicero's remarks on distress and fear, I shall first present an outline of the Stoic framework for the emotions, as it is so relevant to Cicero's work. I shall draw on the work of Brennan (2005), who provides a concise but thorough account of the Stoic system of emotions. The first important Stoic concept, as already noted, is that objects or life events are all considered to be "indifferents." In other words, a dramatic event such as the death of a friend, or objects such as wealth and power lose their value; they are considered to be neither good nor bad. Nevertheless, among the indifferents, some, such as health and shelter, are "preferred" or "promoted" (Brennan 2005, p. 38), and others, such as illness and poverty, are "non-preferred" or "demoted". Even death is considered as indifferent. Stoics may pursue the preferred indifferents, but without desire; and may avoid the non-preferred indifferents with caution but without fear. Thus, rather than desire and fear, the Stoics use the terms "selection" and "deselection" (Brennan 2005, p. 38).

The question arises as to how this ethical system works in practice. Brennan suggests (p. 52) that the "linchpin" of the Stoic system of emotions is the act of assenting. According to the Stoics, humans assent to external "impressions" arising from the senses, or internal impressions arising from memory, thoughts or beliefs. All impressions include a proposition that generates a behavioural response. For example, assenting to the visual impression of a bear close to me generates the proposition that bears are dangerous, and motivates the response of running away. Thus, once an impression is assented to, an impulse for action follows. Graver (2007, p. 91) suggests that the act of assenting is already an impulsion to act or feel, and in the case of fear, an impulsion

[6] "...for the man who is afraid of the inevitable can by no manner of means live with a soul at peace..." (*Tusculans* 2.2).

to feel mental pain. For Inwood (1985, p. 72) assent and impulse are both mental events, assent causing a related impulse. This is the basis for Inwood's significant remark that the importance of Stoic assent is that it becomes the "locus of moral responsibility" (p. 72), given that assent is under voluntary control and rational beings are responsible for the consequences of their decisions. Thus, in the case of emotions, the associated impulses are towards what is judged to be good or bad (Brennan 2003, pp. 265–269). The emotions are therefore, a specific type of belief, for instance the belief that a given impression is good, which results in intentional actions. In other words, an assent has "evaluative content" (Brennan 2005, p. 94) (that is, an evaluation is made as to whether a given object is good or bad), followed by an impulse to act or refrain from acting (for instance, reaching out in the case of desire or avoiding the object in the case of fear).

Sorabji (2000, p. 3) suggests that the Stoic mechanism of emotions involves two judgments, not just one: first the judgment that a given object has negative or positive attributes; and second, that it is appropriate to behave accordingly (e.g. moving towards the positive object or away from the negative one). This is illustrated by Cicero's concept of 'distress' in the *Tusculans* when he says: "But when our belief in the seriousness of our misfortune is combined with the further belief that it is right, and an appropriate and proper thing, to be upset by what has happened, then, and not before, there comes about that deep emotion which is distress" (*Tusculans* 3.61). However, for the Stoics, emotions are always irrational, either because assent is given to an inappropriate impression (for instance, that illness is to be feared), or because the individual gives assent due to his "weak and unstable disposition" (Brennan 2005, p. 95). The Stoics classified emotions based on their value (positive or negative), and their timing (present or future). This results in four types of emotion, namely, pleasure (good at present), desire (good in the future), pain (bad in the present), and fear[7] (bad in the future).

[7]The Stoics sub-classified emotions into sub-species. Thus hesitation, panic, terror, superstition and several others derive from fear (Brennan 2005, p. 95).

In contrast to the notion that emotions are always irrational, the wise Stoic always makes rational judgements, and assents provide the impulses of *eupatheia*, or rational emotions, which are volition (a rational desire), caution (a rational fear), and joy (a rational good). Pain is absent since this is an emotion the wise Stoic never feels. A third set of impulses in the Stoic ethical system is referred to as "selections" or "deselections". These impulses occur when assent is given to objects considered to be 'genuine' indifferents and that reaching or avoiding them is regarded to be a rational action, such as reaching for food. Using the rational emotions of *eupatheia*, the Stoic sage reaches the ideal of *apatheia*, a state free of emotions (Sorabji 2000, pp. 194–196).[8]

In the *Tusculans* Cicero criticised the ethical systems of Aristotle and Epicurus, and strongly defended the Stoic concept of emotions. Following the Stoic tradition, he considered that both distress and fear are based on the false belief that there is evil at present or in the future, respectively.[9] Thus emotions are for Cicero mental disturbances disrupting peace of mind, "for they bring distress, anxious and bitter, and crush and weaken the mind with fear" (*Tusculans* 4.34).

[8]The concept of *ataraxia* was discussed in the previous chapter, and a brief discussion of the concept of *apatheia* is in place. *The Greek Philosophical Vocabulary* (Urmson 1990) defines *apatheia* as a state of insensibility for people or objects (p. 26). Epicurus used *apatheia* to denote absence of emotions, and the Stoics used this term to denote freedom from emotion. Similarly, Liddell's dictionary renders *apatheia* as impassibility or insensitivity regarding persons, and in the more restricted Stoic sense as "freedom from emotion" (Liddell and Scott 1996, pp. 174–175). Gisela Striker remarks that the Epicurean concept of *ataraxia* is the pleasure of mental tranquillity, although the individual in this state is still amenable to be disturbed by external events (Striker 1990, p. 100). On the other hand, the Stoic concept of *apatheia* has the meaning of "complete indifference to everything bodily or external," with the consequent freedom from emotion (Striker 1990, p. 101). Thus, whereas *ataraxia* is reached by balancing external problems with pleasant memories and the anticipation of pleasures, *apatheia* is reached by following a value-system based on making correct judgments (Striker 1990).

[9]"...fear and distress are caused by beliefs about what is bad. Fear is a belief that some serious evil is impending, distress a belief that a serious evil is present" (*Tusculans* 3.24); "...for as distress is due to present evil, so fear is due to coming evil, and consequently some said that fear was a special branch of distress..." (*Tusculans* 4.64); and "Anyone who is subject to distress is also subject to fear since the things we are distressed at when they are present are the very things we fear when they are impending" (*Tusculans* 3.14).

3.3.1 The Nosology of Distress, Fear and Anxiety in the Tusculans

The *Tusculans* brought together a wide range of emotions under the genera of distress and fear. As already noted, Cicero remarked on the conceptual relation between distress and fear, and suggested that the treatment should be the same for both conditions.[10] Cicero defined distress as "mental pain" (*Tusculans* 3.23), the product of the false belief that 'bad' is present. He considered distress as the worst of all passions, "a very torture chamber" (*Tusculans* 3.27). Distress is worse than fear, given that the latter "degrades us", whilst the former produces "gauntness, pain, depression, disfigurement…It eats away at the mind and, in a word, destroys it" (*Tusculans* 3.27). Nevertheless, distress and fear cannot be categorically separated in the Stoic fashion, as having fear is usually thought as distressing, whereas suffering distress raises the fear of its continuation into the future. Cicero included in the genus of distress the species of envy, rivalry, jealousy, compassion, anxiety, mourning, sadness, trouble, grief, lamenting, depression, vexation, pining, and despondency. The inclusion of anxiety under 'distress' is explained by the fact that the term 'anxiety' was used in ancient times and up to the nineteenth century (Berrios 1999) as primarily a somatic symptom of distress and fear.[11]

Cicero defined fear as "an opinion that an evil is impending which one thinks intolerable" (*Tusculans* 4.14). It is "a species" of distress similar "in wretchedness" (*Tusculans* 4.64), and consists of being "petrified with anxiety… [by the]…approaching evil" (*Tusculans* 4.37).[12] For all the "foolish" (i.e. those not educated in philosophy), fear is a "punishment" consisting in living in chronic terror (*Tusculans* 4.37). Cicero

[10]This association was noted by Cicero in *Tusculans* 3.22 where he states that distress is used to denote "sorrow, worry, or anxiety in mind", whereas fear "is clearly related to distress" (*Tusculans* 3.23).

[11]Anxiety (*angor*, in Loeb's edition (*Tusculans* 4.28) is defined by Cicero as "oppressive distress" whereas "worry" is defined as "distress accompanied by thinking" (*Tusculans* 4.28).

[12]We may observe here how 'anxiety,' a species within the class of distress, was also used by Cicero as a symptom of fear.

included in the class of fear the species of indolence, shame, terror, fright, panic, petrifaction, agitation, and dread, and described these emotional expressions as being mental, physical or mixed. Thus "shame" is "accompanied by blushing," and "terror" by "paleness, trembling and chattering of teeth," and are both examples of types of fear associated with bodily symptoms. Others are purely mental, such as "fright" which is the "fear of imminent evil"; "panic", a "fear which upsets the mind"; "agitation", a "fear which scatters one's thought;" and "dread," "a long-lasting fear" (*Tusculans* 4.19). Cicero also made the important nosological distinction between *feeling* anxious and *suffering* from anxiety, the former being a transient emotional state and the latter a full-blown sickness (*Tusculans* 4.27).[13] Thus, the treatment of fear depends on whether individuals suffers anxiety only occasionally, or whether they are constantly tormented by this emotional state (*Tusculans* 4.27), and it is the latter that will be the main target of Cicero's philosophical therapy. This temporal differentiation is highly relevant as it provides a heuristic for when to intervene; but also, and perhaps more importantly, because it points to a question that is still significant in contemporary medicine (see Chapter 9): when should an emotional state be considered a "sickness"? For Cicero, an emotion is a sickness whenever it produces mental or somatic symptoms. Thus, fear, anxiety and distress are all conceptually-related sicknesses. In some instances, being in distress may exaggerate or produce new fears, being in fear may produce the somatic concomitants of distress, and anxiety may result from either distress or fear.[14]

Whereas distress and fear are major emotional upheavals in human life, Cicero describes the Stoic sage as living in consistent self-control, a person who "neither breaks down in adversity nor crumbles with fright"

[13]According to Cicero, a "sickness" occurs whenever "the simmering and agitation of mind becomes habitual," and "cannot be removed" (*Tusculans* 4.23). Mental sickness has to be differentiated from an "infirmity of the mind", which Cicero defines as a vigorous opinion, deeply attached and rooted, that some object is worthy of avoidance which is in fact not worthy of avoidance" (*Tusculans* 4.26). Finally, for Cicero "proclivities" refer to the proneness to contract certain sicknesses, for instance, that "some people are more prone to fear than other people" (*Tusculans* 4.28).

[14]"They are in anxiety either from the evils they undergo or from those they anticipate" (*Tusculans* 3.33).

(*Tusculans* 4.37). However, a close reading of the text suggests that cultivating *apatheia* has a steep price, since the Stoic sage lives in what seems to be a paranoid state of constant vigilance of future dangers, perpetually looking for a place "without sorrow or anxiety" (*Tusculans* 4.38). So incessant is this vigilance that "nothing unforeseen can happen to him, nothing which he does not anticipate, nothing strange at all" (*Tusculans* 4.37). This state of unrelenting mental tension is inconsistent with the Stoic concept of *apatheia* as the state of being free of emotions. Cicero's Stoic sage is certainly not living "free of distress" (*Tusculans* 4.38) but rather is constantly oriented towards the future, living in anxious expectation.

In conclusion, Cicero considered distress to be the worst human emotion, and fear to be a type of distress. These are both pernicious emotions given that once they have begun, humans are carried away by them (*Tusculans* 4.43). This explains Cicero's objections to the Peripatetic therapy of taming these emotions (Tusculans 4.45). According to Cicero, both distress and fear have to be eliminated rather than tamed. I shall now move on to describe his general approach to the treatment of emotions.

3.3.2 "Let Us Therefore Look to See What Remedies Philosophy Has to Offer for the Sicknesses of the Mind" (Tusculans 4.58)

The tradition of asserting parallels while distinguishing philosophy from medicine (one for the soul, the other for the body (*Tusculans* 3.5)), had in Cicero one of the strongest advocates. Specifically, he considered the sicknesses of the mind to be "more destructive" than those of the body (*Tusculans* 3.5). For Cicero, a proper discussion of the therapy of emotions using philosophical tools was of the upmost importance.[15] Philosophy is "the medical science for the mind" (*Tusculans* 3.6), and different from the art of medical healing, as it requires the

[15]"all that tends to alleviate distresses, terrors, lusts, [is important] for here is the richest fruit of the whole field of philosophy" (*Tusculans* 1.119).

rational work of self-examination.[16] As part of a tradition of contrasting and comparing philosophy with medicine that began, as we have seen, with ancient Greek philosophers,[17] Cicero stated that philosophy "…is a physician of souls, takes away the load of empty troubles, sets us free from desires and banishes fear" (*Tusculans* 2.10–12). In the previous chapter I discussed Epicurus' concept of philosophy as a healer of the soul, and here we see a similar therapeutic goal for the unorthodox Stoic position conveyed by Cicero and Seneca. In the *Tusculans*, Cicero proposed a set of remedies for most emotions, but mainly for distress and fear. His therapy encompassed a general approach as well as specific remedies for specific emotions (*Tusculans* 4.59). The first step is to identify those individuals amenable to philosophical treatment, as not every person is amenable to therapy. For successful results the sick person must have a wish for and the motivation to be cured (*Tusculans* 3.5), and this requires patients to have insight into their emotional disorder. Therefore, philosophical therapy is not suitable for those that are too insane (*Tusculans* 3.13). The second step for "curative measures" (*Tusculans* 4.59) is to identify the type of disturbing emotion, since the treatment is specific for each of them. In this stage the philosopher-therapist must decide whether to approach all emotional problems in a generic way, discussing their cause as rooted in irrational beliefs, and whether the emotion should be suffered or whether it is necessary to fully remove it.[18]

Cicero was a partisan of the Stoic therapy of removing emotions rather than discussing whether an object should be feared or not. Those afflicted by fear must understand that emotions are based on erroneous beliefs

---

[16] "We must use our outmost endeavour…to have the power to be ourselves our own physicians" ("*tute tibi imperes*") (*Tusculans* 2.47).

[17] Chrysippus, one of the fathers of the Stoic school remarked that "It is not the case that there is a method which we call "medical", concerned with the disease of the body, but no method for the diseased soul. Nor does the latter method fall short of the former…Therefore, just as it is appropriate for the doctor concerned with the bodies to be inside the sickness which befall them and the proper cure for each, so also it falls to the doctor of the mind to be 'inside' both these things in the best way they can" (Chrysippus, *On Emotion*, book 4, cited in Graver (2002, p. 210)).

[18] "Should we be speaking in terms of "the spurning of reason" and "too-vigorous impulse," or in terms of fear, desire, and so on? And is it to appear that the object of one's distress is not a proper thing to be upset about, or that distress should be eliminated altogether?" (*Tusculans* 4.59).

which are under their voluntary control, and this therapy (as analysed in 3.3 below) requires adopting the Stoic way of life (*Tusculans* 3.24). However, Cicero made the important concession that the harsh Stoic therapy only works in "rare cases" and is not available to the "uneducated" (*Tusculans* 4.60). According to Cicero, it is easier to convince people that a given object should not cause distress or fear, than to use the "specific and more reliable" Stoic treatment of removing the emotion by eliminating the false belief (*Tusculans* 4.60).[19] On the other hand, a successful result of the Stoic therapy is that it empowers people to master their emotions and engage in self-therapy (*Tusculans* 2.47). The question to address now is which type of therapy did Cicero recommend for use in distress and fear. Is the strong Stoic remedy the best option, or are there milder and more acceptable alternatives?

3.3.3 Cicero's Therapy for Distress and Fear

> [philosophy] is a physician of souls, takes away the load of empty troubles, sets us free from diseases and banishes fear
>
> Cicero, *Tusculans* 2.4

A central aspect of Cicero's therapy is to clarify the varieties of "distress", which, as mentioned before, include not only fear, but anxiety, worry, anguish and despair as well (*Tusculans* 3.83). These "root-fibres" have to be identified and uprooted, "so that none of them can ever rise again" (*Tusculans* 3.83).[20] Having identified the specific variety of distress, the principal remedy that Cicero suggests for the treatment of distress and fear is to concentrate on the emotion itself and not on its

---

[19]For instance, Cicero would argue that losing a job in a given context is not something to be feared, as there are other, and potentially even better, job options available for the person at risk. For Cicero, this may be more practical than arguing in the Stoic fashion that losing a job is a non-preferred indifferent, since the main goal in life is to attain virtue.

[20]"Yet how numerous are the roots of distress, and how bitter they are! The trunk itself may have been cast down, and still they must be pulled out, every one, by single disputations if need be" (*Tusculans* 3.83).

object (*Tusculans* 4.62).[21] To remove the emotions of distress and fear it is important to understand the limitations of human life, and that misfortunes are beyond human control (*Tusculans* 4.62). The philosopher-therapist has to analyse the concept of fear with the afflicted person in a "manly" way, specifically addressing pain and death, since "these are the two things people fear the most" (*Tusculans* 4.64). This treatment may help in convincing the 'patient' that there is nothing major to endure. However, to fully remove the emotion patients have to understand that their emotions are under their voluntary control and that it is up to them to remove them completely.[22] But in addition to this Stoic approach, Cicero also discussed a broad menu of additional remedies which is examined below.

To be effective, the philosopher needs to determine which remedy to use. To this end, Cicero considered how rhetoric and dialectics could help. He made an analogy between philosophical therapy and his own profession as a lawyer. In court, lawyers do not always use the same discourse but change it depending on several variables, such as the context, the character of the client, the problem at hand, and the range of potential solutions. Similarly, the philosopher must have the knowledge and capacity to deliver soothing remedies, and the ability to implement the intervention at the proper time based on the patient's emotional status.[23] Thus, philosophical therapy is 'tailor-made', "…for not every distress is assuaged by one method" (*Tusculans* 4.59). Rhetoric and dialectic are non-Stoic techniques of addressing the patient's weaknesses and strengths, scolding in case of weak behaviour and praising in case of adequate emotional endurance (*Tusculans* 4.65). It is also explained to the patient that the misfortunes of life are common to humankind and regularly produce distress and fear. The patient is presented with

[21]"the methods which enable a person to bear present afflictions will also enable him to think little of those in prospect" (*Tusculans* 4.64).

[22]"The entire theory of emotion can be summed up in a single point: that they are all in our power, all experienced through judgment, all voluntary. It is this error, then, that must be removed, this belief that must be taken away" (*Tusculans* 4.65).

[23]"…but we adapt the line we take to the occasion, to the character of the dispute, to the personality of the litigant; we act similarly in the alleviation of distress, for we have to consider what method of treatment is admissible in each particular case" (*Tusculans* 3.79).

examples (*exempla*) of others who have undergone similar misfortunes and is guided by the philosopher towards accepting these emotions as typical conditions of human life.

A more philosophically ambitious remedy consists in meditation about one's fears and their objects (*Tusculans* 4.64). Fear is presented to the patient as an emotion that signifies no real danger, and is described in a negative way, such as the result of being inconstant and feeble. Moreover, the object of fear is treated with scorn. This technique is used to guide people into a philosophical path of self-knowledge, as they learn to recognise their emotions as irrational, and of self-restraint, as they learn to despise the object of fear and better control this emotion. This therapy is especially useful for those with a "poor constitution" who are fearful "by nature" or have a proclivity for fear (*Tusculans* 4.80).

While being critical of the Cyrenaics,[24] Cicero fully embraced their pre-rehearsal technique, which is based on the concept that fear is triggered by the unexpectedness of an event. Pre-rehearsal therapy depends on the hypothesis that practice in anticipating future mishaps will decrease the severity of fear and anxiety. The practice involves imagining the worst outcome for a dreaded event, thinking over it repeatedly.[25] Pre-rehearsal requires mental preparation for every circumstance in life that may pose a danger.[26] For example, Cicero suggested thinking that one's wife and children may be all dead when one returns from a trip: if this calamity does happen, one will be mentally ready and the magnitude of the blow will be diminished; but if the calamity does not take place, one should still consider the exercise a "gain" (*Tusculans* 3.30). Cicero's adaptation of Cyrenaic pre-rehearsal consisted of regular

[24]The Cyrenaic school of philosophy was founded in the fourth century BCE and evolved from the Socratic tradition. The aim of this school was achieving sensual pleasure, which was considered to be more fulfilling than mental pleasures. This school provided an example of 'positive hedonism' in contrast of the 'negative hedonism' of the Epicureans (see previous chapter).

[25]"One looks far ahead to misfortunes that are to come, and this makes their arrival easier to bear" (*Tusculans* 3.29), and "Foresight and mental preparation can do a great deal to lessen the pain [by] rehearsing every event in human life" (*Tusculans* 3.30).

[26]"This indeed is wisdom in its noblest and most godlike form: to scrutinize human life and understand it deeply, not to be surprised by anything that happens; and never to think that something cannot happen merely because it has not happened yet" (*Tusculans* 3.30).

meditation about the following possibilities: (1) that every misfortune will help getting stronger against future evils; (2) that it is important to understand the limitations of the human condition, and that death is inexorable; (3) that the suffering produced by a foreseen misfortune will be diluted by long practice; and (4) that nobody should feel guilty about misfortunes that were properly rehearsed, when nothing can be done about them (*Tusculans* 4.34). Cicero concluded that by using pre-rehearsal nobody should feel distressed, as this technique encourages reviewing the nature of human life and thereby gaining in wisdom.

Several conceptual and empirical limitations of the pre-rehearsal technique require discussion. First, pre-rehearsal may be conceptualised as an expression of fear, since by practicing this technique the individual is regularly thinking about future dangers. As discussed in the previous chapter, Epicurus criticised this technique stating that regularly thinking about future calamities is already making the fear perpetual, and he considered it ridiculous to suffer over something that may never happen.[27] Second, we may argue that accepting that tragedies are part of human life does not necessarily protect a person against suffering anxiety and fear. Finally, fearful individuals who are much given to worry, already practice a type of pre-rehearsal 'by default', since they are continuously thinking about the misfortune potentially awaiting them. For these individuals, pre-rehearsal, is a manifestation of worry that is in need of philosophical therapy.

Cicero tried to neutralize Epicurus' criticism of the pre-rehearsal technique by underrating the magnitude of the future evil. Thus, an Epicurean "misfortune" becomes Cicero's "regular restrictions under which we humans live", "the changefulness of life," and "the weakness of humankind" (*Tusculans* 3.34). Cicero concludes, perhaps unwisely, that by using pre-rehearsal we not only gain in wisdom, but "we are never sad at all" (*Tusculans* 3.34). The Epicurean alternative to pre-rehearsal, he argues, is the therapy of 'evasion', which consists on focusing on past pleasures. Cicero considered this technique as no more than

[27]As rendered by Cicero in the *Tusculans*, Epicurus remarked that "It is foolish to rehearse misfortunes which may not yet happened and may not happen at all…they are always in anxiety, either from the evils they undergo or from those they anticipate" (*Tusculans* 3.32).

"womanish behaviour" (*Tusculans* 3.36) in comparison with the 'manly' Cyrenaic attitude of confronting the potential mishap, and he criticised 'evasion' on the basis that it is not always possible to wilfully choose the object of happy recollection.[28]

Following the Stoics, Cicero also claimed that distress and fear are amenable to the "very effective" cure "of the passage of time" (*Tusculans* 3.35). He suggests that some beliefs may remain for a long time, but once the fear of a negative event is no longer 'fresh' in the mind its magnitude will decrease (Graver 2007, p. 107). Accordingly, this remedy consists in convincing the patient that dread and fear will diminish with time, and that newer life events will help to remove the negative emotions (*Tusculans* 3.35).[29]

Another remedy preferred by Cicero is the technique of "consolation," which in the *Tusculans* refers to the understanding that misfortunes are part of human life. The consolation may be conveyed by a speech or by a written piece to soothe the pain of a current misfortune,[30] something Cicero did himself after the death of his daughter Tullia. The consolation technique consists in removing, restraining or at least diverting distress and fear. Accordingly, if the emotions cannot be removed, they can at least be dampened or restrained so that they do not increase or spread to other objects. The consolation combines remedies from different philosophical schools: the Peripatetic teaching that the misfortune is no great evil, the Epicurean diversion of attention towards good memories, and the Stoic maxim that everything happens according to nature.[31] Comfort is provided by applying the proper words at the right time. The philosopher-therapist not only has to know

---

[28]"For it is not within our power to forget or gloss over circumstances which we believe to be evil, at the very moment when they are piercing us. They tear at us, buffet us, goad us, scorch us, stifle us—and you tell us to forget about them? That is contrary to nature!" (*Tusculans* 3.35).

[29]"For the passage of time is itself a means of cure, a slow one to be sure, yet very effective" (*Tusculans* 3.35).

[30]"And yet it is not the case that consolatory speeches of this kind have no value; indeed, they may well be the most valuable thing of all" (*Tusculans* 3.55).

[31]"In my Consolation, for instance, I combined virtually all these methods into a single speech of consolation. For my mind was swollen, and I was trying out every remedy I could" (*Tusculans* 3.76).

the verbal 'medicine' to be delivered, but also the appropriate moment of delivery (*kairos*) that will produce the greatest benefit.[32] The expertise required for this philosophical therapy cannot be overemphasised. Therapists have to adapt their "speeches to the needs of the moment, the nature of the case, and the persons involved, so also in soothing distress we must consider what sort of cure each hearer is able to accept" (*Tusculans* 3.79).

In conclusion, following Cicero's understanding that emotions take place in specific contexts, and their expression depends on personality traits and life-long habits, the *Tusculans* champions flexible, particularistic philosophical treatments for the management of emotions, especially distress and fear, grounded in generic analyses of their causes. I have discussed how Cicero assembled his own 'drugstore' with remedies borrowed from Peripatetics, Cyrenaics and Stoics. Cicero was not an original thinker, but instead, he was a systematic therapist. He remarked on the importance of analysing, from a philosophical perspective, every "root" of distress to obtain a full understanding of its cause and best treatment. Cicero accepted the rigid Stoic remedy of removing the false belief at the root of fear, but had the flexibility to accommodate other therapies depending on the patient's personality and emotional state. As an astute clinician and a great orator, Cicero emphasised the importance of properly choosing the 'verbal remedy' to suit each patient, the means to convey the message, and the proper timing for applying the remedy. He stressed the importance of understanding that not everybody is amenable to philosophical therapy, and that for some a cure is impossible. Thus, whereas it is necessary for a successful therapy that patients accept the full extent of their problem, the philosopher-therapist has also to accept the limitations of philosophical treatment.

All things considered, Cicero's therapeutic aim was to empower individuals to become their own therapists and to enable them to master their own emotions. His technique may seem to lack internal

---

[32]"But it is necessary, in dealing with diseases of the soul, just as much as in dealing with bodily diseases, to choose the proper time…" (*Tusculans* 3.76).

coherence, but it is because of this non-dogmatic approach and his 'teaching differences' that Cicero's therapeutic advice in the *Tusculans* is so relevant and enduring. In the next section I shall go on to discuss the philosophical therapy of fear proposed by Seneca, another major philosopher of the Roman era, whose *Letters on Ethics* provide an in-depth analysis of fear and its treatment from an eclectic, but also mostly Stoic, perspective. Like Cicero a century before him, Seneca had a preference for Stoic remedies, but his discursive approach is quite different from Cicero's. In the *Tusculans* Cicero addresses a general audience, whereas in the *Letters* Seneca begins a tradition of more personally directed, curative philosophical dialogues between philosopher and patient. This patient is Lucilius, Seneca's friend to whom all the letters are directed, but the real patient, as I discuss below, is the reader.

3.4 Fear in Seneca's *Letters*

> Boys fear trifles, children fear shadows, we fear both
>
> *Seneca, Letters 4.2*

> We are frightened at uncertainties, just as if they were certain.
> We observe no moderation.
> The slightest thing turns the scales and throws us forthwith into panic.
>
> *Seneca, Letters 13.14*

As discussed in the previous section, Cicero was the first known Roman philosopher to strongly argue in favour of using philosophy as a therapeutic tool for distress, fear and anxiety. About a century later, Seneca composed the *Letters on Ethics*,[33] one of the most significant texts ever written on the ethics of emotions, and in which fear is one of the main targets for analysis. One interesting aspect of this work is the freedom with which Seneca discusses his own fears and anxieties, as well as those of his interlocutor, Lucilius. In the *Letters*, Seneca not

[33]This is the title used in the latest translation by Margaret Graver and A. A. Long (Seneca 2015), which I have used in this chapter. The text is also known as *Letters to Lucilius* or *Moral Epistles*.

only shares his emotions, but he also provides a variety of remedies to achieve a tranquil life. I shall later discuss how this tradition of sharing the philosopher's own fears and anxieties with the reader reaches a pinnacle with Michel de Montaigne and his *Essays* in the sixteenth century.

3.4.1 Biographical Notes and Life Context

Seneca was a rich citizen from the imperial province of Andalusia, in Spain, who rose to the Senate and later to the Consulship of Rome (Veyne 2003, pp. 24–26). Interestingly, both Cicero and Seneca had similar careers, both becoming intellectual celebrities. And while they had a major role in Roman culture and politics, both ended their careers in distress and fear for their own lives.

Seneca travelled to Rome to learn the art of rhetoric and to gain a liberal education, but he was converted to the study of philosophy in his early youth, including training in Stoic ethics. Reading philosophy was a spiritual exercise which Seneca always practised (Veyne 2003, p. 58). He was 40 years old when he composed the *Consolation to Marcia* (Seneca 1932), a text written in the Stoic tradition, and he was by then considered one of the main Roman philosophers. It was at this age that Seneca joined the Senate and became a popular figure for his qualities as good orator and lawyer; and it was also at this time that his misfortunes began. Owing to his close connection with the circle of women of the imperial court during the reign of Caligula, he was sentenced to death for adultery. The sentence was subsequently commuted to exile resulting in Seneca spending a lonely eight years on the island of Corsica. Eventually, he was pardoned and returned to Rome. Seneca's star rose with his support for the young emperor, Nero, and he rapidly became the greatest intellectual figure in Roman circles, also amassing a fabulous fortune. It was certainly unusual for a philosopher who professed belonging to the Stoic school, to own one of the most important investment banks in Rome (Veyne 2003, pp. 5–6). Some comments from contemporary philosophers, such as Plutarch, are scathing about the ambiguities both in Seneca's political life and in his philosophical writings. Brennan considers Seneca as "moralizing, maxim mongering", a "curious exponent of tranquillity", and an "overheated advocate of cool" (Brennan 2005, p. 14). Whatever Seneca's misguided political actions, and the contrast between his lofty lifestyle and his philosophical preaching of frugality, he was above all a great writer, with a unique a personal style which never hides his own imperfections (Veyne 2003, p. 29). In 62 AD, recognising the disasters of Nero's policies, Seneca asked to be dismissed from his political duties, which Nero refused to do. Seneca then retired to a villa close to Rome, claiming poor health. It was at this time that he started writing the *Letters*, a text that makes quite explicit the reasons for his decision to retire from politics and to plunge into philosophical studies to strengthen his mind against future calamities. Consequently, he committed to a routine of daily self-training and self-restraint, in other words, a Stoic ascetic path to peace of mind (Veyne 2003, p. 29). In 65 CE, Seneca was forced to commit suicide after being accused of participation in a plot to kill Nero.

3.4.2 The Letters on Ethics

As already noted, Seneca's *Letters on Ethics* (*Letters*) (*L. Annaei Senecae ad Lucilium Epistulae* in the original Latin) were written to his friend Lucilius with the principal aim of addressing Lucilius' (and the reader's) anxieties and introducing him to Stoic philosophy.[34] The *Letters* provide abundant material on the philosophical concept of fear, and illustrate Seneca's unorthodox understanding of the Stoic approach to fear in general, and to the fear of death in particular. In fact, fear is the emotion most frequently discussed in the *Letters*, with explicit reference to fear or anxiety in 45 of the 124 letters.

In general terms Seneca posited that, as humans grow into adulthood, their mental life is shaped by numerous fears, both real and imaginary. Most humans are unable to mentally separate themselves from the objects

[34]Graver and Long state categorically that the *Letters* were not composed to suit a real person, but to convey Seneca's ethical thoughts in a therapeutic way for the posterity. They remark that in Letter 8 (8.2) Seneca admits that "the work I am doing is for posterity: it is they who can benefit from what I write."

of fear, and the mere idea that something bad may happen is frequently sufficient to plunge them into utmost despair. Stressing the significance of fear in human life and how difficult it is to fight it, Seneca claimed, against Stoic ethics that, people should try to avoid "whatever may cause fear" (*Letters* 98.7). His specific advice on how to fight fear, fluctuates between a staunch Stoic position and a more eclectic approach influenced by Epicureanism. His advice on the philosophical therapy of fear was presented in several of his works, but it is in the *Letters* where he examined fear from diverse perspectives, philosophical and personal, that he provides comprehensive and forceful therapeutic suggestions.

3.4.3 The Concept of Fear in Seneca's Letters

Like Cicero, Seneca was not a systematic philosopher. His concept of fear has to be gleaned from different sections of the *Letters*, and interpreted in the context of his understanding of mental sickness. Seneca defines diseases of the mind as "a persistent perversion of the judgment so that things which are mildly desirable are thought to be highly desirable…" (*Letters* 75.11), and emotions as sudden, vehement and objectionable "impulses of the spirit" (*Letters* 75.11). When emotions are not examined and controlled, they may cause physical disease, "just as a catarrh…" (*Letters* 75.11). Seneca makes frequent reference to fear of illness, poverty and violence, and considered fear of death, fear of bodily pain, and fear of lacking pleasures as underlying the fear of aging. According to Seneca, severe worries, once they become chronic, lead to a tortured life.[35] Similarly, repeated attacks of fear may result in a propensity to suffer these attacks following only minor stimuli, causing the affected individual to live in a chronic state of anxiety.[36] Therefore, controlling the inclination towards worrying is one of the biggest challenges to the tranquil life of Stoic *apatheia*.

[35]"… life is not worth living, and there is no limit to our sorrows, if we indulge our fears to the greatest possible extent" (*Letters* 13.12).

[36]"Even in the midst of safety you will have no confidence if your mind has once been given a shock; once it has acquired the habit of blind panic, it is incapable of providing even for its own safety" (*Letters* 104.10).

The process by which Seneca became 'enlightened' about the human mechanism of fear is described in Letter 57. During a rough sea voyage Seneca underwent a "transformation" (*Letters* 57.7). In the midst of the storm he felt "a certain mental thrill…unaccompanied by fear" (*Letters* 52.3), and realised that in that unusual and dangerous context even the most fearless individuals showed changes in skin colour and complexion, accompanied by brow contraction, shudders, and dizziness. Seneca considered this sudden behavioural change as independent of courage or reason. For Seneca, such changes do not amount to fear, but are "a natural feeling that nature cannot rout" (*Letters* 57.4). After the storm was over, Seneca also realised that human fears have specific causes, but the cause of the greatest fear is death. Seneca saw that it is the fear of death that has to be vanquished, and it is only then that other fears will become controllable. The corollary to these discoveries is that according to Seneca, emotions *strictu sensu* have to be distinguished from *propatheia*, those 'pre-emotions' already described by Cicero in the *Tusculans* as "bitings" and "contractions" that occur after a strong impression. "First movements" were for Seneca the immediate bodily responses that occur after a sudden dangerous event but before the intellect is able to make a judgment and provide assent.[37] This is the case with reflex responses such as a startle response to a loud noise or bodily feelings triggered by thunder. These behavioural responses are common to most animals, and there is no belief or assent to danger involved. Therefore, Seneca did not consider these responses as "true" fear, but only as "first movements," that is, unconscious, involuntary and instinctive reactions that cannot be suppressed by training.[38]

[37]It is interesting to contrast Seneca's 'pre-emotions' with William James' concept of emotions. As I shall discuss in Chapter 6, James defined emotions as the feeling of somatic changes. According to James, when we see a bear we feel fear because we run, and not because we believe or think that the bear is a dangerous animal. On the other hand, Seneca considered the behavioural reactions that precede the cognitive evaluation of the object as a mere pre-emotion, a first movement that does not qualify as a true emotion.

[38]"the steadiest speaker, when before the public, often breaks into a perspiration, …some tremble in the knees when they rise to speak; I know of some whose teeth chatter, whose tongues falter, whose lips quiver… nature exerts her own power and through such a weakness makes her presence known even to the strongest" (*Letters* 11.2).

Seneca also analysed the phenomenon of fear at the social level. Thus, he considered that fears can be 'propagated' in a community. Rumours are easily spread among the population and may produce the uncontrollable behaviours of "Panic fear" (*Letters* 13.9), a generalized state of extreme fear that once released becomes difficult to control.[39] Nevertheless, it is fear at the individual level that interests Seneca the most, and having reprised his concept of emotions, we are in a position to discuss his therapeutic approach.

3.4.4 The Therapy of Fear in the Letters

Despite his therapy being mostly based on Stoic methods, and like Cicero, Seneca's conceptual and therapeutic approach to fear was heterogeneous. Unlike Cicero, however, Seneca borrowed extensively from Epicureanism,[40] and although Seneca's therapeutic views are distributed in an unstructured way across many letters, it is possible to discern some systematic themes, provided it is remembered that Seneca was frequently inconsistent in his views and on occasion directly contradicted himself. Where Motto and Clark (1968, p. 38) consider Seneca to be a non-sectarian philosopher, whose philosophical practice consisted in borrowing from different schools whatever he considered most appropriate to support his philosophical speculations, I believe a pattern may be discerned after analysing his writings. Due to Seneca's high number of citations of Epicurus (64 references), Motto and Clarke also describe Seneca as "the Epicurean Stoic" (p. 41). Whatever his philosophical inclinations, Seneca offered numerous laudatory comments about Epicureanism and each of the first thirty letters finishes with an Epicurean maxim and a clear demonstration of how much Seneca valued Epicurus' philosophical teachings.

---

[39]Once an individual is "overwhelmed by the disaster, the rest are overwhelmed by fear, and the possibility that they may suffer makes them as downcast as the actual sufferer" (*Letters* 54.3).

[40]See especially the first 40 letters.

3.4.4.1 Seneca's Concept of Fear During His Epicurean Phase

Although initially in the *Letters*, Seneca's concept of the emotions might be described as diluted Stoicism he rapidly slips into a more accessible Epicurean mode. The first step in Seneca's therapy is to clarify, in the Stoic manner, whether fear is caused by a real object, or whether the cause of fear is "empty", that is, based on a false belief (*Letters* 13.7).[41] Next, he suggests, in an Epicurean fashion, considering whether our body is healthy or sick. If we are physically healthy, then fear "is not an issue" (*Letters* 13.7). Such a state corresponds to the Epicurean state of *aponia* or lack of bodily pain, which together with *ataraxia* or lack of mental pain, creates the maximum state of happiness. In contrast, as I discussed in the section on Cicero, a healthy body was for the Stoics nothing more than a 'preferred indifferent', that is, an object judged to be neither bad or evil but preferred, as being healthy is in accordance with nature.

Seneca next introduces the Epicurean technique of focusing on the present, almost the opposite to the Cyrenaic technique of pre-rehearsal so much valued by Cicero. Seneca's advice is not to be "miserable before it is time,"[42] since feared misfortunes may never happen or at least have not yet happened.[43] When Lucilius worries that misfortune "still is to come" (*Letters* 13.8), Seneca's advice is to ascertain whether mischief is truly forthcoming, "for all too often we worry about what we merely suspect" (*Letters* 13.8).[44] In the initial letters, during this Epicurean phase, Seneca identifies fear of poverty, fear of disease, and fear of the powerful as the main

---

[41]I used the term "diluted Stoicism" because, for the Stoic doctrine, fear is always the result of a false belief and cannot be rational by definition.

[42]"Some evil is probable for the future; it is not proven right off. How many unexpected things have come to pass! How many of our expectations never happen at all! Even if it is to come, what good does it do to anticipate your grief? You will grieve soon enough, when it comes; in the meantime, allow yourself something better" (*Letters* 13.4).

[43]Seneca's remedy is fully Epicurean (compare with Chapter 2): "Some things, then, torment us more than they should, some sooner than they should; and some torment us that should not do so at all: either we add to our pain, or we make it up, or we get ahead of it" (*Letters* 13.5).

[44]"Yes, dear Lucilius, we are too quick to give way to opinion. We do not demand evidence of the things that frighten us, or check them out carefully" (*Letters* 13.8).

human fears,[45] and suggests humans should always try to stay away from the object of fear.[46] Seneca considered poverty and sickness as "silent" fears (*Letters* 14.4), as these do not impact on the senses. On the other hand, the fear of the powerful is "terrifying" because it arrives "with a great deal of noise and activity" (*Letters* 14.4). These are the fears of war, torture and prison, "and everything else that savagery has devised" (*Letters* 14.5).

The question arises as to how to stay safe in a world full of political turmoil. Seneca's answer is first to give no offense to "the populace", the state, or the ruler (*Letters* 14.7); and second, the well-known Epicurean advice of living unnoticed. The danger of the "common crowd" is best avoided by not desiring the same objects as others, thus shunning competition, hatred, envy, and contempt (*Letters* 14.9). And yet, regardless of how much we apply ourselves to allaying dangers by living unnoticed and giving no offense to the powerful, the outcome of our deeds will depend in great part on fortune alone.[47] In other words, circumstances beyond our control will eventually decide the outcome of potential dangers. This important concept will be later adopted by the Stoic philosopher Epictetus who remarked that some things are up to us and we should work on these, but other things are not up to us and we have to accept that there is nothing to be done (Epictetus 1928).

While Seneca explained in several letters what he considered to be the necessary steps to achieve command over fears, he also acknowledges that personal attributes play an important role in how fear impacts upon the individual and how it can be managed. For instance, Seneca wrote that "great and unceasing application to study" (*Letters* 75.15) is important for the proper handling of emotions, but also that human constitutional attributes such as "good fortune with regard to natural gifts" (*Letter* 75.15),[48] are necessary for setting limits to fear. In other words,

[45]Fear of death is implicit in the above list of fears.

[46]"...let us avoid not only danger but also discomfort, as much as we can, and retreat into safety..." (*Letters* 14.3).

[47]"The beginnings are in our power; the results are judged by fortune; to which I grant no jurisdiction over myself. But fortune will bring some trouble, some adversity" (*Letters* 14.16).

[48]"Whatever is assigned to us by the terms of our birth and the blend in our constitutions, will stick with us, no matter how hard or how long the soul may have tried to master itself" (*Letters* 11.6).

to dispel the passion of fear it is not sufficient simply to understand that fears are produced by false beliefs, but having the "natural gifts" of a resilient personality is also required.

Seneca's generic therapeutic approach, in line with the Epicureans, involves teaching limits to desires in order to prevent fear.[49] Given that fear and hope are conceptually related, the therapist has to teach that "you will cease to fear…if you cease to hope" (*Letters* 5.7). According to Seneca the constant movement between hope and fear is a result of an incapacity to live in the present moment. Unlike Epicurus, who found solace in pleasant memories, following Seneca the therapist should stop the patient from dwelling in the past—since memory "recalls the stab of fear"—or thinking about objects far in the future (*Letters* 5.9).[50] Foresight, the greatest attribute of the human condition can be used with great benefit to prevent dangers, but this ability "becomes perverted" (*Letters* 5.8) when it anticipates misfortunes that may never happen.[51] To 'live in the present' it is necessary to cast away any potential pleasure that may bring anxiety, since it is in human nature to always want more.[52] It is also of the essence to be contented with little, and to be weary of fortune, since ambitions lie "wholly toward the future" (*Letters* 15.9).

In a more Stoic vein, Seneca suggested the daily exercise of meditation which he practiced himself every night. The main meditation consists of self-examination with the aim of recognizing and accepting one's failures and progressing along the Stoic path to virtue. Seneca's meditation

---

[49]In *Letters* 14.9 Seneca follows the Epicurean precept of having few desires. Seneca remarks it is a big danger to desire the same objects as the "common crowd" (*Letters* 14.9) since this competition will only bring unsafety. Seneca cites Epicurus' remark that "He enjoys riches most who has least need of riches" (*Letters* 14.17) also adding that "He who feels the need of wealth also fears for his wealth" (*Letters* 14.18).

[50]The main cause of fear is that "we do not adapt ourselves to the present but direct our thoughts toward things far in the future. Thus foresight, which is the greatest good belonging to the human condition, has become an evil" (*Letters* 5.9).

[51]"Beasts avoid the dangers which they see, and when they have escaped them are free from care; but we men torment ourselves over the future which is to come as well as over that which is past. Many of our blessings bring bane to us; for memory recalls the tortures of fear, while foresight anticipates them. The present alone can make no man wretched" (*Letters* 5.9).

[52]"The more you achieve, the more you will have to fear" (*Letters* 19.8).

is to be carried out with extreme honesty. One should study oneself after removing all "ornaments" such as power and wealth (*Letters* 80.10), otherwise our self-concept may depend on what other people value in us, and their opinions are usually biased towards their interests. For Seneca, self-understanding is being conscious of one's mortality, meditating on what is good or bad for us, and deciding on what is worth pursuing in a rational (that is, non-emotional) way (*Letters* 82.6). We should meditate on the fact that fear of death is worse than death itself, and that we are terrified by "phantoms" as well as "real dangers" (*Letters* 104.10). There is no peace of mind once we become accustomed to fearing everything. It is "the habit of thoughtless anxiety" that stops us from thinking in a rational way and being able to distinguish danger from safety and, as a result, we tend to escape from situations when it would be better for us to confront the problem at hand.[53] Therefore, Seneca's meditation practice is aimed at improving our mental strength and resilience rather than following intellectual pursuits. He warned about "tricks of logic" being used as a method of persuasion that death is not an evil (*Letters* 82.8), since in his opinion the practice of logic is not conducive to increasing mental strength.[54] It is courage rather than mental exercises that will prepare us to confront fears. Simple soldiers do not need to understand syllogisms when they hear the final harangue from the Spartan Leonidas: "Eat your breakfast, fellow soldiers; dinner will be in Hades." (*Letters* 82.21). Examples like this were also part of the therapeutic meditation on fear of death, which Seneca suggests is a good theme for the daily reflection. He writes on specific aspects of this fear, for instance, on wanting to live a long life, remarking that this grasping and holding onto life can only result in a chronic state of anxiety.[55] The meditator also has to ponder the fact that living and dying are two faces of

[53]"It does not shun danger but rather takes flight, even though we are more exposed to dangers when we don't face them" (*Letters* 104.10).

[54]"Zeno, of our school, offers the following syllogism: Nothing bad is glorious. But death is glorious. Therefore, death is not bad. Now, that was a big help! You have freed me from fear; after that, I won't hesitate to offer my neck to the sword!" (*Letters* 82.8).

[55]"No one cares how well he lives but only how long—despite the fact that every one of us has the chance to live well, and no one can live long" (*Letters* 22.17).

the same natural process, and that by fearing death we forget to live.[56] Seneca also suggests other remedies, such as philosophical readings on how to manage fears and writing "healthy admonitions". He states in Letter 8 that he is writing for posterity, but it is also likely he was putting to paper Epicurean maxims for his own philosophical benefit.[57]

3.4.4.2 Seneca's Therapy in Action: Letter 24 "Courage in a Threatening Situation"

Letter 24 provides a good example of Seneca's philosophical treatment of fear in action. Lucilius tells Seneca about his worries regarding the outcome of a lawsuit against him. Seneca begins the therapy by assessing his 'patient'. Lucilius is a Roman knight and a writer, the governor of Sicily, and a clever interlocutor. In consequence, Seneca decides against applying the basic remedy of creating hope and providing "comforting expectations" (*Letters* 24.1). Lucilius is too knowing for this 'mild' remedy, and instead Seneca applies the Epicurean strategy of staying in the present moment. The message is that the feared mishap may never materialise, whereas the mental pain (or what Cicero called "distress") is present.[58] The remedy of 'living in the present' is not strong enough to soothe Lucilius, and Seneca turns a variation on the Epicurean *tetrapharmakos* (see Chapter 2) where it is stated that pain is not to be feared because if severe, death is imminent and if it is light, pain may even be pleasurable. Seneca tells Lucilius that "You will soon realize that what your fear is either no great matter or not long lasting" (*Letters* 24.2). If this adaptation of the *tetrapharmakos* is still not successful, Seneca suggests the use of "examples to strengthen you with" (*Letters* 24.3). For instance, some people endure

[56]"These thoughts, and others like them, are what we must ponder if we want to be at peace as we await the final hour. For fear of that one makes all our other hours uneasy" (*Letters* 4.9).

[57]In Letter 8 he states that "I am still plundering Epicurus, in whose work I today found this saying: You should become a slave to philosophy, that you may attain true liberty" (*Letters* 8.7), a good illustration of therapeutic reading and writing.

[58]"...what need is there to take an advance on future troubles, ruining the present with fear of the future? When troubles come is time enough to bear them. Surely it is foolish to be miserable now just because you are going to be miserable later on!" (*Letters* 24.1).

prison and exile courageously, "even gladly" (*Letters* 24.4) and some illiterate soldiers watch their hands "sizzling on the enemy's brazier" without showing any emotion (*Letters* 24.5). Lucilius is still unmoved by stories full of heroism but unable to calm his mind. Seneca's response is that the use of *exempla* is aimed at encouraging Lucilius to understand that he is not brave enough in confronting relatively harmless events. But after this strategy also fails, Seneca suggests to Lucilius that he stay calm since the outcome of dreaded events may be decided by "external factors" not under Lucilius control (*Letters* 24.12), and to meditate on the maxim: "there is nothing to fear in your affairs but fear itself" (*Letters* 24.12). In this way Seneca stresses that like little children who are frightened by "masks,"[59] adults also fear imaginary objects. Making a major turn in the treatment, Seneca's next advice to Lucilius is to confront his fear directly and grasp the notion that "whatever *can* happen…*will* happen" (*Letters* 24.15) (italics in the original). This constitutes a radical strategic change in Seneca's therapy, which began by urging Lucilius to stay in the present and to consider that what is feared may never happen and now changes to encouraging him to accept that the dreaded outcome will indeed happen. Seneca's next advice is a heterogeneous remedy consisting of the Epicurean method of 'diversion', that is, thinking about "people in general", but also that the body is mortal, that life is unpredictable, and that it is better to think that death is nothing to us (*Letters* 24.16). These are all exercises that will "strengthen" Lucilius' mind to cope with daily fears, since what truly underlies all fears is the fear of death. Seneca's treatment of Lucilius' anxiety now enters its final stage, and consists in the analysis of the value of life in the context of great emotional turmoil. He warns Lucilius that committing suicide out of fear is always irrational, since all fears boil down to the greatest of all fears, the irrational fear of death.[60]

[59]"You see with children how people they love and know, people they play with, frighten them terribly if they see them wearing masks: well, the same thing happens with us, who are just slightly bigger children" (*Letters* 24.13).

[60]Seneca proceeds to cite Epicurus in two remarks that are preserved in this text. Both remarks reject suicide as a product of fear of death: "What could be more absurd than to seek death when it is fear of death that has made your life unquiet?", and "So great is the foolishness, no, the madness of human beings, that some are driven toward their death by fear of death" (*Letters* 24.23). Fear of death is specifically addressed below (Section 4.5).

In conclusion, Seneca' therapy of fear in Epicurean fashion uses the important technique of adapting the remedies to the patient, as well as using a variety of methods, such as living in the present, using maxims and *exempla*, diversion of attention and regular meditation on the fear of death, at a midpoint between "excessive love of life and against excessive hatred of it" (*Letters* 24.24). It is interesting to contrast these techniques for addressing fear, with Seneca's Stoic methods. Letter 74, which states that there is no peace of mind in a state of anxiety, and "a life amid anxieties is a life of misery" (*Letters* 74.5) shows Seneca using Stoic rather than Epicurean techniques.[61] In this Letter he considers that the only medicine to end anxiety is to live a virtuous life based on honourable conduct.[62] A life without virtue is worthless, since "every plan is adrift; no good fortune can satisfy us" (*Letters* 74.11). On the other hand, "Virtue rejoices in present goods; has no longing for what is absent; finds nothing meagre that will suffice" (*Letters* 74.12). In living a virtuous life, the Stoic sage shows consistency and harmony in behaviour and is emotionally unperturbed. The wise Stoic is not affected by the loss of children or friends, or by the prospect of death. Fear now becomes "dishonourable" (*Letters* 74.30)[63] since the Stoic has no fear but only 'first movements'.

Nevertheless, Epicurean and Cyrenaic influences still creep in. Seneca admits that only the fool lives in fear, since "what it fears to endure, it endures already through fear" (*Letters* 74.32). Moreover, Seneca still remarks on the importance of living in the present (*Letters* 74.34), and borrows Cicero's technique of 'pre-rehearsal.' Seneca uses the fire that destroyed the city of Lyon as a metaphor for tragedies whose magnitude are greater, the more unexpected they are. Thus,

---

[61]Graver uses anxiety to translate the more generic Latin *malum*, but the Latin *anxietas* is not used here. As I mentioned earlier, *anxietas* had a much stronger somatic connotation than in our current use.

[62]"There is but one road that leads to safety: you must rise above external things and be content with what is honourable. For he who thinks there is something better than virtue, or that anything besides virtue is good at all, exposes his breast to everything fortune can throw at him and waits anxiously for the blows to land" (*Letters* 74.6).

[63]"All anxiety and worry is dishonourable, all reluctance to act; for honourable conduct is sure and unhampered, undismayed, ever standing at the ready" (*Letters* 74.30).

returning to the Stoic therapy, Seneca states that "…we should let nothing catch us unprepared. We should try to anticipate everything and reflect on what's possible rather than what usually happens" (*Letters* 91.4). This can be achieved by being constantly alert even in times of joy and peace, given that even "when all is quite calm, terror emerges" (*Letters* 91.6). Our attitude towards life adopts a suspicious approach to everything and everybody, since "friends turn foes, allies into enemies" (*Letters* 91.5).

With the aim of fighting fear by following the virtuous path of the Stoic sage, in Letter 75 Seneca presents three different stages of human emotional progress. The first and highest stage relates to individuals who are close to Stoic virtue and with no "infirmities of the mind" (*Letter* 75.10),[64] in other words, individuals with no ingrained mistakes when it comes to judging the value of objects as purveyors of fear. These individuals practice diligent scrutiny and self-examination and only pursue what is worth pursuing, that is, Stoic virtue. They will not fear irrational objects, but they have yet to practice a virtuous life. The second stage includes those that are able to control their emotions, although not in a steady manner. Finally, in the third stage, people are afflicted by "faults", since they are unable to manage fear in a rational way. Accordingly, "they are unconcerned about death but still terrified with pain" (*Letters* 75.14). An individual who progresses from the third to the first Stoic stages, will reach a state of having neither desires nor fears; a state of "tranquil mind and independence" (*Letters* 75.11). Through criss-crossing paths, both Cicero and Seneca concluded that the person who is cured of fear will "have absolute power over [them] self" (*Letter* 75.18) and "be master of [them]self" (*Tusculans* 2.47). But to reach this state, it is necessary to cure the mother of all fears: the fear of death.

[64]"an infirmity is a persistent judgment in a corrupted person that certain things are very much worth pursuing that in fact are only slightly worth pursuing" (*Letters* 75.11).

3.4.5 Seneca's Treatment for Fear of Death

For Seneca, fear of death is the greatest suffering of humankind.[65] In his first letters, Seneca provides the Epicurean advice of ignoring death while we are alive (*Letters* 4.2), or if death is close, to consider the duration of life as irrelevant.[66] In this early stage of the *Letters* Seneca suggests that the therapy for the fear of death requires constant reflection, and he paraphrases Epicurus' maxim: "Rehearse for death" ("*meditare mortem*") (*Letters* 26.8). Appropriate reflection will teach us how to die without fear,[67] which involves, first, accepting death as inevitable; and second, understanding that how and when to die is fully in human hands, and in the end, a matter of personal choice. Suicide was for Seneca the great escape in case of extreme distress and fears.[68] He also remarks that extreme fear of death could paradoxically plunge some into suicide. This "craving for death" should be avoided as it is an affliction that is suffered by those that have too much hatred or too much love for life. For most people, for whom suicide is not an option, taming the fear of death requires "long practice" to learn a rational approach to this fear (*Letters* 30.4).[69] For Seneca, the fear of death is conceptually "foolish" (*Letters* 30.10), since fear implies a potential danger, whereas death is a certainty. Philosophy, he claims, will teach students how to

[65] "But of all the suffering crowds of humankind, the greatest is of those who are troubled by the thought of death. That thought meets them at every turn, for death may come from any direction. Like troops passing through enemy territory, they must be looking around all the time, turning their heads at every sound. Unless this fear is driven from the breast, we live with quaking hearts" (*Letters* 74.3).

[66] "No man can have a peaceful life who thinks too much about lengthening it, or believes that living through many consulships is a great blessing" (*Letters* 4.4).

[67] Seneca stated that it is possible to "depart from life contentedly" but that most humans who "ebb and flow in wretchedness between the fear of death and the hardship of life; … are unwilling to live, and yet they do not know how to die" (*Letters* 5.5).

[68] Death may be welcomed, and "even, if circumstances commend that course, to invite it. There is no difference whether death comes to us, or whether we go to death" (*Letters* 49.6).

[69] "…the soul must be hardened by long practice, so that it may learn to endure the sight and the approach of death" (*Letters* 82.15–16).

"depart calmly" (*Letters* 30.4) by training them to speak openly about death, and by encouraging them to reflect on the idea that death is not painful and implies no suffering. This training includes the following exercises: (1) learning how to face incoming death, (2) building courage concerning what is inevitable, (3) understanding that the duration of life is irrelevant for living a virtuous life, and (4) accepting that death may happen at any time. Once this training is successfully completed, students should throw the ladder of their learning away and become their own masters. "The advice I give is a remedy not for this illness only, but for your whole life. It is this: despise death. Once we escape that fear, nothing is ever sad" (*Letters* 78.5).

3.5 Conclusion

Seneca's *Letters* is an invaluable document for understanding the philosophical therapy of fear and anxiety in the Roman Empire. But the range of fears and anxiety-producing situations he described is still relevant today. Fear of poverty, fear of illness, fear of exile, and most of all, the fear of death is as important today as they were two millennia ago. As a result, there are important lessons in his texts for those who are fearful and anxious in current times.

Seneca was principally a Stoic philosopher but his therapeutic approach to fear was eclectic. He mostly adopted the classical Stoic posture of treating any object of fear as an 'indifferent,' and even fear of death was scorned and despised. However, and especially in his early *Letters*, Seneca considered fear to be an emotion that is impossible to ignore, and thus he also provided abundant therapeutic advice. This advice included Epicurean remedies such as living in the present and redirecting attention, but he also advocated the use of pre-rehearsal. Like Cicero a century before, Seneca remarked on the relevance of assessing the patient's personality for the suitability of philosophical remedies. His broad approach to the treatment of fear, also like Cicero's, consisted in teaching differences about the characteristics of the patient and the therapist, and about the treatment itself.

The powerful philosophical and literary value of his *Letters*, with their remedies for fear and distress may relate, among other factors, to the fact that Seneca talks and argues with his friend and with himself, making his readers active students and participants in his own emotional dilemmas. The *Letters* are one of those pieces of antiquity with which we can converse because we may easily identify ourselves with many of the situations of fear and distress he so clearly describes, and find solace and useful advice in them. Seneca tells the reader about his daily emotional problems in a way that resonates with our lives. As Long points out (Long 2006, p. 370) the *Letters* obtained immortality because the text departs in a humanistic way from tradition and context. The *Letters* do not constitute a consistent philosophical treatise on the concept of emotions, as it lacks coherent conceptual structure and has repetitions and contradictions. But these imperfections make the text much closer to life and to our feelings than is the *Tusculans*. Seneca is open to sharing with us his emotional road through life towards self-improvement. Thus, it comes as no surprise that centuries later, Montaigne, the inventor of the auto-biographical essay genre, will consider Seneca as one of his major influences.

According to Sellars the doctrine of *oikeiosis* is at the bases of the Stoic ethical system (Sellars 2014, p. 108). Sellars defined *oikeiosis* as an instinct of self-preservation, with a predilection for what leads to self-preservation and rejection for what is damaging. Self-preservation is an encompassing concept, ranging from the instinct to stay alive shared with all animals to the uniquely human attribute of self-awareness, that is, being conscious about dangers to one's life and about mortality. The emotion of fear is a manifestation of both the drive for self-preservation and the self-reflective attitudes of humans. In some instances, humans show a behavioural response to sudden danger which is non-reflective. These reflexive behaviours were labelled as 'first movements' by Seneca, who did not consider them as true fear. As we have seen, what both Cicero and Seneca were concerned about, and wrote about, are the universal fears of poverty, sickness, and death. Both Roman philosophers followed the Stoic dogma that fear, like all other emotions, is irrational and it has to be removed to achieve *apatheia*. Cicero's treatment was primarily aimed at removing distress, but he pointed to the conceptual connections between distress and fear, making the treatment common to both emotions. Both Cicero and Seneca developed therapies of fear based on the use of words, and not surprisingly, both were excellent orators. Thus, they recommended choosing the right words and deliver the verbal therapy at the appropriate time to allay the distress and fear of the sick person. The power of words over human emotions was known since the time of the Greek Sophists. Thus, in his *Encomium on Helen*, the sophist Gorgias proposed that words have the capacity to take away fear, as they have a power comparable "to that possessed by well-compounded medicines to the body" (Gorgias 1991). For Cicero, words had the potential for curing, or at least soothing, teaching and consoling. He created a Stoic-Platonic therapy consisting in a thorough investigation of the roots of fear, complemented by reading and listening to philosophical maxims, and applying the techniques of self-mastery, memorization and meditation. Seneca considered fear to be the greatest scourge of the human mind, with fear of death underlying all other fears. He proposed a broad range of remedies, from the Epicurean notion of living in the present, to Cyrenaic pre-rehearsal and Stoic cognitive removal of emotions. Neither Cicero nor Seneca introduced novel therapeutic techniques or modified the concept of emotions, which they borrowed from various philosophical schools, and yet the *Tusculan Disputations* and the *Letters on Ethics* are enduring and universal texts. One explanation for this phenomenon is that both philosophers found a way of reaching into the emotions of the reader. We suffer with Cicero the loss of her daughter, and fully understand and identify with his distress. Cicero points, indirectly, to our own distress and suggests different ways to assuage this emotion. Distress is an emotional response to a current misfortune, as well as the pain we feel in respect to future misfortunes. Seneca's *Letters* provide an even more engaging approach to the problem of fear. He preaches and admonishes his friend Lucilius like a harsh Stoic teacher, but simultaneously he relates to us his own fears, with which again we become identified. His advice is for both Lucilius and ourselves and his situation-specific non-dogmatic approach to fear will suit most affected individuals.

Conquering fear is for Cicero and Seneca the main path towards freedom and tranquillity of mind. As Seneca remarks at the end of Letter 75, "What is freedom, you ask? To fear no human being and no god, to want neither what is base nor what is excessive, to have absolute power over oneself. Just being one's own person is wealth beyond measure" (*Letters* 75.18).

References

Berrios, G. (1999). Anxiety disorders: A conceptual history. *Journal of Affective Disorders, 56*(2–3), 83–94.

Brennan, T. (2003). Stoic moral psychology. In B. Inwood (Ed.), *The Cambridge companion to the stoics* (pp. 257–294). Cambridge: Cambridge University Press.

Brennan, T. (2005). *The stoic life: Emotions, duties & fate*. Oxford: Clarendon Press.

Cicero. (1927). *Tusculan disputations* (J. E. King, Trans., Vol. 141). Cambridge, MA: Harvbard University Press.

Epictetus. (1928). Enchiridion (W. A. Oldfather, Trans.). In *Discourses* (Vol. 218, pp. 479–534). Cambridge, MA: Harvard University Press.

Gorgias. (1991). *Encomium of Hellen* (D. M. Macdowell, Trans.). Bristol: Bristol Classical Press.

Grant, M. (1990). *The Hellenistic Greeks : From Alexander to Cleopatra* (New ed.). London: Weidenfeld & Nicolson.

Graver, M. R. (2002). *Cicero on the emotions* (M. R. Graver, Trans.). Chicago: The University of Chicago Press.

Graver, M. R. (2007). *Stoicism and emotion*. Chicago: The University of Chicago Press.

Inwood, B. (1985). *Ethics and human action in early stoicism*. Oxford: Clarendon Press.

Liddell, H. G., & Scott, R. (1996). *Greek-English lexicon*. Oxford: Clarendon Press.

Long, A. A. (2006). *From Epicurus to Epictetus*. Oxford: Clarendon Press.

Montaigne, M. D. (1991). *The complete essays* (M. A. Screech, Trans.). London: Penguin.

Motto, A. L., & Clark, J. R. (1968). "Paradoxum Senecae": The Epicurean stoic. *The Classical World, 62*(2), 37–42.

Nussbaum, M. C. (1994). *The therapy of desire: Theory and practice in Hellenistic ethics*. Princeton, NJ: Princeton University Press.

Patch, H. R. (1974). *The goddess Fortuna in medieval literature*. New York: Octagon Books.

Sellars, J. (2014). *Stoicism*. Durham: Taylor and Francis.

Seneca. (1932). *De Consolatione ad Marciam* (J. W. Basore, Trans., Vol. 254). Cambridge, MA: Harvard University Press.

Seneca. (2015). *Letters on ethics* (M. R. Graver & A. A. Long, Trans.). Chicago: The University of Chicago Press.

Sorabji, R. (2000). *Emotion and peace of mind: From stoic agitation to christian temptation*. Oxford: Oxford University Press.

Striker, G. (1990). Ataraxia, happiness as tranquillity. *Monist, 73*(1), 97–110.

Striker, G. (1995). Cicero and Greek philosophy. *Harvard Studies in Classical Philology, 97*, 53–61.

Urmson, J. O. (1990). *The Greek philosophical vocabulary*. London: Duckworth.

Veyne, P. (2003). *Seneca: The life of a stoic*. New York: Routledge.

4

Montaigne's *Essays*: A Humanistic Approach to Fear

It is fear that I am most afraid of: In harshness it surpasses all other mischances.

Michel de Montaigne, *Essays* (Book I, "On fear") (Montaigne 2003)

4.1 Introduction

Michel de Montaigne, born in 1533 in the Aquitaine region of France, was a classic example of the Renaissance humanist thinker: an excellent rhetorician who mastered the use of the vernacular language as well as Latin, allowing him to study the classical sources of Roman philosophy and translations of Greek philosophers into Latin (Frame 1984, pp. 29–45). Montaigne became a famous writer as a result of a single work, the *Essays*, which contain more than one hundred pieces of differing lengths dealing with a variety of subjects, from a scholarly analysis of a theological work to advice on how to obtain the best breed of horses. The *Essays* are considered the most important work in French philosophy until the Enlightenment, almost 100 years later. The significance of this work lies in the fact that Montaigne experimented with a new way of writing, characterised by analysing a subject from different perspectives and at different times in life.

S. Starkstein, *A Conceptual and Therapeutic Analysis of Fear*,
https://doi.org/10.1007/978-3-319-78349-9_4

Montaigne starts discussing a topic and may digress to something different, or he provides an opinion about, say, fear in the first set of essays, and then radically changes his opinion twenty years later. Since his initial point of view is not deleted, we have the opportunity to examine, directly, the progression of Montaigne's thinking along the years.

The *Essays* provide a vast amount of information regarding the culture and social habits in Renaissance France, as well as philosophical analysis of the most significant human afflictions. I will argue that fear is one of the most important subjects discussed in the Essays, as this emotion was strongly present in Montaigne's life.[1] I will also argue that it is Montaigne's practical approach to living with fears and his attempt at dominating them that makes the *Essays* so attractive. His early life was spent tortured by different fears, which is reflected in many chapters of the *Essays*, and the 'remedies' used by Montaigne are highly instructive and inspiring.

The *Essays* were written during a period of almost 20 years[2] and reflect the early period of Stoicism, a middle period characterised by Epicureanism and Scepticism, and a final period when Montaigne released himself from established philosophical views and provided his own thoughts.[3] Bakewell (2010, p. 303) has suggested that the

[1]It is difficult to introduce Montaigne as a philosopher, as he did not belong to the 'establishment' nor did he want to become a 'professional' philosopher. He was a 'humanist' in the sense of Petrarch and Erasmus, a man of letters, and a politician. Nevertheless, the *Essays* is the work of a profound philosopher, one of the most original thinkers of the Renaissance who understood the human soul as few before or after him. Julie Roberts (2015, p. 246) considers the *Essays* as a "pathographically curative" text, with the effort to examine oneself as one of the main aspects of philosophical therapy. She connects Montaigne's therapy with Foucault's "care of the self" (Foucault 1986). Rachel Starr (2012, p. 436) considers the *Essays* as the pinnacle of "humanistic psychotherapy."

[2]After publishing the first edition in 1580, Montaigne continued adding material, which creates some confusion, as he did not correct his previous concepts even when they were in contradiction with the new ones. The additions from 1580 to 1588 are marked with a "B", whereas the additions from 1588–1592 made in the 1588 'Bordeaux copy' (first published in 1595) are marked with a "C". I have used Screech's translation (Montaigne 2003), but also added material from Frame's translation whenever I considered the concept to be more clearly conveyed (Montaigne 1965). Reference to specific essays will be given to by volume and number, and page numbers within specific essays will be referred to by volume, essay, and page number. Letters A, B and C are used, when necessary, to indicate the different editions.

[3]The presence of clearly demarcated philosophical stages in Montaigne's intellectual evolution has been contested by a number of authors, and is extensively discussed in Bermúdez (2015, pp. 54–61). Frame (1955, pp. 5–7) describes three periods in Montaigne's philosophical

Essays do not propose specific theories or grand metaphysical statements; the text is full of contradictory remarks due to Montaigne's epistemological and personal changes over time. This is most evident in his treatment of fear, and Montaigne should figure prominently in any work discussing the philosophy of this emotion. First, even though the *Essays* is not an academic work on fear, it provides a unique discussion of how the therapies of fear proposed by the different Hellenistic Schools of philosophy were applied in the life of a prominent humanist at a time when there were obvious reasons for being in fear, such as the ravages of the Wars of Religion in France and the horrors of the plague, which decimated entire populations. Montaigne himself was also on the brink of early death after suffering a serious concussion.

Another unique attribute of the *Essays* regarding fear is that the text is written primarily about the author.[4] Thus, the work could be considered as mere anecdotal evidence, but Montaigne's description of his own fear is used as a springboard to analyse the phenomenon of fear from different philosophical perspectives in a novel non-dogmatic style. Montaigne openly tells the reader about his main fears, especially poverty, pain and death, and the major impact this emotion had on him. We read of Montaigne's fear of illnesses, which led to him being a valetudinarian, the miraculous' cure of these fears after contracting a real and serious illness, his reaction to the terrors of the plague, his at times desperate search for a solution to his fears in philosophical writings, and finally, the creation of a unique type of therapy, free from conceptual restrictions; a therapy 'all his own,' which consisted of self-reflection, self-knowledge, and acceptance as the main attributes.

---

development: the first one ("Stoic period") extended from 1572 to 1574; the second one ("Sceptical period") extended from 1575 to 1577, and the final period ("Epicurean period") extended from 1578 until Montaigne's death in 1592.

[4]This type of autobiographical writing was not new (Montaigne's *Essays* was preceded by Augustine's *Confessions* and Petrarch's *Secretum*), but Montaigne's text is unique in the frankness of personal descriptions, in which a reader of any place and period may be easily reflected.

4.2 The *Essays* as a Narrative of Fears

It may seem paradoxical that a text that addresses fear as one of the main topics only includes the word "fear" in the title of one of its 106 essays. In several of the essays of Book I,[5] Montaigne conveys fear indirectly through narrating heroic feats from Roman and Greek history. In these narrations, which aim at displaying the virtuosity of Antiquity, Montaigne depicts Greek and Roman soldiers as showing great contempt of death. These stories may be interpreted in different ways, such as presenting the Stoic perspective of the 'early' Montaigne, and a contrast with the non-virtuous behaviour of his contemporaries in the wars of religion. Readers may feel dwarfed by these stories, and find it impossible not to compare their own relatively pedestrian fears with the heroic feats of the ancients. Montaigne also tells narratives about individuals that were savagely tortured, and the detail he provides may produce a feeling of great fear and horror. We are time and again forced to a labour of self-reflection regarding our own capacity to face fear in similar circumstances.[6] Thus, the therapeutic aspect of these early essays lies in contrasting our petty fears against the courageous behaviour of the heroes of antiquity, and they also provide a guide for those who have to face fear of death and may find Montaigne's examples inspirational. However, as much as we would like to imitate them, the *Essays* use cases that are exceptional in the history of humanity (e.g., Alexander, Caesar, Socrates, and Solon). All these examples aim at the extirpation of fear, but this 'remedy' is not available to most mortals. It was also not available to Montaigne himself, who was at that time beset by all kinds of fears, as I shall discuss later.

[5]Fear is a main theme in I.6 "The hour of parley is dangerous", I.11 "On prognostications", I.16 "On punishing cowardice", I.19 "That we should not be deemed happy till after our death", I.20 "To philosophise is to learn how to die", I.21 "On the power of imagination", I.33 "On fleeing from pleasures at the cost of one's life", I.39 "On solitude", and I.57 "On the length of life".

[6]This sounds anachronistic, but the extrapolation of the *Essays* into contemporary life is commonly practiced and for good reasons (Lazar and Madden 2015, pp. 1–2), as fear is one of the most primitive human emotions, the phenomenology in terms of feelings and behaviour has not changed in its conceptual essence, and the main causes of this emotion are perennial, such as the fear of death, poverty, sickness and wars.

There is another indirect way in which fears are conveyed to the reader, and this is an original move on Montaigne's part. Humbly initially, but with much more confidence in the later essays of Books II and III, we see Montaigne embarked on a major exercise of self-analysis, where he discloses *his* humours and *his* opinions, as well as his own fears and worries. Montaigne brought a great innovation to the understanding and mastery of fear, that is, his narration in the first person of his own pilgrimage to subdue his fears. Already in the note "To the Reader", Montaigne states, with complete honesty, that he is not serving his own reputation as he presents himself with all his weaknesses for the benefit of "friends and kinsmen" (p. 1). Montaigne wants to be regarded "in [his] simple, natural, everyday fashion" (p. 1), with his virtues and weaknesses. And the benefit to the reader is certainly great, as Montaigne offers several useful remedies in his description of his own fight against fears and worries. Although Montaigne's fears are of course intrinsic to his life experience, his personal accounts often resonate with his reader's experience, by way of identification or comparison, allowing the reader to acquire understanding, repose and companionship.[7] We are not alone with our distressing fears, and Montaigne, so open to accepting differences, that is, without being dogmatic or doctrinaire, is one of our best guides. I shall next discuss Montaigne's fears in more detail.

4.3 Montaigne's Collection of Fears

Montaigne stated that what he feared most was fear itself (C.1.18.82). Such is the rather enigmatic and catching phrase inserted in the short essay appropriately entitled "On fear". The brevity of this essay is puzzling, since, as I have discussed, fears had a significant role in Montaigne's life; yet he does not provide, in this early essay a comprehensive discussion of his own fears and the methods he used to tame

---

[7]Scholar (2010), remarks that the *Essays* "haunt its readers" by the free-thinking style of Montaigne's writings. Montaigne was a scholar, but fiercely anti-dogmatic, anti-authoritarian, and able to make "all questions accessible to his readers" (Scholar 2010, p. 7).

them during his life. On the contrary, the essays "On sadness" and "On fear" mostly provide a rather shallow discussion of the Stoic concept of fear (see previous chapter), providing examples of automatic behaviours after a great fright, such as physical paralysis, loss of basic instincts of self-preservation, and even suicide. Thus, the sudden announcement of bad news may cause one to be "struck with alarm" (A.1.3.8); people become paralysed, unable to respond, until they suddenly burst into "tears and lamentations" (A.1.3.8). In line with Seneca's notion of 'first movements', Montaigne states that the first reaction to a sudden alarm is a reflex behaviour.[8] The 'Stoic sage' becomes pale and tense following a sudden loud noise, although without assenting to this event as dangerous. After paying his respects to the Stoics whom he initially followed, Montaigne rebels against this school as being too dogmatic. The Stoic attitude and strategies to fight fears are for Montaigne impracticable and inhuman. Fear "penetrates through to the seat of reason… infecting and corrupting it", and it is too strong to be dominated by the rational arguments of the Stoics (C.1.12.49). As discussed in Chapter 3, Cicero made a similar criticism, and yet both Montaigne and Cicero were strongly influenced by Stoicism. Cicero's remedies were mostly Stoic, whereas Montaigne was still providing Stoic advice during his most anti-dogmatic period.

A possible explanation for Montaigne's association of fear with first and violent movements is that he used the French *peur* (the French title for this essay) with the connotation of extreme fear. Montaigne begins this essay by stressing he is not a "natural philosopher" (i.e. a physician), and therefore he is not interested in the biological mechanism of fear. Montaigne considers fear an "odd" emotion since it may drive a person insane: fear engenders "fits" of mad behaviour, and a "terrifying confusion" even in the steadiest of men. Captains in battle behave in a crazy way after being seized by the terror of a minor threat, some of them even dropping dead on the spot. Behavioural changes elicited by fear become unpredictable, with some people fleeing and others becoming

[8]"When he is threatened with a blow nothing can stop a man closing his eyes, or trembling if you set him on the edge of a precipice…" (A.2.3.388).

unable to adopt behaviours of self-preservation. In another essay ("On coaches"), Montaigne divides fear into that caused by lack of judgment, as in first movements, and that caused by lack of courage and provides the example of his fleeing from battlefield, which he did with a rational fear, "without ecstatic terror" (B.3.6.1018). When faced with the fear of death, some people behave in the most heroic manner as if pushed by "some celestial impulsion" (1.18.83). These fears may also be contagious, taking hold of whole battalions or populations, a fear Montaigne terms "Panic terrors" (C.1.18.84). Whereas this is not the most interesting essay dealing with fear, we can already appreciate the variety of behaviours fear may produce among humans.

A strong reason for Montaigne's 'fear of fear' is that he was besieged by truly frightening events, as already mentioned, living amid the war of religions and the plague. But Montaigne's anxiety is not only accounted for by the causes above. In "On coaches" he acknowledges that he lacked the strength to tolerate deep fear, stating that if he should be hit by such an emotion he would never recover from the experience. Montaigne was not so much concerned about negative events, but rather about the emotional impact these could have on him. This explains his statement that he liked the Spanish saying, "God save me from myself" (C.3.13.1234), that is, from his tendency to catastrophize.[9] Montaigne stated that his main fears were sickness, poverty and death, and these fears are addressed in different essays.[10] Montaigne had a chronic fear of sickness, being convinced of suffering "rheums, fluxions of gout, diarrhoeas, coronary palpitations and migraines" (3.13.1235). His most dreaded fear was of having kidney stones, the disease that killed his father. Montaigne eventually did develop kidney stones, but even while suffering the extreme pains produced by this illness, he found the experience liberating. His fear of the illness and constant worrying was a permanent weight on his mind; after developing the illness the agonising uncertainty lifted, and he was 'free' to face the consequences. Earlier,

[9]"Anyone who is afraid of suffering suffers already of being afraid" (3.13.1243).

[10]The main essays discussing the fear of death are "Constancy" (1.12), "That the taste of good and evil…" (1.14), "That to philosophise is to learn to die" (1.20), "Solitude" (1.39) and "The inconsistency of our own actions" (2.1).

Montaigne's fear of poverty tortured him at the time when his fortune was greatest. He tamed this fear when he decided to delegate the management of his finances to others. This was not a rational confrontation with this fear, but effective avoidance behaviour. Finally, his omnipresent fear of death diminished when he was very close to death after suffering a severe head injury. Montaigne had to 'taste' what it might be like to be dead to appease his fear of death. I shall now address in more detail the causes of fear as described in various essays, and prepare the ground for Montaigne's therapeutic advice.

4.4 The Maddening Thoughts of Fear and the Power of Imagination

Montaigne starts Essay 14 by paraphrasing Epictetus' view that humans are "tormented not by things themselves", which for the Stoics have no intrinsic value, "but by what they think about them", that is, the value that is invested in a given object (A.1.4.52). But even during his 'dogmatic' phase, Montaigne challenged this Stoic doctrine stating that emotional events may be too strong and unable to be intellectually manipulated. If, as the Stoics state, emotions are a matter of rational assent "why do we not act as their masters and accommodate them [i.e. the interpretations] to our advantage?" he asks (A.1.4.52). In another early essay, Montaigne disagrees with the Stoics that the technique of premeditation (see previous chapter) may help to allay fears. Montaigne considered that the anticipation of misfortune may produce fears which many times exceed the suffering produced by the dreaded mishap, an effect which demonstrates the powerful influence of imagination on human emotions.[11]

Among the intellectual powers, Montaigne considered a person's imagination to be the strongest source of fears. He stressed that imagination may generate self-fulfilling prophecies: once the idea of a bad outcome

[11]The topic on the futility of premeditation is discussed in-depth in the penultimate essay "On physiognomy" (3.22).

comes to mind, the trouble will most probably happen. And Montaigne himself was a victim of his own extreme susceptibility to imagining all sorts of negative incidents, which produced in him great fear and anxiety.[12] He was convinced that a strong imagination could produce severe disease and sexual impotence.[13] When Montaigne writes that one "fellow often has stone in the mind before stone in the kidney" (A.2.12.547), implying that it is enough to imagine suffering a disease to already feel it, he may well be referring to himself. In fact, as already noted, Montaigne feared distress and fear more than bodily problems.[14] He complains about being unable to find peers with whom to have an interesting conversation, which he needed as a distraction. If left alone, he would fall into imagining maddening thoughts.[15]

Imagination lured Montaigne into retirement and tortured him afterwards. He decided on an early retirement from a promising political life to spend more time alone. Montaigne was averse of taking any risks needed to foster his advancement, and curved all political ambitions. Instead he wanted to retire quietly and privately, living in idleness, to care for himself, to be concerned with himself, and to think about himself. He soon realised, however, that his idealised retreat was not heaven but a hell in which his imagination "bolted off like a runaway horse", producing "chimeras and fantastic monstrosities, one after another, without order or fitness" (B.1.8.31). One of these "fantastic monstrosities", as mentioned earlier, was his imaginings of being affected by all kinds of diseases. After hearing the story of a neighbour having consumption, Montaigne would start coughing. He was unable to tolerate the anxiety of waiting for the outcome of any feared event. He lived in anguished expectation, often "torn between fear and hope" (B.2.17.732).

---

[12] "I am one of those by whom the powerful blows of the imagination are felt most strongly. Everyone is hit by it, but some are bowled over" (A.1.21.109).

[13] "When I contemplate an illness I seize upon it and lodge it within myself" (C.1.21.109).

[14] "Once the pain has gone I am not much depressed by weakness or lassitude. I know of several bodily afflictions which are horrifying even to name but which I fear less than hundreds of current disturbances and distresses of the mind" (C.3.13.1245).

[15] "Then, there is no madness, no raving lunacy, which such agitations do not bring forth" (A.1.8.30).

Doubt paralysed him, and he was unable to make simple decisions.[16] The torture of uncertainty was too unbearable, and Montaigne faced a present misfortune better than its anxious expectation.[17]

This seems to be a portrait of a pathologically fearful person, and it is legitimate to wonder whether Montaigne is able to provide rational and sound advice on how to manage fear. Would it not be better to be guided by physicians, who especially since Galen, have been dealing with pathological emotions using their herbal remedies? I believe, for reasons I discuss below, that Montaigne was in a solid position to provide useful advice on how to deal with fear. First, because Montaigne suffered from a broad variety of fears, he had a first-hand understanding of how big a torture this emotion can be, and more importantly, he also found the way out of this excruciating pain (although with some relapses as I shall discuss later). During the ten years he lived self-confined to his tower, Montaigne conducted a rigorous self-analysis. He examined his fears with brutal honesty, as he hated lies, and especially lying about oneself. Montaigne examined his fears from different angles using tools of the different philosophical schools, and applied philosophical remedies to himself. This combination of deep self-examination and broad knowledge of the Hellenistic schools, Roman philosophers and poets, as well as a dedicated practice to philosophical therapy, placed Montaigne in a strong position to give advice on the therapy of fear, using himself as an example.

Regarding the role of medicine for treating human sickness, it is impossible, here, to exaggerate Montaigne's contempt for doctors, which is so overtly expressed in several of the essays. The reason for this strong rejection is unclear, but it may be related to Montaigne's own hypochondriasis and his fear of doctors. He hated the incumbent profession of medicine, and yet he had to accept contact with doctors because of his physical infirmities.

---

[16]"Resigned to any outcome whatsoever once the dice have been thrown" (B.2.17.732); and "Few emotions have ever disturbed my sleep, yet even the slightest need to decide anything can disturb it for me" (B.2.17.732).

[17]"In events I act like a man: in the conduct of events, like a boy. The dread of a tumble gives me more anguish than the fall" (B.2.17.733).

4.5 Fearing Doctors

Montaigne considered successes in medical cures to be due to mere luck, given that in his opinion, the foundations of medicine were "too fragile" (A.1.24.143), and doctors too dogmatic. He "despised" medicine when in good health[18] and rejected it when ill,[19] but this was in part due to fear of doctors, their medications, and their prognoses.[20] Montaigne claims that contempt for medicine was a family trait, and that nobody in his family, from his grandfather onwards wanted any contact with physicians.[21] His father was "horrified" by doctors, and the only one of his brothers who relied on medicine was the youngest to die. A more personal reason for his dislike of medicine was Montaigne's hypochondriasis. He was aware this was a product of the imagination,[22] and that doctors tricked people to produce their cures.[23] In any case, and despite all the medical promises, he asserted that we are made for growing old and weaker, and falling ill (B.3.13.1236).

This rejection and fear of doctors was not simply the result of Montaigne's imagination, given that in Sixteenth century France the practice of medicine was not legislated, and quacks and barbers were practicing as physicians (Roberts 2009, p. 722). This was a time of

[18]"...thank God we have nothing to do with each other" (A.1.24.143).

[19]"I tell those who urge me to take medicine at least to wait until I am well and have got my strength back in order to have the means of resisting the hazardous effects of their potions" (A.1.24.143).

[20]"Can I feel something disintegrating? Do not expect me to waste time having my pulse and urine checked so that anxious prognostics can be drawn from them: I will be in plenty of time to feel the anguish without prolonging things by an anguished fear" (B.3.13.1243).

[21]His father lived to 74 years, a grandfather to 69, and a great-grandfather to almost 80, "none having swallowed any kind of drug" (A.2.37.864).

[22]"How many men have been made ill by the sheer force of imagination? Is it not normal to see men bled, purged and swallowing medicines to cure ills which they feel only in their minds?" (A.2.12.547).

[23]"Why do doctors first work on the confidence of their patient with so many fake promises of a cure if not to allow the action of the imagination to make up for the trickery of their potions? They know that one of the masters of their craft told them in writing that there are men for whom it is enough merely to look at a medicine for it to prove effective" (A.1.21.116). Thus, the trickery of doctors consisted in using medications as strong placebos to cure imaginary illnesses, as well as convincing patients that their drugs were curing an otherwise irreversible condition (Justman 2015).

radical changes in the training and practice of medicine (Justman 2015, pp. 496–498). The teaching of medicine was becoming institutionalised in universities, and physicians began to be accepted in new medical corporations in most major French cities (Brockliss and Jones 1977). On the other hand, trained medical practitioners faced strong competition from unqualified healers, barbers and apothecaries, as well as students and itinerant quacks (Brockliss and Jones 1977, p. 230). Whoever the provider happened to be, there was more luck than rational knowledge in the practice of medicine, and even those physicians trained at reputed universities were practicing on shaky theoretical grounds. Montaigne was aware of the rudimentary empirical basis of medical practice, which he strongly criticised (C.3.13.1243).[24]

Most of the population in rural and urban regions had scarce resources to pay the fees of trained physicians and had to resort to charlatans and quacks. Once in the hands of a physician of whatever type, the patient had to follow the prescribed regime, which included frequent visits to ensure the proper taking of medications, follow-up examinations, and changes to the treatment if necessary (Brockliss and Jones 1977, p. 284). This interaction continued until the patient was cured or dead. Montaigne disliked what he considered a lack of moderation in medical practice, as well as what he perceived as efforts from physicians at bringing not only illnesses but also good health under their supervision. With interesting foresight, Montaigne asked the rhetorical question as to whether doctors themselves have long and happy lives that demonstrate the benefits of their own medicine (A.2.37.866).

In conclusion, we can see in Montaigne's contempt witness to the professionalization of medicine, with its increasing influence upon human life. Although the progress of medical treatment over subsequent centuries has undoubtedly had enormous benefits for humanity, Montaigne was astute enough to see this empowering of medicine as the beginning of the medicalization of human life, and how great a role fear played in its further development. On the other hand, Montaigne's

[24]Robert (2015, pp. 721–744) has analysed the subtle way in which Montaigne ridiculed both physicians and patients for engaging in fully unproven expensive treatments.

great foresight was one of his main sources of fear and suffering, as I shall now discuss.

4.6 Fear, Fortune and Foresight

In the third essay of Book I ("Our emotions get carried away beyond us"), Montaigne already argues against the human tendency to look forward into the future, oblivious of what is available at present. Fear, he says, is one of the main reasons that "impel us towards the future" (B.1.3.11).[25] This may explain the human fondness for prognostication, the main subject of another early essay. Montaigne considers prognostication to be a "mad curiosity" (A.1.11.42), since many plans and projects, no matter how many precautions are taken, depend in great part on fortune.

After his Stoic period, Montaigne became convinced that it is fortune rather than foresight that rules human destiny. Nevertheless, he considered that the force of habit could tame the negative impact of fortune. The technique of habit-creation was very important because as he claimed with typical flourish, proper habits are more necessary for a happy life than the "whole of philosophy" (A.1.23.129). This is because he thought that habits and customs, if properly developed, are able to reduce the severity of fear (see further discussion below). To support his view, Montaigne comments on Roman emperors who became accustomed to ignoring conspiracies against them rather than being enslaved by fear.[26] On the other hand, Montaigne considered that philosophical knowledge "is a dangerous sword" (A.1.25.158) which may wound the unprepared. Philosophical training is not for everybody and philosophical techniques against fear, such as pre-rehearsal, may help some people but hurt others.[27] Montaigne admired those "souls" that were trained in good

[25]"… they rob us of feelings and concern for what now is, in order to spend time over what will be – even when we ourselves shall be no more" (B.1.3.11).

[26]"The continual suspicion, which leads a Prince to distrust everyone may torment him strangely" (A.1.24.145).

[27]"So vain and worthless is human wisdom: despite all our projects, counsels and precautions, the outcome remains in the possession of Fortune" (A.1.24.143).

habits, with luck having nothing to do with the capacity of enjoying a life without fears, "calm, unruffled and contented" (B.1.42.290). Achieving this serenity is independent of social position, he thought, as even in the case of the king, "when surrounded by his armies, anxiety and fear can have him by the throat" (B.1.42.291).

One's social position does not spare one from disease, the pains of old age, or paralysing fear (A.1.42.292). As Montaigne grew older, he became used to planning for the short-term only, an Epicurean strategy against fear and worry.[28] By not having great ambitions or long-term plans, he avoided the consequent anxiety of seeing them to fruition. Following this change of habits, Montaigne's worrying diminished, and he started coming to terms with the idea of dying.[29] One objection to this rather selfish strategy to fight the fear of having one's plans cut off by death is that it evades the possibility of strengthening oneself against the daily fears, a fearful 'shrinking' of the soul. In his late essays in Book III, and especially in "On physiognomy" Montaigne attacked the Stoic technique for fighting fears, preferring a more natural approach, such as the lifestyle of his farmers, who lived almost indifferent to death even during the plague. Unfortunately for Montaigne, he did not have the farmers' temperament, and his fear of poverty, pain and death remained with him for most of his life.

4.7 "Our Main Enemies Are Held to Be Death, Poverty and Pain"

In the essay entitled "That the taste of good and evil things depends in large part on the opinion we have of them" (1.14) Montaigne provides a philosophical analysis of his main fears. He initially follows the Stoic stance that life events, even dying, have no intrinsic value, and

[28] "The longest of my projects are for less than a year; I think only of bringing things to a close; I free myself from all fresh hopes and achievements" (C.2.28.797).

[29] "My old age…deadens within me many of the desires and worries which trouble our lives: worry about the way the world is going; worry about money, honours, erudition, health… and me" (C.2.28.797).

any emotional attribution depends on our personal interpretation. After all, Montaigne says, whereas death is for some "the dreadest of all dreadful things," for others it is "the only heaven from life's torments" (A.1.14.53). In the same essay, Montaigne provides several examples of impressive fearlessness in the context of imminent violent death, and ends with the pleonasm that the number of individuals wishing for death (for various reasons) is so vast that "I would find it easier to list those who did fear death" (A.1.14.57). His own name would have certainly figured in the latter category. Even in the last (and emotionally steadiest) period of his life, worries weighed heavily on Montaigne, and a "thousand things" caused him "to hope or to fear" (B.3.9.1076). Let us now examine these fears in more detail.

4.7.1 Poverty

Once again, in fleshing out his account in light of his own experience, Montaigne relates three different stages in relation to his fear of poverty. During the first period, he depended on others for his income and spent money "easily and cheerfully" (1.14.66). His needs were frugal, but in case of need he could always borrow from friends. Montaigne admitted that "thrifty" people would never tolerate this state of financial uncertainty. In the second stage, after he had accumulated a good fortune, Montaigne admits that he became too "attached to it" (1.14.68). During this period, like many who value material wealth beyond other goods, he was tormented by the idea of poverty, fearing all kinds of events that would find him bereft of money. These fears plunged him into "painful anxiety" ("the heavier the money, the heavier my worries" (1.14.68)), and Montaigne tried to hide the extent of his wealth from others. He worried about being robbed when taking his safe-box on a journey; but if the strong-box was left at home, he would suspect everyone in his château (C.1.14.68). He suffered when he had to spend, and became a miser. After several years of fearing poverty while he was earning a fortune, Montaigne entered his third and last stage during which he quietly, and without anxiety, tried to balance earnings with expenses. Bringing a more reflective perspective on his situation, Montaigne accepted that it was impossible to provide for all the negative events in life (C.1.14.70), and that there was no guarantee he would live to spend the money he had accumulated. He accepted that exceptional life circumstances may happen, and lived without worries, "from day to day" (B.1.14.70).

4.7.2 Pain

Fear of pain and disease also tormented Montaigne during most of his life. Montaigne considered pain as "the worst disaster that can befall our being" (A.1.14.59). He acknowledged his extreme fear of pain[30] and was ambiguous about how much pain he could tolerate.[31] Montaigne wanted to be "either totally well or totally ill" (B.3.9.1072), unable to endure uncertainty. "I am no [Stoic] philosopher" (C.3.9.1076) he stated in his last years, honestly accepting his low tolerance for pain. Montaigne never pretended, in Stoic fashion, that pain is an 'indifferent' when in fact it is cruel and that suffering, consequently, is unstoppable. Nevertheless, Montaigne follows the Stoics when accepting that it is up to the individual to confront pain with boldness, or if courage is not available, to exit life.[32]

It may be argued that fear of illness, as a type of 'natural' premeditation technique, has the positive aspect of emotionally preparing a person to confront the worst outcome in the best way possible. Here we need to remind ourselves of the Epicurean criticism (see Chapter 2) that it is irrational to suffer in the present about misfortunes that may never happen. Fear of illness is not simply a matter of benign rehearsal but a source of great distress. During the past five centuries the objects of fear have certainly changed (kidney stones have quite an easy treatment currently), but fear of illness still affects many people (Barsky 1988).

[30]"I am the most ill-disposed toward pain" (C.1.14.69).

[31]"When my condition is bad I cling violently to my illness: I abandon myself to despair and let myself go towards catastrophe" (B.3.9.1072).

[32]"Death is the only guarantor of our freedom, the common and ready cure of our ills" (A.1.14.53). Montaigne acceptance of suicide is not explicitly stated in the text, perhaps due to fear of the Inquisition.

As Montaigne states (C.3.9.1075) pain and disease were feared doubly for being indicators of impending death, and I shall now discuss Montaigne's greatest fear.

4.7.3 Death

Fear of death oppressed Montaigne for most of his life. Bakewell (2010) suggests that Montaigne's obsession with death was due to reading about death from a young age, whereas Frame (1984, pp. 20–21) suggests that Montaigne's persistent preoccupation with death resulted from close and consecutive deaths. In a period of ten years Montaigne lost his beloved friend La Boetie, his father, an uncle, his youngest brother, and two daughters. But it is possible that Montaigne's fear of death may have deeper roots. Even before those events he was obsessed with death as expressed in behaviours such as investigating the cause of death of different people (including philosophers), their facial expression, and their last words (A.1.20.100). He studied the death of prominent individuals from history books, and one of his literary wishes was to write "a compendium with commentaries of the various ways men have died" (C.1.20.100). Montaigne's fear of death was already prominent during his early adulthood. Amidst happy times with friends, for example, he was struck by moments when he would be suddenly absorbed by thinking that in similar situations, somebody like him died after a short fever. Montaigne denied being a melancholic but rather claimed he was just "an idle dreamer" (A.1.20.97). However, these dreams were rarely about the joys of life and mostly about death (A.1.20.97). Even when in good health Montaigne was terrorised by death and was convinced his life would be short (A.1.20.97). Yet he took some temporary comfort from the Stoic maxim that a good life is not measured by its length but by its good use (C.1.20.106). Montaigne considered that a good death consisted in no suffering, and he wished for a sudden death, as in this situation "we have no time to feel afraid" (A.1.20.100). On the other hand, reaching old age, he speculated, may lessen the fear of death, given that the loss of our youth is more grievous than death itself (B.1.20.101). Finding peace of mind was certainly not a minor challenge for Montaigne.

In general terms, Montaigne considered that one of the main reasons for fearing death is that humans are unconvinced of their own mortality (A.1.13.684), believing themselves to be special creatures, the axis around which life events rotate (A.1.13.684). Therefore, death comes as a sudden surprise, as "a great event" in Montaigne words (A.1.13.685). In his opinion, this abrupt awareness of one's own mortality is most commonly observed among scholars, who believe they are endowed with special mental capacities, as well as among the wealthy, who believe they are responsible for the lives of many people. Unfortunately, "None of us gives enough thought to his being only *one*" [italics in the original] (C.1.13.685), that is, just another individual among millions of mortals. Here, Montaigne's writing is self-referential, being himself a scholar and wealthy. He is oblivious to the dispositions of the elderly, who after leading good lives, have to deal with their painful physical decay and increasing loneliness. For the elderly, rather than a sudden visitor, the process of dying is a faithful companion.

Montaigne's obsession with fear of death is also exemplified by his behaviour during the plague that desolated Bordeaux. He was ashamed by the way he waited in "ecstatic dread" for the evolution of "a slightly sore finger" into the initial symptom of the plague (B.3.12.1186), at a time when his farmers were preparing their own sepulchres with a natural acceptance of their destiny. Later in life Montaigne appreciated the greater courage of the "common people" (A.1.14.53), who would die peacefully while putting their affairs in order, preaching, conversing with friends and even joking. Dying is a short process, perhaps no more than "a quarter of an hour of pain" (C.3.12.1190), and yet the scholar's preparation for dying is counted in years. Montaigne, the scholar, spent years preparing himself for death. He tried to obtain through bookish learning the courage that his poor farmers obtained spontaneously, accepting death as a fact of life. This remark educates the reader in understanding that fear of death is not necessarily tamed by erudition, or nowadays, by an increasing collection of psychotherapies, but by the unselfish "matter of fact" lifestyle of those that will never figure in prominent places. Friedrich (1991, pp. 258–262) values Montaigne's insight that it is nature rather than any ethical philosophy that can best master the fear of death. By accepting what is natural in life there is no need for Stoic straining.

4.8 Montaigne's Therapy of Fear

Nobody should expect a scholarly exposition on the therapy of fear in a text so chaotically organized as the *Essays*, and it is necessary to examine each essay with care to gather together Montaigne's views and advice on how to best treat fear. It is also necessary to distinguish suggestions made in the different editions of the essays, as they run in parallel with major changes in his philosophical thinking. This complexity of interleaving time periods is also a bonus, because, as mentioned earlier, it provides explicit evidence of the philosophical evolution of Montaigne's approach to fear, while at the same time alerting the reader to his desire not to erase earlier understandings.[33] Because Montaigne went through different philosophical periods with influences from different philosophical schools, the remedies he suggested are diverse. In the end, his approach provides alternatives for people to choose the therapy that agrees best with their personality, an approach that thereby refuses dogmatic or one-size-fits-all cures. This is the humanistic preservation of the tradition started by Cicero and Seneca of adapting the philosophical treatment of fear and distress to each individual using specific remedies (see previous chapter). I shall discuss later (Chapter 9) the marked difference between this individualised technique and the current medicalised management of fear and anxiety, according to which therapies are chosen based on objective but generic psycho-physiological facts. I shall now examine the main remedies suggested in the *Essays*.

4.8.1 Premeditation

In the early essays, Montaigne valued the Stoic exercises of premeditation of future misfortunes and of treating death with contempt. At this stage, Montaigne also devalued "ordinary people" (A.1.20.92) since, in his opinion, they were unable to meditate about death. These people, he thought, froze in panic as soon as the

[33]It may also be the case that Montaigne had no firm opinion about the best 'remedies' for fear, and left different options open.

word 'death' was mentioned, and became irrational when stricken by the "pain and terror" of having been diagnosed with an incurable illness (A.1.20.92). Death cannot be ignored, as it may happen at any moment and in the most unthinkable ways. Montaigne's youngest brother, after all, died after a blow from a tennis ball! And yet, when distress is absent, 'ordinary' people "go…trot…and dance" (A.1.20.95) oblivious of the final human fate. But "it is madness to think that you can succeed [in mastering your fears] that way" (A.1.20.95) as death will eventually catch up with everyone, says Montaigne, plunging everyone into despair. Therefore, early in the *Essays* Montaigne suggests fighting the fear of death using the strategy of premeditation: "we must start by providing for [death] earlier" (A.1.20.95). Montaigne suggests getting used to death by constantly thinking about it in the Stoic fashion, even "in the midst of joy" (A.1.20.95). Any day could be the last one and we must be on guard, given that meditating upon death "beforehand [sic] confers great advantages" (A.1.20.101). It is therefore necessary to prepare for reversals of fortune, "picturing future ills in comfort" (A.1.30.273). Montaigne supported the Stoic doctrine that "to practice death is to practice freedom" (A.1.20.96), since only after conquering the fear of death we can live free of anxiety and anguish (C.1.20.101). Therefore, Montaigne practiced continually thinking about death, with the aim of "taming" his fears, and avoiding a life of "continual terror and frenzy" (A.1.20.97). He suggested befriending death to the extent of having nothing else in mind (B.1.20.95). Premeditation should not be constrained by too laborious exercise; rather, it has to flow naturally as a gentle and not a strenuous practice. Those who become anxious to do well will suffer more than they will benefit.[34] Montaigne's premeditation is an epiphany of heavenly thoughts. Unless the soul is trained for the moment of death, fear will allow no rest. But once the fear is conquered "it is impossible for anxiety, anguish, fear or even the slightest dissatisfaction to dwell within her" (A.1.20.101).

---

[34]"The anxiety to do well…puts the soul on the rack, break it, and make it impotent" (Montaigne 1965 1.10.26, Frame's translation).

But, personally, beyond advice on how to best conduct premeditation exercises, Montaigne himself was living in terror, to the point that he would not be "certain of getting back home" if he was just "one league" away (A.1.20.98).[35] And after engaging in the strenuous Stoic practice towards happiness, why was the beggar at his door merrier and healthier than he was (A.1.39.273)? In light of these contradictions, Bakewell suggests that Montaigne started using the Epicurean method of "diversion." By means of diversion, a fear is re-fashioned into a positive emotion, such as thinking about a sweet past event. Bakewell further suggests that it was especially in old age that Montaigne used diversion against the fear of ageing and death.

After all the years of reading the Stoics, Epicureans and Sceptics, Montaigne's discovery was that philosophical learning increased his knowledge but did not change his feelings and emotions. He could not find in philosophical books a remedy for his fears, a good reminder of Cicero's remark that the philosophical therapy of fear and distress is not for every person (C.3.12.1176) (see also Chapter 3). Whereas philosophical learning should help in arming oneself against future dangers, it may "imprint on our thoughts" (B.3.12.1176) even more fear against which the "subtle arguments" aimed at protecting us are insufficient. As a result, Montaigne distanced himself from the Stoics and his earlier support for the method of premeditation[36] and instead approached the Epicureans, affirming the view that "anticipating the injuries of Fortune, depriving ourselves of such good things as are still in our grasp" (A.1.39.272) is inappropriate therapy. Montaigne rejected "that curious desire to anticipate…and prepare" for every misfortune, even those that "may never touch us" (B.3.12.1189). He discovered the importance of self-knowledge for mastering emotions, rejecting the "excessive concerns [and] useless thoughts" of philosophical maxims (C.1.3.11). Humans have a rich nature, and yet we have to go "borrowing and begging" (C.3.12.1175); we are greedy for excessive

---

[35]Bakewell states that premeditation did not liberate Montaigne from his fears, but actually served to imprison him (Bakewell 2010, p. 3).

[36]"Do we ask to be whipped right now…just because it may be that Fortune will, perhaps, make you suffer a whipping some day?" (B.3.12.1189).

knowledge, which will "cost us dear" (C.3.12.1175), since some of this philosophical knowledge is not nourishment but poison. The first book of the *Tusculans*, devoted to the fear of death, did not help Montaigne face death more courageously, but on the contrary, imprinted this fear even deeper. Whereas Montaigne was unsuccessfully fighting his fear of death by the rehearsal of maxims and Stoic precepts, his farmers learned from life the courage to face death, from actions that "are purer and more unbending than those which we so carefully study in our schools" (B.3.12.1178). Montaigne discovers that philosophy has to imitate what he saw as the natural way of life, which will teach us "how we should live and die, manage our goods, love and educate our offspring and maintain justice" (B.3.12.1188).

In conclusion, Montaigne wanted to free himself of fears and worries, and live the simple life of his farmers: "Death… [should]…find me planting my cabbages, neither worrying about it nor the unfinished gardening" (A.1.20.99). Montaigne was (apparently) ready to die without regrets.[37]

4.8.2 Acceptance

At this later stage, Montaigne also considered 'acceptance' of one's own destiny an important remedy for fear. Bakewell (2010, p. 102) suggests that the technique of acceptance has its origin in the Stoic '*amor fati*' (love of fate), conceding to whatever destiny brings (C.1.20.101). To accept the dangers of life and not to resist them is one of the most effective protections against fear, and the most conducive attitude to achieve peace of mind. During the peak of the war of religions Montaigne's neighbours fortified their houses with strong defences, out of fear of being invaded. This strategy backfired, as those fortified mansions became highly suspicious because they were thought to hide treasures. Montaigne did not improve his defences "fearing that its strength could be turned against me" (C.2.15.700). His château may have been

[37]"No man has ever prepared to leave the world more simply nor more fully than I have. No one has more completely let go of everything than I *try* to do" (C.1.20.98) [my italics].

less conspicuous, but was invaded nonetheless. With great *sangre froid*, Montaigne received his assailants without showing, he says, a hint of fear and accepting whatever the outcome should be. This made the invaders believe there was nothing of value there, and they left. A similar event took place when Montaigne was travelling on horseback and was assailed by robbers. He was left unscathed after showing a cool and fearless demeanour, simply resigned to his fate.

Acceptance of misfortunes and death is a natural condition of life, without the need for Cicero's philosophical artifice of uprooting fears. This explains why Montaigne's farmers died "with as much constancy as the philosopher" (B.3.12.1176). Montaigne suggests there is no great therapeutic value in Stoic exercise or even in learning Epicurean maxims (C.3.12.1177) if the habit of acceptance is not practiced. The best example is again found in the "simple people" (C.3.12.1177), those ignorant of philosophical discourse in whom acceptance comes as a natural attribute.[38] As eloquently stated by Bakewell "philosophy looked more like a way of teaching people to unlearn the natural skill that every peasant had by birthright" (Bakewell 2010, p. 10). After all, in keeping with the realities of the time peasants could not expect much from life, not even a long life, and someone in Montaigne's aristocratic position could readily construe from this that they were contented with little.[39] It is the philosopher, with all his ethical and moral dogmas, who paradoxically, it seems, most strongly resisted the idea of death and was in need of treatment. Montaigne considered that Seneca's daily exercises, designed to fortify against the fear of death, were a manifestation of non-acceptance of death. In his final years, Montaigne welcomed death but without trying to bring it on. He was enjoying each day, living in the moment, as I discuss below. He finally accepted death and

---

[38]"How many country-folk do I see ignoring poverty; how many yearning for death or meeting it without panic or distress? That man over there who is trenching my garden has, this morning, buried his father or his son" (B.3.12.1178).

[39]This description seems to idealise and romanticise the behaviour of the 'lower classes', but this is what Montaigne was contemplating, what he saw in his own estate. Although he cannot know what was going on in the minds of his peasants and he employs a clumsy generalisation I believe that this image can be read as being used to contrast different human responses to fear and to show that fear can be successfully dominated.

experienced some "pleasure" (B.3.9.1099) in exploring the 'feelings' of dying by letting himself fall into states of a "powerful sleep", devoid of pain or suffering. He just wanted to find a place "entirely to my taste" (B.3.9.1112) where he could die a peaceful death.

The basis of Montaigne's acceptance technique was Pyrrhonian scepticism, and the use of *epokhé* or suspension of judgment. According to this sceptical view, the outcomes of many events in life are difficult to foretell, and having fear or hope produces mental suffering. Therefore, the Pyrrhonian sceptic achieves *ataraxia*, or tranquillity, by suspending judgment about the eventual outcome of unpredictable events. Even a predictably bad outcome may turn out, on some occasions, to be a good.

Montaigne's famous motto "Que sçais je?" ("What do I know?") is considered to be an expression of his Pyrrhonism (Frame 1955, p. 75), but Bermúdez Vázquez (2015, pp. 54–62) suggests that the motto implies a search for knowledge, closer to those of Socrates and Cicero, over the Pyrrhonian "inevitability of uncertainty" (p. 17). This point is not a mere interpretive dispute, but has therapeutical implications. I believe Bermúdez Vázquez is wrong, and that the *Essays* have many examples where Montaigne does not want to commit himself to obtaining knowledge or passing judgment, such as on the questions: is it better to live longer? Should death be feared? Is poverty something to be shunned? Rather than embarking on a quest for knowledge, Montaigne's motto is an expression of consent, a "why should I know?" that permits immediate acceptance and moving on with life. As Bermúdez Vázquez himself acknowledged, the quest for certainty produces anxiety, and conceptualizing things as good or bad produce disquietude. Montaigne does not want to know; he wants to live.[40]

[40]Hartle (2013, p. 17) also believes in a more opinionated than a non-judgmental Montaigne, stressing that throughout the *Essays* Montaigne constantly makes judgments of all sorts. This is certainly true, except for the questions that obsessed Montaigne the most: the fears of sickness poverty and death. When discussing Montaigne's scepticism in relation to Sextus Empiricus, Bermúdez Vazquez remarks that "philosophical speculation leads only to confusion because of the inevitability of uncertainty. It produces anxiety rather than peace of mind" (p. 17).

4.8.3 Living in the Present

In his early essays, Montaigne discussed the notion that fear and worrying are a worse torture than the dreaded misfortune. He begins the essay, appropriately entitled "Our emotions get carried away beyond us" (B.1.3.11), by praising those who criticise the tendency to "always gaping towards the future" (B.1.3.11) without enjoying the present.[41] He calls this tendency an "aberration", but acknowledges that it is produced by "Nature herself" (B.1.3.11) on behalf of self-preservation. In later additions to this essay, Montaigne acknowledged that we have to fight this instinct by concentrating our attention in the present while ignoring past and future; otherwise "we are never 'at home': we are always outside ourselves" (B.1.3.11).[42] The technique for living in the present requires first developing self-knowledge, that is, awareness of one's emotions and the capacity to work on them, as well as the understanding that most external objects and events are not within our power. It also requires mastering one's thoughts, focusing on the present and doing what is strictly necessary, whilst ignoring any superfluous projects. There is no dwelling in the past or worrying about the future, and, apparently neither guilt nor fear.

Montaigne also considered that living in the present requires the capacity for caring for oneself. Living in a state of anxiety "about the future" (C.1.3.11) and having "excessive concerns" only increases our vulnerability in the present. Staying in the present also requires avoiding boredom, given that idleness leads to our concentration drifting into fears and preoccupations (A.1.8.30). In this situation Montaigne recommends writing down those grotesque imaginations that we think about when idle and bored. Thus, when we read them later, we feel ashamed of ourselves and our ridiculous fears. Furthermore, keeping a diary

[41]"Fear, desire, hope, impel us towards the future; they rob us of feelings and concern for what now is, in order to spend time over what will be – even when we ourselves shall be no more" (B.1.3.11).

[42]This has obvious Buddhist resonances, and may be related to Montaigne's admiration of Pyrrhonism, which has many affinities with Eastern thought (Beckwith 2015). Pyrrho's main concepts as reported by Sextus Empiricus had been translated into French about 20 years before the first edition of the *Essays* (see Calhoun 2015).

with our fears will teach us how many fears have no foundation and consistency and how much we have suffered in vain. Eventually, late in life, Montaigne learned how to be fully in the present, and he closes the *Essays* thus: "When I dance, I dance. When I sleep, I sleep; and when I am strolling alone through a beautiful orchard, although part of the time my thoughts are occupied by other things, for part of the time too I bring them back to the walk, to the orchard, to the delight in being alone there, and to me" (B.3.12.1258).

4.8.4 The Force of Habits

Montaigne wrote that one of the reasons the Spartans did not fear death was because they were used to it. The graveyards were outside the temples, so that children became accustomed to see the dead "without feeling terror" (A.1.20.99). He complains that in his time everything related to death was being concealed from the public, giving the impression that death was something unusual (A.1.20.99). Montaigne considered that creating the habit of accepting mortality and of facing fearful situations would be instrumental in reducing fear. For him, the remedy of habit creation is better than "the whole of philosophy" (A.1.23.129). On the other hand, and following Epictetus, Montaigne suggested that other habits are not so helpful, such as becoming too attached to family, property, and health. After reaching 'old' age, Montaigne suggested that we seek a "room, just for ourselves" (A.1.39.270) where away from daily restrictions we can read and meditate about living in the present, in loneliness, "as though we had no wife, no children, no possessions, no followers, no menservants" (A.1.39.269). Showing some prejudices against the values of community engagement and solidarity, Montaigne's withdrawn attitude strongly resonates with the Epicurean 'living unnoticed'.[43] Montaigne recommends that we must meditate on what is good for us,

[43]Montaigne's purported unnoticed way of life was only partially true, since while trying to stay away from the daily nuisance at his chateau, he would eagerly seek the company of the few erudite Montaigne had in esteem to engage in conversation, and more reluctantly, work for the king on political missions.

which requires "disentangling" (A.1.38.271) ourselves from demanding relationships. These are "violent traps" which do not allow reflection on what is truly good for us. It is only by meditating about our emotional weaknesses that we can provide ourselves with adequate medicines for our fears and worries (A.1.39.273). We should reflect on having an occupation "neither toilsome nor painful" (A.1.39.273) which depends on our capacity to work peacefully. Solitude will also allow us to search for faith in God, which will provide the best way of life.[44] Thus, in case of misfortunes, we may always have the resources to find refuge in the strength of our inner life. This strategy is different from that of the bookish scholar, who works continuously in isolation because he is unable to enjoy the present moment.

Montaigne said that he had a "hard skin", or as contemporary parlance would have it, a thick skin, against violent emotions (B.1.2.10). However, it was by self-examination and meditation that he was able to achieve that strength. But how hard Montaigne's skin actually was may be questionable, as he says that "the sight of another man's suffering produces physical suffering in me…A persistent cough tickles my lungs and my throat…when I contemplate an illness I seize upon it and lodge it within myself" (C.1.21.109).

The question remains as to how successful Montaigne was in taming his fears. Even in the last essays Montaigne was feeling distressed about minor mishaps; his mind stuck to the problem at hand. This led to a state of inertia that Montaigne was unable to control, in which his worries continued to grow (B.3.9.1076). As discussed earlier, Montaigne was prone to catastrophizing, a manifestation of a personality that could not accept a minor setback.

4.8.5 Self-Examination

Alone in his garret Montaigne embarked in an exercise of self-examination. He discovered how disturbed he was by his emotional instability (C.2.1.377), and the variability in his psychological attributes.

---

[44] "The greatest thing in the world is to know how to live to yourself" (A.1.39.272).

He examined himself from different perspectives and found in himself "every sort of contradiction" (B.2.1.377). He felt either fearful or courageous, depending on the combination of his own personality and the context, and he made progress in discovering differences in the way he reacted to fearful situations: "the most universal article of my own logic is DISTINGUO"[45] (capitals in the original) (2.1.377). This mental exercise of noting differences, rather than forcing oneself into a unique way of feeling emotions or responding to given situations, is very innovative and liberating. Unfortunately, Montaigne did not provide any more details about his DISTINGUO, except his confession that he accepted his virtues and defects after examining them in a very honest way.

What is the role of philosophy in Montaigne's self-examination, and how successful was philosophical analysis in taming his fears? Montaigne is sceptical that this technique can properly deal with emotional problems, stating that it may only be useful for those who are already "in control" of their souls (emotions and mind) (A.2.12.619). But even a philosopher may become a "madman" when afflicted by strong emotions, bodily injuries, and "gastric vapours" that confuse the soul. Montaigne's progress in self-examination allowed him to accept that he was unable to control external events. He remarks that he is able to control his emotions, a doubtful confession given that he also admitted to being anguished by suspense, "torn between fear and hope" (B.2.17.732). Also, as already discussed, Montaigne was annoyed by minor upsets, and was unable to tolerate doubt and fear (B.2.17.732). But this emotional instability was due to the mutability of contexts and personal events inherent to human life. Montaigne had varying views on himself, his soul twisting in different directions. Thus, "every sort of contradiction can be found in me" (B.2.1.377), including drastic changes in mood and behaviour. His DISTINGUO was a symbol of his attention to differences and changes in human emotions.

---

[45]This is clarified in a footnote by Screech (Montaigne 2003) as "I make a distinction," a term used in formal debates to reject or modify an opponent's assertion.

4.9 Dying Without Fear

Dying without fear was for Montaigne one of his major challenges for, as we have seen, he was obsessed with death. In his late essays, he stressed that an important mistake of philosophers is to confound death as the "End" of living, with death being simply the end of a biological cycle (C.3.12.1191). For Montaigne, "*How to die*" [italics in the original] is no more than a section of a bigger chapter on "*How to Live*" (C.3.12.1191). If we manage to learn how to live with equanimity and mental tranquillity, death will be peaceful. Against Cicero and the Platonic tradition, Montaigne eventually came to the view that a life tortured by premeditation cannot teach us how to die peacefully. The challenge is therefore, not how best to prepare for death, but how to live a more fulfilled life.[46] Montaigne suggested a life with no sophistications, of always striving for simplicity and respecting different personal tastes and habits. People should be educated following "differing routes, to what is good for them, each according to their nature" (C.3.12.1191).

But when life is unbearable, and everything fails, suicide becomes an option. The Stoics accepted suicide in a few circumstances such as irreversible illness, extreme poverty, social degradation and ostracism. The option of suicide and having no fear about it, reduces the fear of suffering from those calamities. Montaigne, following the Stoic lead, condoned suicide, although his position seems at times contradictory. In the essay entitled "A custom of the Isle of Cea" Montaigne presented the Stoic doctrine on suicide with approval: "death [by suicide] is the prescription for all our ills" (A.2.3.393). Living in anguish is a sign of cowardice, and there is no difference between one's life ending or ending one's life (A.2.3.393). Even when "enjoying good fortune," we are responsible for deciding when it is time for us to depart from life. This initial posture in favour of suicide seems to be rapidly dismissed by citing Christian texts condemning suicide. It is only up to God to decide

[46]"Life must be its own objective, its own purpose. Its right concern is to rule itself, govern itself, put up with itself" (C.3.12.1191).

about the end of life, and those who are stronger will fight adversity and misfortunes since "life is our being and our all" (A.2.3.397). But after this religious interlude Montaigne subtly returns to a defence of suicide, claiming that although it is uncertain what life events justify suicide, this is "a reasonable exodus" (A.2.3.397).

Before concluding this section, I would like to take stock on Montaigne's therapy of fear. Montaigne stated that everybody can see him reflected in his book as well as his book reflected in him. The meaning of this is that for Montaigne the writing of the *Essays* was a therapy which helped him mature as a scholar as well as a person. He grew with the book in difficult times of wars and the plague. The *Essays* discuss many fearful and horrific events, but also 'showed the fly out of the bottle', as Wittgenstein would later put it (Wittgenstein 2001, p. 309),[47] by providing examples of great courage, thus indirectly teaching how to face great fears and stressful life events. Moreover, Montaigne also discussed explicit therapies of fear as described above. But there is another dimension from which we can learn a great amount about how to deal with fear, and this is conveyed at a second level, in Montaigne's own life. Montaigne, as we have seen, was haunted by fears of all sorts, to the extreme that the best therapy, which he followed until a few years before his death, was the remedy of 'ignorance.' Basically, he did not want to be told about any problems occurring in his household, not even minor ones. What is strange about this great difficulty in facing fear is that Montaigne was well trained in Stoicism, Scepticism and Epicureanism, but none of these Hellenistic philosophies was able to reduce his strong tendency to fear. He is certainly inconsistent in his narration of his own fears, with sections in which he recognizes all types of fears and how he is paralysed by them, and sections when he claims to be free of this malady. For his readers, this is therapeutic in itself, as we can reflect ourselves in the *Essays*. Our own fears, waxing and waning but never totally dominated, push us in pursue of any treatment available. Currently, we have an assortment of therapies for fears, from the orthodox psychotropic medication, to a rainbow of psychotherapies, alternative medicines,

[47]The number following the year corresponds to the remark in *Philosophical Investigations*.

oriental philosophy and meditation, among others. In this context, it is not surprising to see the 'self-help' sections of bookstores being the most visited shelves. In other words, we may see ourselves reflected in Montaigne's own fears, since he had so many of them. And we may also see ourselves, like Montaigne, in pursuit of a therapy that may be helpful, and varying with time and circumstances. We may certainly criticise the inconsistency of Montaigne's approach, but many generations during five centuries since his *Essays* were published have been inspired by Montaigne's text. He was able to find the appropriate way to talk to his readers, by conversing about himself, showing with brutal honesty not only his intimate fears and their embarrassing consequences, but sharing the variety of therapies he tried, and his fluctuating states between feeling fully healed and accepting that his fears had no ultimate solution.

4.10 Conclusion

Montaigne's *Essays* is a work of major importance for the philosophy of fear. Fear was one of the main problems in the life of this great humanist and philosopher, and his analysis and treatment of the emotion is unique because he was among the first philosophers to openly discuss his own fears and the variety of philosophical therapies he used—sometimes successfully, sometimes not—to subdue them. The first step in the therapy resides in reading about these fears and understanding that we are not alone in this suffering, in the same way that Montaigne found therapeutic value in writing about his fears. Reading and writing have an important cathartic value. The second step of premeditation was initially considered by Montaigne as having great value. By constantly thinking about the worst outcome of a potential misfortune we believe we shall tame the impact of the mishap if this occurs. However, as discussed in the previous chapter, engaging in premeditation is nothing but a particular way of manifesting fear.

Montaigne considered Epicurean therapy to be clearly more useful. Live with little, have few expectations and no ambitions, dwell in sweet memories in times of suffering, and above all 'live unnoticed,' as Montaigne tried to do by secluding himself in his garret. But this strategy did not work either, as during the long periods of reflection, he was invaded by all sorts of monstrous thoughts. Montaigne found a more viable alternative in the sceptical Pyrrhonian tradition. His dogmatic approach to life started to fade, and he found peace of mind in the alternative of remaining uncommitted to life events. Yes, things could look bad, but the outcome could be good. Death itself may not be so tragic an event as is experienced in his near-death experience and the sweetness of falling asleep after a tiring day. The *Essays* express an open-minded, particularistic and anti-dogmatic approach to life and that is a big part of the appeal of the text. 'What do I know?', his motto, reflects his open-mindedness and receptiveness to improving his emotional well-being and increasing his knowledge and joy of life, by accepting his life as it enfolds.

Less than fifty years later the humanist tradition lost most of its influence, unable to hold its own against the new science. The Cartesian revolution, its philosophical counterpart, will present emotions in a mostly mechanistic way, something predicted by Montaigne when he referred to "the chop-logic which has captured all the [philosophical] approaches" (A.1.26.180). Fear is reduced to interactions between soul and body, and mainly explained in neuro-mechanical terms. This dramatic change in understandings of fear will be discussed in the next chapters.

References

Bakewell, S. (2010). *How to live—Or a life of Montaigne in one question and twenty attempts at an answer*. Great Britain: Chatto & Windus.

Barsky, A. J. (1988). *Worried sick: Our troubled quest for wellness*. Boston: Little, Brown and Co.

Beckwith, C. I. (2015). *Greek Buddha: Pyrrho's encounter with early Buddhism in Central Asia*. Princeton: Princeton University Press.

Bermúdez Vázquez, M. (2015). *The skepticism of Michel de Montaigne* (Vol. 216). Switzerland: Springer International Publishing.

Brockliss, L., & Jones, C. (1977). *The medical world of early modern France*. Oxford: Clarendon Press.

Calhoun, A. (2015). *Montaigne and the lives of the philosophers: Life writing and transversality in the Essais*. Newark: University of Delaware Press.

Foucault, M. (1986). *The care of the self* (H. Hurley, Trans., Vol. 3). New York: Vintage Books.

Frame, D. M. (1955). *Montaigne's discovery of man: The humaization of a humanist*. New York: Columbia Unversity Press.

Frame, D. M. (1984). *Montaigne: A biography*. San Francisco: North Point Press.

Friedrich, H. (1991). *Montaigne* (D. Eng, Trans., P. Desan, Ed.). Berkeley: University of California Press.

Hartle, A. (2013). *Montaigne and the origins of modern philosophy*. Evanston: Northwestern University Press.

Justman, S. (2015). Montaigne on medicine: Insights of a 16th-century skeptic. *Perspectives in Biology and Medicine, 58*(4), 493–506.

Lazar, D., & Madden, P. (2015). *After Montaigne* (D. Lazar & P. Madden Eds.). Athens, GA: The University of Georgia Press.

Montaigne, M. (1965). *The complete essays of Montaigne* (D. M. Frame, Trans.). Stanford: Stanford University Press.

Montaigne, M. (2003). *The complete essays* (M. A. Screech, Trans.). London: Penguin Books.

Robert, J. (2015). Pa/enser bien le corps: Cognitive and curative language in Montaigne's essais. *Journal of Medical Humanities, 36*, 241–250.

Roberts, H. (2009). Medicine and nonsense in French Renaissance moch prescriptions. *The Sixteenth Century Journal, 40*(3), 721–744.

Scholar, R. (2010). *Montaigne and the art of free-thinking*. Oxford: Peter Lang.

Starr, R. (2012). Should we be writing essays instead of articles? A psychotherapist's reflection on Montaigne's marvelous invention. *Journal of Humanistic Psychology, 52*(4), 423–450.

Wittgenstein, L. (2001). *Philosophical investigations* (G. E. M. Anscombe, Trans.). Oxford: Blackwell.

5

Thomas Hobbes and Fear: The Political Use of a Human Emotion

> Of all passions, that which enclineth men least to break the Lawes, is fear. Nay…it is the onely thing… that makes men keep them.
>
> *Leviathan, 2.27.464* (Hobbes 1996)

> The origin of all great and lasting societies lay not in mutual human benevolence but in men's mutual fear.
>
> *De Cive 1.2.23* (Hobbes 1972)

5.1 Introduction

Montaigne masterfully described the diversity of human fears and their origin, and provided advice on how to deal with them based on his personal experience. Montaigne speaks to the individual, to the afflicted person, and only wrote about the connection between fears and society at large when discussing the ravages of war or the torturing of people in public, which he detested (see Chapter 4). What is missing in Montaigne is a discussion of how social structures, such as absolutist

S. Starkstein, *A Conceptual and Therapeutic Analysis of Fear*,
https://doi.org/10.1007/978-3-319-78349-9_5

governments and the whims of sovereigns silenced, by the use of force, any possibility of expression of civil discontent. Montaigne's world was one of inner analysis of how to come to terms with one's fear of death, rarely discussing the types and causes of social fears. Sixty years after the publication of Montaigne's *Essays*, the English political philosopher Thomas Hobbes (1586–1679) published *Leviathan*,[1] a work with important insights concerning the social and political aspects of fear.[2] Hobbes is not much interested in the details of individual fears, but rather in explaining fear as the crucial human emotion when it comes to understanding the origin of social institutions. Hobbes, like Montaigne, lived at a time of religious wars and was witness to major civil and religious turmoil. Hobbes's reaction to social chaos was to propose a solid political system that would prevent social unrest, a system based on fear, and more specifically on the fear of violent death. Hobbes's most influential work, *Leviathan* (published in 1651, when he was 63 years of age) discusses the organization of a civil state at a time when England was in the midst of a civil war and Hobbes, himself, was exiled in Paris. The main argument of the book is that without a government with the power to enforce a legal system, the life of the citizens will be sordid, full of fears of becoming victims of a violent death, and with no hope of developing science and culture.

This chapter will examine the dynamic interaction between individual fear and social practices. I will first analyse how his understanding of individual fear of a violent death and anxiety about future misfortunes led Hobbes to propose a civil state ruled by a powerful sovereign, "a mortal God" (the Leviathan) with the capacity to decide on both civil and religious matters. Secondly, I will argue that a powerful state does

---

[1]In keeping with previous editions, the Oxford version used in this chapter (Hobbes 1996) numbers each head paragraph with a new run of Arabic numerals for each chapter. Thus "1.15.34" means Part 1, Chapter 15, head 34.

[2]In his book on fear, Corey Robin considers Hobbes as the philosopher who formulated the most coherent political account of fear, as well as a "great visionary" on the problem of social and political fear (Robin 2004, p. 29).

not help to reduce human fears and anxieties; rather it only modifies the characteristics of fear, from those of an acute emotion related to the danger of imminent death, to a subtler one, a state of chronic anxiety related to the punishments that await those not abiding by the dictates of the sovereign. Thirdly, I will discuss Hobbes's reference in *Leviathan* to the myth of Prometheus and to the *Book of Job*, the first as a metaphor about the sufferings of those who live focused on the future, and the second as an allegory for what awaits those who defy the power of the Leviathan. Finally, I will analyse the conflict between institutionalised religion and the Hobbesian commonwealth for a monopoly on one of the main societal pillars: the fear of death.

5.2 Hobbes: A Story of an Anxious Life

This work is not specifically about the influence of the personal life of philosophers in their works, but for Hobbes, like Cicero, Seneca and Montaigne before him, biographical details seem to have a large influence on his thought. It would be counterproductive to ignore the strong influence of political upheaval during Hobbes's life, as well as what we know of his own personal characteristics in his political writings. Pointing wryly himself to this influence in his autobiographical poem, Hobbes noted that his life was marked by fear while still in utero. His mother was pregnant when the mighty Spanish Armada was on its way to England, spreading terror on the population. Thus:

> For fame had rumour'd, than Fleet at Sea,
> Wou'd cause our Nations Catastrophe;
> And hereupon it was my Mother Dear
> Did bring forth Twins at once, both Me, and Fear
>
> (Martinich 1999, p. 356)

Hobbes's life was also marked by the fear of imprisonment, poverty, and assassination. He had to flee different countries on several occasions, and his books were burnt in public. He claims that he only found some solace at the end of his long life:

> I've now completed my Eighty four year,
> And Death approaching, prompts me not to fear.
>
> (Martinich 1999, p. 356)

Hobbes had a sad childhood, with a violent and alcoholic father who eventually abandoned his family in poverty. Hobbes was frightened by the plague that affected Oxford when he was studying there, and being of a weak constitution, he was the target of abuse by peers. Hobbes was also frightened by the religious wars that were ravaging Europe. In one of his earliest writings he warned Englishmen visiting Rome to pass unnoticed and to refrain from discussing religious matters or even speaking English to avoid the risk of being sent to the Inquisition (Martinich 1999). In 1640 one of Hobbes's early writings upset the English parliament, and fearing for his life, he fled England for the Continent. Twelve years later, he had to escape Paris, returning to England because of fear of being murdered.

Both fear and power are the driving forces behind Hobbes's politico-philosophical works, and fear had primacy over any other emotion in his writings (Pettit 2008, p. 99). Hobbes wrote that fear was the origin of religions, and in *Leviathan* he defined religion as "*Feare*, of power invisible, feigned by the mind, or imagined from tales publicly allowed" (1.6.86). Given this and other anti-religious statements, it is not surprising that Hobbes was harshly criticised by Roman Catholics and Protestants alike—reason for further fear. In 1683 copies of both *De Cive* and *Leviathan* were burnt by the public hangman in Oxford, as these works were considered heretical and blasphemous, and a danger to both church and state. Hobbes came under investigation by the English Parliament for atheism and was accused of treason by his former friends (Martinich 1999). He lived under the fear of life imprisonment or exile until the end of his life (Martinich 1999).

Besides political dangers, Hobbes was obsessively concerned with his health to the point of becoming a valetudinarian (Mintz 1970, p. 19). He was extremely methodical in his habits, exercising on a regular basis and singing popular songs with the idea of improving his lung capacity (Martinich 1999, p. 294). As summarized by Martinich in his biography of Hobbes, "much of Hobbes's life had been a struggle for survival…Much of what he did was motivated by fear" (p. 357).

5.3 Leviathan

Leviathan is considered one of the most important texts ever written on political philosophy (Newey 2014, p. 1). The main themes pertain to individual safety, political strife and social instability, and the role of religion in social life. *Leviathan* was written in the middle of the Seventeenth century in the context of wars ravaging Europe. Several countries, such as Holland, experienced major civil conflicts which ended with the assassination of political leaders (Harrison 2003, p. 9), and by the time *Leviathan* was published, Hobbes was in exile in Paris due to being on the 'wrong' side of the English civil war. After the English king was executed, "nothing was safe or certain" (Harrison 2003, p. 10). As Harrison points out, *Leviathan* was written to answer the deep challenges of civil turmoil and war, and to provide a philosophical-political analysis of how individual and social fears are crucial elements for the constitution of strong civil regimes which Hobbes personified in the shape of the biblical monster, the Leviathan.

The "terrible" power of the Leviathan was already manifest in the frontispiece of the first edition of the book, which included a banner with a paragraph from Job 41:31–4: "There is no power over earth that compares to him", the Leviathan, "a creature without fear…king over all the sons of pride". The Leviathan is presented in the Introduction as a being created not in a natural way like humans, but artificially, as "the great LEVIATHAN called a COMMONWEALTH, or STATE" (Leviathan, pp. 12–13), aimed at protecting all citizens within the community. 'Sovereignty' is the "artificial soul" that gives life to the Leviathan, whose body is composed of magistrates working as "artificial joints"; the mechanism of providing rewards and punishments constitute the "nerves"; the strength of the monster is "wealth and riches"; the safety of the citizens is the Leviathan's occupation; its "memory system" is in charge of providing counsel and advice, whereas its "reason and will" provide a legal system which determines health and death. The members of the Leviathan are fastened by contracts and covenants.[3]

In *Leviathan* Hobbes speculated that human societies evolved from a primitive "state of nature", in which humans lived devoid of laws and social organisation, pursuing a self-interested life while trying to avoid a violent death. Given the high risk of death in the hands of other fellow-humans, and motivated by fear, individuals organised themselves in a Commonwealth governed by a powerful and absolute ruler.[4] Hobbes considered this political order as the only possibility for providing the necessary safety for scientific and social progress. The Leviathan (Commonwealth) will reciprocate for civil obedience by assuring the rights of property, of self-preservation, and by providing a more contented life. I will now discuss the elements central to the process of social organization described in *Leviathan*, which include the state of nature, the rights of nature, and the laws of nature.

5.4 The State of Nature: From Individual to Social Fears

Hobbes describes the state of nature as the condition in which humans live in a condition without laws or government, having to fight for survival (Newey 2014, p. 1). Life in the state of nature is characterised by insecurity, where human behaviour is dominated by the instinct of self-preservation. Hobbes considered that mutual aggression among humans is the result of natural and insatiable appetites (Hobbes 1889) (*Elements* I.14.11), and the emotion of irrational vanity, which he termed "vainglory." The only defence available to an individual comes from that individual's own powers, and scarcity of resources leads to war of all against all. In this context, when individuals are dominated by the

[3]Contracts refer to the transfer of individual rights to the Leviathan, with the assumption that citizens will obtain safety in return. The promise of reciprocal benefits between citizens and state constitute a covenant (Hobbes 1889) (*Elements* 1.8–9).

[4]As noted by Kavka (1986, p. 80) fear of death is a "vital premise" for Hobbes's argumentation about anarchy and the state.

need to defend themselves against others, there is no pleasure in life. There is also no culture, given that people are preoccupied with increasing their physical power and protecting their belongings. Life is short, there is no society that can protect the individual, and violent death is frequent as crime is rife.[5] In this context, humans become acutely aware of their mortality which engenders a state of anxiety (Ahrensdorf 2000, p. 580), a chronic suffering which can only be tamed by a powerful ruler. Other examples of the state of nature are not so gloomy, and propose a collective arrangement in which people could be in peace in the context of fewer fears, where people would help rather than attack each other.[6]

Hobbes's understanding of the state of nature was strongly criticised by contemporary critics, but according to Schochet (1967, p. 428) these critics were wrongly interpreting Hobbes's state of nature as a real historical account when in fact it was just "a logical and reductionist device" to demonstrate the need for an absolute government. Hobbes suggested three arguments against the state of nature being a 'peaceful' state. First, he considered that life has no final goal, and that the essence of life is being in constant motion towards different desires.[7] There is no *finis ultimus*, and each individual moves and fights for their own aims and objectives, the main one being to preserve their own life. Second, Hobbes posited that living a fulfilled life not only implies enjoyment

[5]In the state of nature people "avoid that which is hurtful; but most of all that terrible enemy of nature, death" (*Elements* I.14.6). It is interesting that here, Hobbes seems to consider any death as an enemy of nature, like a target to be vanquished, rather than a natural and irreversible event. This use of rhetoric, I believe, helps to construe fear of death as the most catastrophic event of human life. In other words, if death is rationally considered as the end of life, it can be accepted by some without much fear, such as in the case of the Stoics of antiquity. On the other hand, Hobbes considers death (or at least violent death) as an enemy to be avoided (see also footnote 220).

[6]Examples, proposing a mythical "golden age" of civilization abound in the works of many philosophers, from Seneca to Suarez (Zagorin 2009). Any later social contract philosophers, like Locke and Rousseau, had more benign understandings of the state of nature.

[7]"For there is no such *Finis Ultimus* (utmost aim) nor *Summum Bonum*, (greatest good) … Felicity is a continuall progresse of the desire, from one object to another…" (*Leviathan* 1.11.2), "for as to have no desire, is to be dead" (*Leviathan* 1.8.35).

in the present, but also the certainty of having pleasure in the future.[8] This creates anxiety, as in the state of nature nothing is assured when the only certainty is daily danger.[9] This need for pleasure and safety generates a "restlesse desire of Power after power, that ceaseth onely in Death" (*Leviathan* 1.11.2). Third, humans are the result of their natural attributes and education. They have different personalities and intellectual capacities, resulting in different opinions and the concomitant risk of conflict. But what is common to humans is the desire for power and safety, and in the quest for these elements, physical, emotional and intellectual differences become balanced, as people are equal in the threat they pose to each other (Bagby 2009, p. 103). For instance, not everybody is vainglorious, seeking wealth and honours, but in the state of nature the righteous are unable to live peacefully given their ignorance of the intentions of others in a context of scarcity, the state of nature becoming a state of constant war. Conflict is unavoidable and the only way of stopping the state of war is by the controlling power of a strong sovereign (Bagby 2009, p. 101).

Hobbes suggested that all humans in the state of nature have equal capacities, although their attributes may differ. Thus, a physically weak person is compensated by a cleverer mind compared with that of a stronger person.[10] In the state of nature humans are equal in their abilities, in needs and desires, and in fears and anxiety, as they desire the same objects and have similar capacities to obtain them (Mintz 1970, p. 31). With resources being finite and scarce, there is constant competition for power, and the "contention, enmity and war" (*Leviathan* 1.11.3) is the expression of the fight to subdue one another. In this condition, the main fears are the fear of a violent death and the fear of being oppressed by others. These fears are the chief reason why people

---

[8]"That the object of man's desire, is not to enjoy once onely, and for once instant of time; but to assure forever, the way of his future desire" (*Leviathan* 1.11.2).

[9]Hobbes' concept of anxiety is of an indefinite worry for the future (the "Anxiety of the time to come" (*Leviathan*, Section 2, Religion, 52), whereas fear is defined as an "*Aversion* with opinion of *Hurt* from the object" (*Leviathan* 1.6.25) (italics in the original).

[10]"…there is no reason why any man, trusting to his own strength, should conceive himself made by nature above others. They are equals, who can do equal things one against the other" (Hobbes 1972) (*De Cive* 1.3).

are willing to submit to a powerful ruler, a Leviathan, bringing order by way of its capacity to enforce protective laws.

5.4.1 Criticism of Hobbes's State of Nature

There are some obvious difficulties with Hobbes's account of the state of nature. In the first place, he had no empirical evidence to propose a "nasty" and "brutish" state of nature. However, he had a political reason, given the violent events of the English revolution and the need to put a limit on the chaos engendered by rebellion. If a warring state of nature never existed, it had to be invented to justify the construction of the Leviathan. Hobbes had to create the notion of a context of chronic fear of a violent death to make individuals' submission to an all-powerful sovereign plausible.

The arguments supporting a bleak state of nature are also questionable. We may accept that for the non-believer life may not have an ultimate goal, and that some people often seek assurances about the future, though the notion that these traits are common to all individuals is far from convincing. But the third argument concerning the inherent equality of individuals is even more questionable: what does it mean for humans to be "equal"? Hobbes himself stated in the Introduction to *Leviathan* that whereas humans have the same type of emotions, they differ in the objects that trigger these emotions. Some people have fear of death, whereas for the vainglorious, death is less relevant than achieving power and honours. Hobbes suggested that the pattern of humans' emotional responses depends on both intrinsic and extrinsic factors, such as the psychological constitution of the individual, their education, and their social context. In *Elements* (1.14.3) Hobbes stressed the "great difference" among humans in terms of their leading emotions, with some being "vainly glorious," regardless of the strength of their objective powers, and others being "moderate" in their desires. Nevertheless, for the Hobbesian state of nature to function, all humans have to be similar in mind and body, since all have to develop a similarly intense fear of death (Gold and Pearce 2015, p. 187).

There is here another interesting contrast between Montaigne and Hobbes's concepts of human nature. Montaigne's *Essays* (Montaigne 2003) provides examples of numerous psychological changes in different people, across different stages in life and under different circumstances, whereas Hobbes suggests a more mechanistic human whose behaviour and emotions are determined by universal scientific laws. The scientifically styled discourse of Hobbes, such as the regularity of putative laws, depends on regularities in human behavioural and emotional responses to contextual stimuli. This concept of homogeneity and regularity of human behaviour is a necessary factor for the plausibility of universal acceptance of living under the laws of a strong sovereign, which will in return remove the fear of living in social anarchy and of a violent death. This uniformity of human life, however, is apparently not available in the state of nature, since life in this state is complicated by the fact that, according to Hobbes, human behaviour can be difficult to predict.[11] Quite often, human actions have inscrutable reasons, given the tendency to deceive, to rely too much on others, or to be frightened by multiple causes. To understand human reasons, says Hobbes, "is to decipher without a key" (*Leviathan*, Introduction, p. 20). It is the complexity of human behaviour as a result of causes not always easy to understand that makes the state of nature so unpredictable and dangerous. This inscrutable human behaviour will complicate the maintenance of civil order under the Leviathan, since to rule a commonwealth effectively, the sovereign has to understand the actions of "not this, or that particular man; but Man-kind: which thought it be hard to do, harder than to learning any language, or Science" (*Leviathan*, Introduction, p. 18).

5.5 The Rights of Nature

According to Hobbes, in the state of nature, humans have the right to defend themselves, and this right to preserve one's life is the principal right of nature. Hobbes based this right of self-preservation on

[11]"the characters of man's heart, blotted and confounded as they are, with dissembling, lying, counterfeiting, and erroneous doctrines, are eligible onely to him that searcheth hearths" (*Leviathan*, Introduction, p. 20).

empirical factors, such as the instinct for self-preservation and fear of death.[12] Other rights of nature are the rights to freedom and to social equality. Individuals have the right to be free from oppression and to defend their lives by killing if necessary.[13] As Zagorin (2009, p. 28) clearly states: "For Hobbes, natural rights are not the creation of natural law but a primordial entitlement grounded in the most basic instinct and reasonable desire of human nature, the passion and wish to go on living."

5.6 The Laws of Nature

Hobbes defined a law of nature as "a Precept, or general rule, found out by Reason, by which a man is forbidden to do, that, which is destructive of his life, or taketh away the means of preserving the same; and to omit, that, by which he thinketh it may be best preserved" (*Leviathan* 1.14.64). In other words, the rules of nature are rational rules of life with moral content that pre-exist civil legislation enacted by governments. As remarked by Hobbes, the laws of nature, rather than 'laws' in their judicial connotation, are "theorems" concerning self-preservation (*Leviathan* 1.15.80).

According to Zagorin, Hobbes's conception of the laws of nature should be understood against the Platonic and Sophist tradition of separating nature, which is universally normative and permanent, from *nomos*, which as already mentioned, is a set of customs that consist of what is variable and different in human legal practices (Zagorin 2009, p. 5). In contrast, for Hobbes, the laws of nature operate like a covenant or contract arrived at by all humans due to the desire of

[12]The right of nature is "the liberty each man hath to use his own power, as he will himself, for the preservation of his own nature, that is to say, of his own life, and consequently of doing anything which, in his own judgment and reason, he shall conceive to be the aptest means thereunto" (Hobbes 1972) (*De Cive* 1.7).

[13]"Therefore the first foundation of natural Right is this, that every man as much as in him lies endeavour to protect his life and members" (*De Cive* 1.7).

self-preservation. It is the fear of death that will unite people in curbing their desires and accepting a common sovereign (Johnston 1986, p. 46). Hobbes proposed twenty laws of nature aimed at promoting safe and productive social practices, as well as harmonizing the individual interest for self-preservation with the equivalent interests of other individuals. The principal law of nature is that humans have to pursue peace, but when conditions make this impossible to achieve, they should be ready for war.[14] The second law of nature is to renounce our rights as much as others do for the sake of peace, and the third is that people should perform their covenants (Springborg 2007, p. 225).

The laws of nature are weak when it comes to enforcement, as they are controlled only by people's mutual confidence in each other, which for Hobbes is no more than mere words, "too weak to bridle men's ambition" (*Leviathan* 1.14.68). These virtuous laws are ineffective "without the fear of some coercive power" to enforce them (*Leviathan* 1.14.68). Fear of a violent or early death, the need for enforceable laws, and hence the need for a political structure sufficiently powerful to compel compliance with these laws, underlie the creation of the Leviathan. Under the power of the Leviathan, humans will be disposed to obedience because of the threat of punishment.[15] Hobbes's Commonwealth was not designed to suppress all freedom, but to curtail some liberties by the institution of a 'civilized' fear. This is no longer the panic fear of the state of nature, but a fear shaped by the imposition of laws. The aim of the Leviathan is to produce a proper balance between bodily safety and the understanding of human frailty (Cooper 2010, p. 3). Citizens are free to decide on their actions, although fear of punishment should convince them to live within legal boundaries.

[14]"...to seek peace and follow it"; otherwise, "By all means we can, to defend our selves." (*Leviathan* 1.14.64).

[15]Laws are "mere words", and "Covenants, without the Sword, are but Words, and of no strength to secure a man at all" (*Leviathan* 2.17.85).

5.7 Hobbes's Concept of Human Emotions

For a better understanding of the conceptual position of fear in Hobbes' political system, a brief discussion of his concept of emotions is in order. In resonance with Stoic accounts, Hobbes described emotions as "perturbations of the mind" given that they impede proper reasoning (Hobbes 1972) (*De Homine* 12.1). Emotions push individuals towards short-term gains, whilst reason aims at long-term benefits.[16] Hobbes considered that the best legal system should be based on reason and not be influenced by emotions, as only a rational system can guide humans into a state of peace and mutual defence (*Elements* 1.1). Nevertheless, "mental perturbations" are important in the construction of a powerful social system, as the government is primarily structured around the fear of punishment. Among human emotions, fear was for Hobbes the most relevant for enforcing a given social system. He describes fear as the state produced by impending evil, continually alternating with the emotion of hope (i.e. the state of avoiding evil). In *De Cive*, Hobbes stresses the important social role of fear, as being the only 'antidote' against vainglory and excessive ambition, and the fact that the political power of the sovereign is built on social fears rather than on mutual good will (*De Cive* 1.2).

5.7.1 Hobbes's Concept of Fear

For Hobbes, as we have seen, the significance of fear is mainly related to its social role. In *De Cive* he provided the usual description of fear as the expectation of a future evil, but he elaborated on the conceptual association between fear and related behaviours and emotions that are relevant in social interaction. Thus, Hobbes described the emotions of distrust, suspicion, and "taking heed" as related to fear. Fear is an emotion pervasive in simple daily behaviours such as locking the door when leaving

[16] "...appetite seizeth upon a present good without foreseeing the greater evils that necessarily attach to it" (*De Homine* 12.1).

home, as well as in more complex state policies, such as patrolling the frontiers or training the police force. According to Hobbes all deliberation stops when safety is at stake, "for security is the end wherefore men submit themselves to others" (*De Cive* 5.3). Out of fear, most humans will abide by a strong ruler capable of protecting their goods and life. Those individuals who, on the other hand, are strongly motivated by natural pride and by a thirst for glory will be subdued by the terror of the Leviathan. It is fear that creates the necessity for the Leviathan, and fear is what keeps it alive.

5.7.2 Fear in the State of Nature and Fear Under the Leviathan

In the state of nature fear is rife as the risk of death is high given that the only protection from violence is one's own power. The laws of nature provide implicit rules of behaviour with the aim of preventing individuals from injuring one another. For Hobbes, as already noted, one limitation of these laws is that they can only be imposed by the force of a "coercive power" (*Leviathan* 1.14.68) thus ending the omniscient fear of the state of nature. When the Leviathan assumes the shape of military dictatorships or totalitarian governments, the expression of fear ranges from that of minorities living in "panic terrors," to whole societies living under the intense grip of this emotion. Hobbes himself fostered the role of fear under the Leviathan by strikingly suggesting that pacts arranged under the influence of fear, such as having to pay ransoms to thieves, have to be respected. There is only one exception to full obedience to the positive laws of the Leviathan, and this is when a person is physically threatened. In this situation, a person is permitted to commit acts that would otherwise be punished, such as killing in self-defence, if necessary. On the other hand, crimes committed due to 'religious fear' (e.g. due to superstition) should always be punished. I shall later describe the conflicting interaction between religious institutions and the government of the commonwealth.

The question now arises as to whether the Leviathan provides peace of mind to the individual, or whether it only changes the cause and expression of fear without diminishing its strength. According to Hobbes, respect for laws and pacts of non-aggression allows individuals, and society at large, to divert their energies from protecting their lives and fighting wars to the healthier development of commercial, cultural and scientific activities. Nevertheless, as Hobbes admitted, even when abiding by the laws and covenants of the Leviathan, "The Passion to be reckoned upon is Fear" (*Leviathan* 1.14.70). In an organized society fear is still present, albeit in subtle ways since the prospect of suffering injuries or death is more predictable than in the state of nature. In *De Cive* (1.14.2) Hobbes remarks that a state of constant fear is unsustainable, as people would be unable to "endur'[d] each others looks," making any civil transaction impossible. Nevertheless, he considered that being acutely scared, or "affrightened", should be distinguished from fear where the latter is understood under the wider concept of "a certain foresight of future evill" (*De Cive* 1.14.2), that is, in terms of the variety of behaviours that may result from "rational" fears.

In contemporary western life fear permeates human decision-making processes, from major life decisions (such as migrating due to lack of jobs, social corruption or political violence), to much subtler expressions of fear, such as bolting doors before going to sleep or placing valuables in safe boxes. Humans no longer live in the 'fight or flight' condition of the state of nature, but in a more complex society, practised in the arts of simulation and dissimulation (Bodei 1995, p. 110). In modern western society, fear is expressed in the emotions and behaviours of distrust, suspicion, and careful attention, as humans not only want to avoid future dangers, but also the very emotion of fear.

In *Leviathan*, Hobbes considered curiosity, prudence and foresight as relevant expressions of fear, deserving independent analysis. Showing how much he sees the world through the lens of fear, Hobbes claimed that far from a benign desire for knowledge, curiosity results from the "great anxiety about future time" (*Leviathan* 1.12.51) generated in the state of nature,[17] and refers to the desire of understanding

[17]"Anxiety for the future time, disposeth men to inquire into the cause of things: because the knowledge of them maketh men the better able to order the present to their best advantage" (*Leviathan* 1.11.51).

the causes of one's own "good and evil fortune" (*Leviathan* 1.12.52). Prudence is, for Hobbes, a necessary condition for ruling families and kingdoms, and is essential to the preservation of one's life, given that "human desires have no limits" (*Leviathan* 1.11.1). Due to the need for sustenance and protection, humans live in "a perpetuall solicitude of the time to come" (*Leviathan* 1.12.52). This is the origin of foresight, the capacity for proper planning, which in the state of nature is of critical value for the provision of food, shelter and safety against beasts and humans. But foresight is a double-edged sword, since this is the same human attribute that provokes anxiety about potential misfortunes, such as illness, poverty and death. Thus, prudence and foresight come at a price.

In Chapter 12 of *Leviathan* ("Of Religion") Hobbes analysed the causes of fear and anxiety by comparing humans to lower animals. He noted that humans have the intellectual capacity and curiosity to search for the causes of life events, and consequently to make predictions. Because they lack foresight, "beasts" just enjoy the day, whilst humans, knowing the causes of events and having the capacity to formulate predictions, fall into a state of chronic anxiety when facing a future that appears bleak. For humans, it is not enough to feel safe, but to remove anxiety they also need to believe they will be safe in the future.[18]

Recognising the fact that foresight is fallible as well as the impossibility of completely allaying the anxiety of future dangers, Hobbes states that humans fall "in an estate like to that of *Prometheus*" (*Leviathan* 1.12.52, italics in original), the Titan of the Greek mythology who forever enchained to Mount Caucasus, was left to predict his chronic evils. I shall discuss, below, the importance, according to Hobbes, that myths have in triggering human emotions. The myth of Prometheus is a clear allegory of the disadvantage of having 'too much' foresight, and given its prominent position in *Leviathan*, it deserves specific discussion.

[18]Every human "…continually endeavoureth to secure himselfe against the evill he feares, and procure the good he desireth, not to be in a perpetuall solicitude of the time to come" (*Leviathan* 1.12.52).

5.8 Prometheus: The Negative Consequence of Challenging the Sovereign

Hobbes introduces the myth of Prometheus when discussing the human state of anxiety and the quest for safety.[19] Reference to the myth is included in Chapter 12 of *Leviathan*, in the section entitled "The natural cause of religion, the anxiety of the time to come" in which Hobbes elaborates on the origins of religion, the causes of human anxiety, and the importance of abiding by the laws of the Commonwealth. This short but significant section makes reference to the benefit that science may bring to humankind, but also the chronic anxiety that may result from excessive foresight. Furthermore, the myth of Prometheus also illustrates the ominous consequences that await those who defy the Leviathan.

Aeschylus' *Prometheus Bound*[20] is an allegory of human progress based on Prometheus'[21] gift of fire to humans, fire which he stole from Zeus, the King of the Gods. With the benefit of fire, humans were able to develop technology and science, starting an age of progress. The myth begins with an act of transgression (stealing a treasure from the Olympian god) for which Prometheus was punished to suffer for life.[22] He was bound to the Caucasus, and underwent the perpetual torture of having his liver repeatedly gnawed by an eagle during the day, and regenerating by night. Prometheus' punishment went further than this, as he was left to eternally anticipate this terrible fate. Prometheus' suffering was made more severe by the expectation of daily torture rather than by the pain inflicted by the eagle, an example of mental pain being

[19]"So that every man, *especially those that are over provident*, are in a state like that of Prometheus" (*Leviathan* 1.12.52) [my italics].

[20]The myth of Prometheus is described by various Greek poets and philosophers. I have decided to use Aeschylus' version (Aeschylus 1961) given that this is one of the most commonly associated with Hobbes' *Leviathan*.

[21]The meaning of Prometheus in Greek is 'fore thinker'.

[22]Prometheus is always looking to the future in a state of anguish "for pain present and pain to come", "no torment will come unforeseen", and "whatever comes, brings fear" (Aeschylus 1961) (*Prometheus* 441, 461).

greater that physical pain. In a similar vein, Hobbes states that a "man which looks too far before him, in the care of future time, hath his heart all the day long, gnawed on by feare of death, poverty, or other calamity; and has no repose, nor pause of his anxiety, but in sleep" (*Leviathan* 1.12.52). As discussed in the previous chapters, a similar concept of the dangers of looking into the future is found in Epicurean ethics and in Seneca.

Michaelis (2007, pp. 115–123) has suggested that the inclusion of the myth of Prometheus in *Leviathan* highlights the state of chronic anxiety that humans suffer due to their always uncertain future. Unlike Ahrensdorf (2000, p. 580), who considers ambition to be the major cause of civil strife, Michaelis suggests that the main source of social conflict lies in the constant need of safety. She bases her hypothesis on the fact that Hobbes's account does not mention the stealing of fire from Zeus, an act of major defiance against the mighty ruler of Olympus. This is a striking omission, as the dire consequences of challenging the sovereign is a central theme of *Leviathan*. Michaelis suggests that by omitting discussion of the act of challenge Hobbes changed the focus of the myth towards the ominous consequences of always looking towards the future.

Vasalle suggests that the Promethean myth has been classically interpreted as a metaphor for the anxiety and anguish that humans suffer when exposed to dangerous life events, which *increase* their desire for greater foresight (Vasalle 2010, p. 28). The quest for knowledge about the future turns into a vicious circle, since greater foresight exposes humans to a wider horizon of dangers that they are unable to dominate, which in turn results in more anxiety (Vasalle 2010, p. 23). This is the fate of poor Prometheus after he has stolen fire, fully able to foretell his future but unable to change it. Similarly, among humans, anxiety is generated by the conflict between having a clear perception of the future and our limited capacity to avoid unwanted events (Vasalle 2010, p. 30). Prometheus does no suffer from fear, which in *Leviathan* is conceptualised as the prediction of an objective evil, but from anguish, which is a state of paralysing anxiety due to the anticipation of undefined calamities (Vasalle 2010, p. 30). This concept of anguish will be developed centuries later by Sigmund Freud under the syndrome of "neurosis anxiety" (*Angstenurose*) (see Chapter 8).

In Aeschylus' play, the Chorus asks Prometheus:

> *Chorus*: Did your offence perhaps go further than you said?
> *Prometheus*: Yes: I caused men no longer to foresee their death.
> *Chorus*: What cure did you discover for their misery?
> *Prometheus*: I planted firmly in their hearts blind hopefulness.
> *Chorus*: your gift brought them great blessing.
> *Prometheus*: I did more than that: I gave them fire…and with it they shall master many crafts.
>
> (Aeschylus 1961)

It is interesting that in Aeschylus' version of the myth, the gift of fire comes only in third place of significance, after the gifts of "blind hopes" and ignorance of death. That all three elements are of crucial importance for the political system proposed by Hobbes in *Leviathan* will be discussed below. It cannot be denied that technology and science are both relevant for improving humans' standard of life, and both are missing in the state of nature. They also allow for making more accurate predictions about the future, with the concomitant anxiety if the prediction happens to be of negative events. In seventeenth century England, at the time when *Leviathan* was published, there was a major interest in medicine and surgery, with a high regard for medical care. Thomas Sydenham, the most prestigious physician of the century, was a pioneer in establishing medicine on a solid scientific basis (Merton 1938, p. 24). Physicians became the objects of respect and fear, as they had the capacity not only to heal but also to diagnose incurable illnesses. Thus, science may be construed as a double-edged sword, providing humans with technological advances while simultaneously delivering more accurate predictions of the calamities awaiting them. It is in this context that Prometheus' present to humans of "blind hopes" becomes valuable. For most mortals, Prometheus' gift of blind hope is a fitting remedy for the fear and anxiety produced by foresight. Even the Olympian gods may benefit from blind hopes: "when Io, a goddess punished by Zeus," asked Prometheus when her curse would come to an end, he responded that "not to know this [i.e. her fate] is better for you to know" (*Prometheus* 834). Ignorance of the future to come is for Prometheus better than knowledge. A good illustration of Prometheus' curse is provided by Montaigne and his fear of illness. Montaigne lived in a state of chronic anxiety about having kidney stones, the cause of his father's death. He eventually did develop the disease, as already discussed in Chapter 4, but discovered he was able to cope quite well with the illness, his previous dread being worse than his current sufferings.

Montaigne's experience and Prometheus' myth expose the ethical and epistemic dilemma of how much knowledge is necessary for a life with (relative) tranquillity of mind. Hobbes denied that the peace of mind (the "*Finis ultimus*" or "*Summum Bonum*") of the "old Morall Philosophers", in reference primarily to Epicureans and Stoics, is achievable (*Leviathan* 1.11.47). He inverts Stoic ethics, according to which reason subdues the passions, by making fear the main psychological condition for achieving a paradoxical 'tranquil' life under the Leviathan. Hobbes also rejected the *katastematic* or static pleasures of the Epicureans, considering instead that human happiness resides not in enjoyment just "for one instant of time", but in the future as well (*Leviathan* 1.11.47).

In Aeschylus' *Prometheus Bound*, the main gift to humankind was suppression of the capacity to foretell death. Fear of death, the emotional axis of *Leviathan*, is a factor of chronic anxiety, because, as already noted, humans live in "a perpetuall solicitude of the time to come" (*Leviathan* 1.12.52).

Hobbes presents the reduction of fears as one of the major benefits of living under the Leviathan, but this seemingly straightforward conclusion needs unpacking. One of the problems of increasing one's sense of safety is that this feeling may undermine the very usefulness of the fear of death as a bulwark against insurrection.[23] Ahrensdorf (2000, p. 581)

[23]Ahrensdorf even suggests that Hobbes tried to blur the fear of death to such an extent that death could be considered an almost avoidable event, a sickness to be cured by the Leviathan. Ahrensdorf makes reference to Hobbes's statements such as death being "the chiefest of natural evils" (*De Cive* 1.7), and "the terrible enemy of nature" (Hobbes 1994) (*De Corpore Politico* 1.1.6).

suggests that, ironically, providing too much safety empowers the individual to reflect on the inexorability of death, and rationally suppress the fear of death. Relieved of this fear, those individuals seeking glory may challenge the political system.[24] As suggested by Strauss (1963, p. 17), the origins of law and the state are not found in a rational understanding of the human condition of death, but the "aversion from death", a fear of a violent death, which, Strauss claims, is at the basis of morality.

The striking Promethean gift becomes a poisoned apple for the Leviathan, as the man prepared to die will not be beaten cheaply, Montaigne (see Chapter 4) dedicated a chapter of his *Essays* to warning against excessive severity in punishments, since those that have nothing to lose (or, in this case, to fear) pose the greatest danger to the government. On the other hand, Bagby suggests that for Hobbes, one of the main problems impacting on social life was not that humans are always fearful, *but that by nature they are not fearful enough* [italics in the original] (Bagby 2009, p. 106). Hobbes considered fear of death the main deterrent for war, and therefore, lack of fear was for Hobbes one of the main causes underlying civil conflicts.

Finally, we should not omit the by now obvious construction of the myth of Prometheus as a reminder for those who dare to defy the power of the Leviathan. Prometheus is described in Aeschylus' myth as defiant, proud and imprudent, as well as lacking in self-control. He tricked Zeus, ruler of Olympus, and was heavily punished for his deed. Prometheus was sentenced to the eternal knowledge that "whatever comes, brings fear" (*Prometheus* 461). The same future awaits those who do not abide by the laws of the Commonwealth. In *De Cive* Hobbes states that societies are constituted either for gain or glory (*De Cive* 1.2). If it is for gain, a pact is necessary to avoid violent death and war. This may work for the fearful, but may be useless for the vainglorious, who

[24]"...a generall inclination of all mankind, a perpetuall and restlesse desire of Power after power, that ceaseth only in death. And the cause of this, is...because [man] cannot assure the power and means to live well...without the acquisition of more" (*Leviathan* 1.11.46).

are not frightened by death. It is "mutual fear" and not the good will of humans that will produce "great and lasting Societies" (*De Cive* 1.2).

In conclusion, Hobbes's *Leviathan* oscillates between the need to provide safety as a better alternative to the state of nature, and simultaneously, to keep a level of chronic fear (Ahrendorf's "subjective insecurity," p. 30) high enough to maintain obedience to social pacts and covenants (Ahrendorf's "objective security," p. 30) but not so high as to incite defiance. Thus, for the ordinary individual, Hobbes provides a mixed bag of recommendations: being prudent but not over-prudent; having foresight, but not in excess; and enjoying life, with an adequate dose of fear, based on the security provided by the Leviathan.

It is intriguing that in *Leviathan*, Hobbes makes reference to diametrically opposed characters, such as Prometheus and Job. Prometheus is antithetical to the citizen Hobbes desires for his commonwealth, since nobody should dare to defy the commands of the sovereign. On the other hand, the *Book of Job* is an important allegory of the life of those citizens, who regardless of how righteous their lives may be, are nevertheless at the mercy of the powerful ruler.

5.9 The Fears of Job

The main emotions depicted in the Book of Job are fear and terror.[25] There are many different interpretations of this text, but it is generally accepted that the Biblical story addresses the question of why the righteous suffer, and centres around Job, a pious man whose fear of God leads him to constantly worry about sins his family may commit. In the eyes of God Job is a man of full integrity and honesty, but the Accuser (Satan) objects that Job's piety is no more than egotistic behaviour aimed at obtaining God's protection. Should God cease to protect him, Job's piety would immediately vanish. God allows the Accuser to put Job to trial, a process which is carried out mercilessly. After the killing

[25] I used Mitchell's translation of *The Book of Job* (Mitchell 1987).

of his family and the loss of his wealth, his "worst fears have happened", and Job falls in a state of terror and despair (*Job* 6.2):

> If ever my grief were measured
> or my sorrow put on a scale,
> it would outweigh the sands of the ocean…
> …For God has ringed me with terrors,
> and his arrows have pierced my heart.
> …all hope has been driven away.

With his family gone, his wealth lost, and his health dissipated, Job should have nothing to fear. And yet, even after these horrible sufferings Job maintained his submission to God. In response to one of his friends' comments about how to show respect to God, Job states (9:3):

> …no man can argue with God
> or answer even one of a thousand accusations.
> However wise or powerful, who could oppose him and live?
> …He makes me gasp with terror;
> He plunges me in despair
> For in strength, He is far beyond me.

Thus, there can be no rational arguing with God, and there is no rational explanation for Job's suffering. In the context of *Leviathan*, the *Book of Job* provides a dramatic allegory about the brutal power of Hobbes's sovereign. Hobbes refers to the *Book of Job* as a reminder that the problem of human vainglory threatening the state may be easily crushed by the sovereign, and Newey considers the whole of *Leviathan* as a "parody" of the *Book of Job* (Newey 2014, p. 178). Cooper (2010, pp. 244–245) argues that the reference to Job is to illustrate God's natural prerogatives over humans, since even the virtuous may suffer his omnipotence. Hobbes's reference to Job is both a reminder of the limitations of human life as well as an extrapolation of the power of celestial God to the sovereign of the commonwealth as the mortal God on earth.[26] There is no succour for the believer in God or the commonwealth from either of these "Gods", as they are not bound by any promises (Newey 2014). Disobedience will be punished, and obedience will be rewarded by protecting their lives.

5.10 Civil Versus Religious Fears

The myth of Prometheus and the *Book of Job* refer to an essential theme in Hobbes' political system, namely, the role of myths, superstition and the fear of death. As already mentioned, the construction of Hobbes' social pact depends on keeping the fear of death as omnipresent. One of the problems of myths, superstition, and even of religion is that their roots extend deep enough to remove the fear of death and the instinct of self-preservation (Johnston 1986, p. 108). According to Johnston, Hobbes proposed that there are two types of individuals, those with poor education who are easily influenced by superstition and those rational citizens whose religious beliefs concur with those of the state. This creates a contrast between the rational and irrational, between science and superstition, and between fear of the laws and fear of imaginary spirits (Johnston 1986, p. 109).

The problem for the sovereign is that according to Hobbes, most of the world is populated by irrational people, in whom the fear of death is not strong enough to subdue their behaviour. Therefore, it is necessary for the preservation of the commonwealth that all superstitions such as the belief in supernatural creatures be eliminated. In other words, the creation of angels and saints will undermine the terrestrial fear of death by pointing to a power greater than that of the sovereign of

[26]This is conveyed in *Leviathan* (2.31.188): "And Job, how earnestly does he expostulate with God, for the many Afflictions he suffered, notwithstanding his Righteousnesse? This question in the case of Job, is decided by God himselfe, not by arguments derived from Job's Sinne, but his own Power." In the biblical story, the Leviathan is described as a powerful beast, "Nothing on earth is his equal—a creature without fear. He looks down on all that are haughty; he is king over all that are proud" (*Job* 41:1–34). Hobbes construed the Leviathan as a monster subdued by God's omniscient power and transformed the Leviathan into a powerful ruler not to be understood, but to be feared and obeyed.

the commonwealth.[27] As clearly rendered by Johnston (1986, p. 111), the fear of spirits as an expression of irrational myths and superstition (especially those of the Catholic Church) "destroys the ultimate basis of sovereign power…by virtue of his right to determine whether they [the citizens of the commonwealth] will live or die".[28] A religion that creates myths and superstitions, and fear for the afterlife, which is stronger than the terrestrial fear of death, provides a major challenge to the Leviathan. Peace under the ruler of the commonwealth will not be maintained if fear of death is replaced by fear of the irrational. If fear of death is removed, "the whole basis of sovereign power and civil peace is destroyed" (Johnston 1986, p. 121).

It is fully consistent that the philosopher who despised the "Morall Philosophers" of antiquity would construe the fear of death as a *necessary* emotion for achieving social peace. From alternative perspectives, Epicurus attacked both the fear of superstition and the fear of death in his quest for *ataraxia*, Seneca fought against the fear of death with all the philosophical remedies available to him (whether Epicurean, Cyrenaic or Stoic), and Montaigne's *Essays* provide a therapeutic narrative about his lifelong battle against the fear of death. But these philosophers were not Hobbes's main target. Since in his view their moral philosophy had been long ago been replaced by institutionalised religion, it is religion independent of the civic rulers that receives the brunt of Hobbes's attack. The main argument of the section in *Leviathan*, "Of a Christian Common-Wealth", is that the Bible prepares people for becoming obedient to God (and the *Book of Job* is a good illustration of this), but the second principal argument is to show that individual salvation occurs through obedience to the earthly sovereign.

[27]"…the Canonization of Saints, and declaring who are Martyrs…induce simple men into an obstinacy against the Laws and Commands of the Civill Sovereaigns even to death…" (*Leviathan* 2.47.383).

[28]"If this superstitious fear of Spirits were taken away, and with it Prognostiques and Dreams, false Prophecies, and many other things depending thereon, by which crafty ambitions persons abuse the simple people, men would be much more fitted that they are for civill Obedience" (*Leviathan* 1.2.7–8).

Johnston (1986, p. 140) suggests that Hobbes's reinterpretation of the Bible was based on his materialism and his mechanistic concept of the world.[29] Hobbes's adoption of materialism was in opposition to the more popular spiritualism, which accepted the reality of Angels and spirits as immaterial substances. Mintz asks (but does not answer) the important question: why did Hobbes reject spiritualism and adopt materialism at a time "when the notion of spirit as real held a firm grip on the mind of men"? (Mintz 1970, p. 66). I believe the answer to this question is found in the criticism to Hobbes's materialism by Bishop Bramhall, cited by Mintz, who considered that by denying spiritual entities Hobbes "taketh away God himself…And to say that an Angel or Spirit is an incorporeal substance, is to say in effect, that there is no Angel or Spirit at all" (Mintz 1970, p. 67). In other words, by denying the existence of Angels and Spirits, and even a veiled rejection of an immaterial God, Hobbes was simultaneously investing the sovereign of the commonwealth as the terrestrial God. Hobbes is thus removing a crucial problem for a subdued commonwealth, that is, disobedience to the terrestrial laws created by the possibility of an eternal heavenly life.

Surrendering the greater good of eternal life is for the religious majority far worse than giving up the lesser good of life on earth (Olsthoorn 2014, pp. 150–151). Once the possibility of torments in hell or the benefit of a heavenly life is averted, the citizens of the commonwealth will be more interested in life on earth, and the fear of death, as a pervasive emotion, can be manipulated. This is clearly articulated in *Leviathan* (2.38.238): "It is impossible a Common-wealth should stand, where any other than the Sovereign, hath a power of giving greater rewards than Life; and of inflicting greater punishments, than Death." The cause of 'religious fears' lies in people's credulity: "So easie are men to be drawn to believe anything, from such men as have gotten credit with them; and can with gentlenesse, and dexterity, take hold of their fear, and ignorance" (*Leviathan* 1.12.56). Hobbes not only rejects the

[29]Hobbes's materialism is thoroughly discussed in Mintz's *The Hunting of Leviathan* (Mintz 1970, p. 63). Materialism is the theory that everything that exists in the world is body, and entities considered immaterial such as space and time are attributes or "phantasms" of the mind, itself a material phenomenon constituted by physical motion.

irrationality of superstitious fears and miracles, angels and spirits, that are part of the common practice of Christianity, but also states that the only God to be obeyed is the Sovereign of the commonwealth.

In summary, Hobbes's materialism follows Epicurus' efforts to explain religion as originating from ignorance of the causes of natural phenomena. Hobbes rejected the institution of religion given that it has the potential to undermine the role of the sovereign as all powerful ruler of the commonwealth. On the other hand, the rejection of religious fears is tamed by the fact that religion also provides relief to anguish as well as an increased sense of safety (Ginzburg 2008, pp. 7–8; Vasalle 2010, pp. 27–29). In the Hobbesian social system, the sovereign has the role of a mortal god and has the final decision even about religious policy (*De Homine* 15.3). The sovereign exerts a tight control over religion by deciding on what constitutes a sin, how to interpret the Bible, and how to teach about the afterlife (Ahrensdorf 2000, pp. 580–583). With full control of secular and religious matters, the sovereign gains complete influence over the fears and anxieties of citizens.

5.11 Conclusion: Hobbes's Therapy of Fear

Why discuss Hobbes, a political philosopher, in a thesis whose main focus is to provide a philosophical analysis of fear from a therapeutic perspective? The answer is quite simple. Humans live in social systems which greatly shape their aspirations, goals, and emotions (see Chapter 9 for a discussion of the social construction of fear). Fear is not felt in a vacuum, but in the context of a complex pattern of life, produced by multiple causes, and expressed in a myriad of ways.[30] The relevance of *Leviathan* is that this is among the first philosophical texts to provide a systematic argument concerning the crucial role of fear in

[30]Blits (1989, p. 417) considers that "more than any philosopher, Thomas Hobbes emphasises the determining power of fear," as it is "both the sole origin of civil society…and the only reliable means of its preservation."

shaping human social life, and how political and religious systems are designed to manipulate this emotion.

By way of contrast, the philosophers I have so far discussed, namely Epicurus, Cicero, Seneca and Montaigne have a personal, individualised, approach to fear. Epicurus lives in the Garden in the outskirts of Athens, Cicero wrote the *Tusculans* in his villa while having philosophical discussions with friends, Seneca wrote his *Letters* as an epistolary exchange with a dear friend, and Montaigne composed the *Essays* while isolated in his chateau. In humans, fear is primarily a social emotion strongly dependent on the socio-political context. It is because of the fear and anxieties that usually accompany a political life that Epicurus proposed his *lathe biosas*; Cicero considers the distress of a political life as one of the most damaging emotions; Seneca has to provide repeated therapeutic advice to Lucilius about retiring to avoid political misfortunes; and Montaigne, after being elected on two occasions as Mayor of Bordeaux, mostly wanted to "glide rather lightly over the surface of this world" (*Essays* C.3.10.1135). The reductionist conception of fear as expressed in Hobbes's laws of nature provides a stark contrast, a mere deterrent for a civil war based on allaying the fear of a violent death. Hobbes teaches how to fight vainglory with sword and fear, whereas Montaigne teaches how not to be vainglorious without the need of violent methods, in a truly humanistic way. Hobbes is not interested in discussing his own fears as Montaigne does, but in how fear, anxiety and terror create a modern absolutist political system, and how fear may be used politically to force obedience to the sovereign.[31] Hobbes reduces human life to a state of chronic fear and anxiety to avoid a violent death.

Hobbes's work is significant and insightful for the way it shows up the role of fear in social life and how fear can be manipulated to shore

[31]Guinzburg claims that this form of manipulation is rife in contemporary states: "We live in a world where states threaten terror, spread terror, are sometimes the target of terror. A world inhabited by those who try to steal the venerable, powerful weapons of religion, as well as by those who use religion as a weapon. A world in which huge Leviathans either move frantically or squat waiting. A world not too different from the one Hobbes imagined and dissected" (Ginzburg 2008, p. 14).

up power (insights that many cotemporary rulers seem to use to their advantage). On the other hand, Hobbes's remedy leaves much to be desired, since it basically consists on a strong state able to reduce anxiety to 'tolerable' levels, a society in which both life and death occur in a rather predictable way, and in which the 'horizon of expectations' is stabilised by fear. As a tool for social control, fear is applied in 'appropriate' doses under a system of rewards and punishments. In his Manichean approach to human life, Hobbes considers that tranquillity of mind is best provided by living in the relative peace of complete submission to the Leviathan. The price to be paid for living under this watchful monster, however, is chronic anxiety about being punished for transgressing its laws, a subtle but pervasive fear that has the potential to gnaw at human souls' day and night. The Hellenistic high values of *ataraxia* and *apatheia* have no place in Hobbes's absolutist system, and the therapies of Montaigne, as humane antidotes against fear, are ignored in the quest for building a strong social structure based on fear and terror.

References

Aeschylus. (1961). *Prometheus bound and other plays* (P. Vellacott, Trans.). London: Penguin Classics.

Ahrensdorf, P. J. (2000). The fear of death and the longing for immortality: Hobbes and Thucydides on human nature and the problem of anarchy. *American Political Science Review, 94*(3), 579–593.

Bagby, L. M. J. (2009). *Thomas Hobbes: Turning point for honor*. Lanham: Lexington Books.

Blits, J. H. (1989). Hobbesian fear. *Political Theory, 17*(3), 417–431.

Bodei, R. (1995). *Geometría de las Pasiones, Miedo, Esperanza, Felicidad: Filosofía y uso Político*. México: Fondo de Cultura Económica.

Cooper, J. E. (2010). Vainglory, modesty, and political agency in the political theory of Thomas Hobbes. *The Review of Politics, 72*, 241–269.

Ginzburg, C. (2008). *Fear, reverence, terror: Reading Hobbes today*. San Domenico di Fiesole: European University Institute.

Gold, R., & Pearce, J. (2015). *Ferox* or *Fortis*: Montaigne, Hobbes, and the perils of paradiastole. *Philosophy and Rhetoric, 48*(2), 186–210.

Harrison, R. (2003). *Hobbes, Locke, and confusion's masterpiece: An examination of seventeenth-century political philosophy*. Cambridge: Cambridge University Press.

Hobbes, T. (1889). *The elements of law natural and politic* (F. Tönnies, Ed.). London: Elibron Classics.

Hobbes, T. (1972). *Man and citizen (Thomas Hobbes's De Homine and De Cive)* (B. Gert, Ed.). New York: Humanities Press.

Hobbes, T. (1994). *Human nature and De Corpore Politico* (J. C. A. Gaskin, Ed.). Oxford: Oxford University Press.

Hobbes, T. (1996). *Leviathan* (J. C. A. Gaskin, Ed.). Oxford: Oxford University Press.

Johnston, D. (1986). *The rhetoric of Leviathan: Thomas Hobbes and the politics of cultural transformation*. Princeton: Princeton University Press.

Kavka, G. S. (1986). *Hobbesian moral and political theory*. Princeton: Princeton University Press.

Martinich, A. P. (1999). *Hobbes: A biography*. Cambridge: Cambridge University Press.

Merton, R. K. (1938). Technology and society in seveteenth century England. *Osiris, 4*, 360–632.

Michaelis, L. (2007). Hobbes's modern Prometheus: A political philosophy for an uncertain future. *Canadian Journal of Political Science, 40*(1), 101–127.

Mintz, S. I. (1970). *The hunting of Leviathan*. Cambridge: Cambridge University Press.

Mitchell, S. (1987). *The book of job* (S. Mitchell, Trans.). Pymble: HarperCollins Publishers.

Montaigne, M. (2003). *The complete essays* (M. A. Screech, Trans.). London: Penguin Books.

Newey, G. (2014). *The Routledge guidebook to Hobbes' Leviathan*. London: Routledge.

Olsthoorn, J. (2014). Worse than death: The non-preservationist foundations of Hobbes's moral philosophy. *Hobbes Studies, 27*, 148–170.

Pettit, P. (2008). *Made with words: Hobbes on language, mind, and politics*. Princeton: Princeton University Press.

Robin, C. (2004). *Fear: The history of a political idea*. Oxford: Oxford University Press.

Schochet, G. J. (1967). Thomas Hobbes on the family and the state of nature. *Political Science Quarterly, 82*(3), 427–445.

Springborg, P. (2007). *The Cambridge companion to Hobbes Leviathan*. Cambridge: Cambridge University Press.

Strauss, L. (1963). *The political philosophy of Hobbes: Its basis and its genesis* (E. Sinclair, Trans.). Chicago: The University of Chicago Press.
Vasalle, A. (2010). Prometheus bound: Curiosity and anxiety for the future time in Hobbes' Leviathan. *Humana-Mente, 12*, 23–42.
Zagorin, P. (2009). *Hobbes and the law of nature.* Princeton: Princeton University Press.

6

Descartes and the Mechanization of Fear

There is something surprising in misfortunes, even those that have been foreseen, of which I am mistress only after a certain time; my body becomes so strongly disordered that several months are necessary for me to restore it, and those months hardly pass without some new subject of trouble. Princess Elisabeth of Bohemia, "Letter to Rene Descartes", 22 June 1645.

(Descartes 2015; AT 4:233)[1]

The greatest souls of which I speak draw a satisfaction in themselves from all the things that happen to them, even the most annoying and insupportable… just as the greatest prosperity of fortune never intoxicates them or makes them insolent, so too the greatest adversities are unable to defeat them or render them so sad that the body, to which they are joined, becomes sick. Rene Descartes, "Letter to Princess Elizabeth of Bohemia", 18 May 1645.

(Descartes 2015; AT 4:200)

[1] I have used the recent translation by Michael Moriarty for the Oxford World's Classics edition (Descartes 2015). Numbering corresponds to the Adam and Tannery (AT) edition of *Oeuvres*.

S. Starkstein, *A Conceptual and Therapeutic Analysis of Fear*,
https://doi.org/10.1007/978-3-319-78349-9_6

6.1 Introduction

Seven decades after the publication of Montaigne's *Essays*, and following Hobbes's focus on the political importance of emotions there was a major shift in the conceptualization and philosophical treatment of emotions. The French philosopher Rene Descartes revolutionised the established concept of body-soul interaction and inaugurated a tradition of reductionism in the conception of emotions based on psychophysical theories that are still extant in the current neurosciences (Gross 2007). This change is evident in Descartes's last work *On the Passions of the Soul* (PS) (Descartes 2015), considered one of the major works on the epistemology of emotions in philosophical history (James 1999).[2]

During the seventeenth century the philosophy of the passions was dominated by the Aristotelian scholasticism as revised by Aquinas (Hatfield 2007, p. 6). The soul was considered to consist of 'higher' faculties, such as the intellect and volition, controlling the 'lower' sensitive appetites, and moved by either 'irascible' passions (e.g. hope, despair, fear, courage, anger) or 'concupiscible' passions (e.g. love, hate, desire, aversion). In other words, external objects perceived by agents were assessed intellectually in terms of their value to the agent, which assessment may result in a passion.[3] Passions were therefore defined as responses of the appetites to perceptions judged intellectually to be good or evil (Dixon 2003, p. 54). The passions were not isolated from the body, but included in the sensitive soul as states of "the soul-body composite" (James 1999, p. 65). Descartes was among the first philosophers to break with this scholastic concept of the passions by proposing that the passions are produced by bodily movements, but are unable to directly move the body (Hatfield 2007, p. 11). This novel concept was based on Descartes's hypothesis that the soul and body are independent

[2]The seventeenth century was rich in treatises on theoretical aspects of emotions (Boros 2006, p. 125). The ideal of modernity was the mechanical science, which greatly influenced medicine and philosophy. The latter is evident in the works of Hobbes and Descartes (see Hatfield 2007, for a thoughtful discussion).

[3]In this chapter I use the term 'passion' rather than emotion given that Descartes uses 'emotion' in a technical way, different from passion.

ontological entities, rather than the soul being the form of a biological entity as in the Aristotelian tradition. The challenge for Descartes became how to explain the interaction between these ontologically different entities.

A second major departure from the Aristotelian tradition was Descartes's proposal of an undivided soul replacing the Aristotelian concept of a soul divided into nutritive, sensitive and intellectual parts. These are the philosophical bases of the Cartesian "revolutionary analysis of the activities of thinking" and a new conceptualization of the passions (James 1999, p. 90). The Cartesian 'revolution' also implied a major break from the humanist tradition of Erasmus, Petrarch and Montaigne, with roots in Cicero and Seneca, which considered the passions as disorders to be treated by the philosopher as 'physician of the soul'. Descartes's philosophy of the passions had a different aim, mostly focused on validating his dualistic[4] approach to soul and body functions using the passions as a heuristic tool. Descartes understood non-human animals as essentially mechanical objects, whereas humans were considered to be constituted by both a body, working like clockwork, and an incorporeal soul. The passions, produced by bodily movements on the soul, are therefore, uniquely human.

In this chapter I shall critically examine the new construct of the passions inaugurated by Descartes and its impact on the concept and treatment of fear. I shall also discuss how Descartes's treatment of the passions and fear in particular, fail on two grounds. First, his concept of the passions is flawed by conceptual limitations which extend beyond the well-known problems with dualism. Second, his therapy 'in action', specifically as it was delivered to Princess Elisabeth of Bohemia, was highly problematic. I shall discuss the therapeutic methods used by Descartes and the poor results of this intervention. This particular case is not merely anecdotal evidence against his view because Descartes' work, the *Passions of the Soul* published in 1649, is in great part the result of his interaction with Princess Elisabeth who was an acute critic

[4]That is, soul and body are conceived of as different substances: the former as *res cogitans* and the latter as *res extensa*.

of his epistemology of the passions. I will also contrast Descartes's mechanistic approach to fear with the Hellenistic and humanistic tradition discussed in Chapters 2, 3 and 4, and as a forerunner of the conceptualization of fear in biophysical terms.

6.2 The Passions of the Soul: Text and Context

As in the case of his near contemporaries, Montaigne (1533–1592) and Hobbes (1588–1679), events in the life of Descartes (1596–1650) had a strong influence upon his theory of the passions. His main work on the passions, *The Passions of the Soul*, was written at the request of Elisabeth, Princess of Bohemia (1618–1680), with whom Descartes had frequent correspondence. His letters to Princess Elizabeth include important material for understanding his conception of the passions, and how this was put into practice. Additionally, they also provide relevant information on Descartes as a 'therapist', since he was the main advisor to the Princess on how to manage her distress and anxiety.[5]

Princess Elisabeth was a precocious and gifted intellectual, with a strong interest in languages, theology, mathematics, philosophy, astronomy and physics (Gaukroger 2002, p. 385). On the other hand, she was not immune to the major upheavals that surrounded her life, and showed a personal proclivity to fear and distress. Elisabeth met Descartes when they were both living in the Low Countries, where she became very interested in Cartesian geometry and moral philosophy.[6] She corresponded with Descartes until his death, and they exchanged impressions about different subjects, including her emotional problems (mostly anguish and worry caused by political and personal misfortunes).

Descartes acted as Elisabeth's 'physician of the soul', suggesting different remedies for her emotional disturbances, including her distress

[5]See the important book by Genevieve Lloyd (2008) (which is discussed below) and an interesting analysis of Descartes as Elisabeth's physician in Shapiro (2011).

[6]In one of the first letters, Elisabeth asked Descartes to tell her "how the soul of a human being… can determine the bodily spirits and so bring about voluntary actions" (6 May 1643; AT 3.660).

and fears, but as we shall see, with unclear success. In a letter dated 10 June 1643 (AT 3:683) Elisabeth complained about how impossible it was for her to develop the habit of meditation based on Descartes's technique as described in his *Meditations* (Descartes 1984). In the Introduction to this text Descartes suggests meditating on the subject at hand by withdrawing oneself from sensory stimulation and prior opinions. Two years later,[7] Descartes explained to Elisabeth, who was suffering fever and exhaustion, that the main cause of her ailment was sadness provoked by major family setbacks. He suggested the remedy of bringing "contentment in your soul," stressing he was not "one of those cruel philosophers" (a clear reference to the Stoics), for whom all passions should be eradicated. However, Descartes considered it typical of "vulgar souls" to surrender to the passions. In contrast, the virtuous soul may initially suffer passions, but it will in the end master them using reason. Furthermore, virtuous people "steel themselves" to patiently bear bodily pain, and may even feel pleasure from having their courage tested. These are virtuous people who never show despair or depression even among the "greatest misfortunes". Elisabeth tacitly accepted the Cartesian soul/body division, also stating that her body was imbued "with the weakness of my sex" (24 May 1645; AT 4:207). She struggled to control her anxiety and distress, as manifested by continuous worrying and somatic symptoms of anxiety. Elisabeth begged Descartes for a remedy that would cure "my body along with my soul." Eventually, this 'remedy' came in the shape of a treatise on the passions, the last work Descartes wrote in his life.

Descartes suggested to Princess Elisabeth that the best way to allay distress is to "turn [the] imagination" aside from the current problem and to forget about it unless "compelled by practical necessity". This old Epicurean technique of distraction was further emphasised by Descartes's suggestion to think only "about what could bring…contentment and joy" given that this habit would allow the person to judge life events "without passion". He advised the Princess to get rid of sad thoughts by using reason only, and to avoid "serious meditation on

[7]Letter dated 18 May 1645 (AT 4:200).

intellectual matters." Instead, Descartes suggested that she should "gaze at the green of a wood, the colours of a flower, the flight of a bird, and such things as require no attention…thinking of nothing" (May or June 1645; AT 4:218).

Elisabeth was apparently pleased with this advice, initially finding in it an "antidote for my melancholy" (Letter 22 June 1645; AT 4:233). On the other hand, she was unable to follow the Cartesian "precepts" of vanquishing passions by the use of reason (see below), and the technique of distraction eventually failed.[8] She could not separate her bodily symptoms from "the idea of a particular matter". The technique of premeditation (see Chapter 3) suggested by Descartes also failed to produce improvements. Even when able to foresee forthcoming misfortunes, Elisabeth was emotionally impacted by the effect of "surprise", and only the passage of time soothed her despair. She conceded that she was not getting better, as she was unable to be as rational as Descartes (Letter 22 June 1645; AT 4:233). As astutely stated by Nye (1999, p. 47) "The context of Elisabeth's virtue is life in time, life in history, a life from which Descartes has removed himself".

Descartes acknowledged that some passions cannot be avoided (Letter June 1645; AT 4:236),[9] but suggested that a good sleep can restore "calm to our minds" and insisted that Elisabeth pursue the venerable exercise of diversion with more energy.[10] A month later (Letter 21 July 1645; AT 4:251) Elisabeth was still ailing with fear and distress. Any letter received was a cause for anxiety, with great fear that it might contain "distressing news" (AT 4:251). Descartes suggested that

[8]"The slightest period of inactivity causes [my mind] to fall back on the reasons it has to feel distressed, and I am afraid that, if I do not keep it active while taking the Spa water, it will become more melancholy" (Letter 22 June 1645; AT 4:233). Elisabeth is speaking about her soul in the third person, as an entity she is unable to govern.

[9]"I know well that it is virtually impossible to withstand the initial turmoil that new misfortunes bring about in us, and indeed that it is normally the finest minds that have the most violent passions."

[10]"This is done by concentrating on all the benefits we may derive from the thing that the day before we were treating as a great misfortune, and by diverting our minds from the evils we had imagined in it".

responding with anxiety upon receiving bad news had become for her a habit.

Descartes also suggested a therapy he would strongly reject a few years later, advising the Princess to read the ancient philosophers as a useful strategy against her distress. More specifically, he recommended that she read Seneca's *On the Happy Life*, in which the Stoic philosopher explains that the pursuit of virtue through reason is the main path to happiness (AT 4:251).[11] Elisabeth found Seneca's book full of "fine sentences and maxims" on which to meditate, but in Cartesian fashion, she found the Stoic philosopher "without any method" in writing his ideas (Letter 16 August 1645; AT 2:268). Furthermore, she did not benefit from the Stoic approach of detachment from emotions. According to Descartes, Seneca should have discussed "the principal truths" for the practice of a virtuous life, regulating but not rejecting the passions (4 August 1645; AT 4:263). Thus, after the failure of the Stoic literature strategy, Descartes insisted on using his "three rules of ethics" as described in the *Discourse on the Method* (Descartes 1991) (Letter 4 August 1645; AT 4:263). These precepts consist in first, using reason in every situation and taking care in making sound judgments; second, avoiding "being led astray" by the passions, given that virtue consists of staying firm on consistent resolutions to do what is rational; and third, being contented with one's life, getting used to have fewer desires, and doing only what is in one's power.[12]

Elisabeth disagreed that happiness does not require anything beyond our control, as poor health clearly impacts the capacity to enjoy life (Letter 16 August 1645, AT 2:268). She implied that whereas the philosophers could 'play' Stoicism to their advantage, this was not available to the unsophisticated life "of a ruler, a commander, or courtier."

[11]"One of these means, and among the most useful, it seems to me, is to examine the writings of the ancients on this subject, and to attempt to go beyond them by adding to their precepts; for in this way we can make their precepts fully our own, and prepare ourselves to put them into practice" (Letter 4 August 1645; AT 4:263).

[12]Nye (1999, p. 53) has rendered Descartes' maxims in an eloquent way: "Happiness is contentment, contentment comes from being virtuous, and virtue is nothing but a firm will to carry out whatever one understands is best as long as one has used one's reason to try to discover what is best."

As for the Cartesian rules of ethics, the Princess conceded that it is best to know the real value of things before making decisions,[13] but that this requires "perfect and infinite knowledge" which is not available "when we live the active life."[14] Elisabeth pre-empted a response by Descartes that if a mishap happens when we have taken all possible precautions we should still be happy, by flatly saying "that [being happy] never happens, when things do not work out." She presented Descartes with a 'real life' dilemma about how to behave, when for instance, there is a danger and we have to decide on whether to save ourselves or others. Both behaviours could be equally defended as being rational, especially when the behaviour is innate. Furthermore, Elisabeth asked whether innate behaviours should be corrected, and if so, how. Finally, she was not convinced that passions are "disorders" of the soul, and challenged Descartes to justify his suggestion that all passions should be subject to reason. She demanded from Descartes a definition of the passions, since *she* was by then interested in pursuing the origin of her distress and wanted to better understand the mechanism of the passions.

In a letter dated 25 April 1646 (AT 4:403), Princess Elisabeth complained, again, about being unable to employ the Cartesian remedy of using reason to subdue her morbid passions. She was unable to manage her distress by using her will, and found no help in PS.[15] In a letter dated November 1646 Descartes advised Elisabeth (in a rather circular way) that to achieve happiness it is necessary to "avoid all passions associated with those things that may upset us." This was the last epistolary exchange about Elisabeth's emotional problems. She might have felt frustrated by Descartes's insistence in using reason to fight

[13]"It is true that a habit of valuing goods in proportion to their capacity to contribute to our contentment, of measuring this contentment by the perfections that give rise to pleasures, and of judging these perfections and pleasures dispassionately will protect them from many mistakes" (Letter 16 August 1645; AT 2:268).

[14]Elisabeth (perhaps ironically) refers to living the life of a human engaged in court and household matters, with all its contingent problems, unlike the protected and semi-secluded life of a philosopher.

[15]"For how can we foresee all the accidents that can occur in life, when they are impossible to count? And how can we help ardently desiring things that necessarily tend to our preservation as human beings (such as health and the means of life) which, nonetheless, do not depend on our will?" (25 April 1646; AT 4:403).

her emotional suffering, and the use of reason to subdue the passions remained one of the main themes in the last section of PS.

In conclusion, the epistolary exchange between Princess Elisabeth and Descartes is essential to understanding the origins of PS as well as understanding Descartes's philosophical therapy. Lloyd and Nye have both provided thoughtful analyses of this exchange, with emphasis on the different therapies Descartes recommended to Elisabeth. Nye stresses the 'asymmetry' between the philosopher and the Princess, with Descartes always trying to impress his 'patient' (Nye 1999, p. 47). Lloyd points out that Descartes never acknowledged his failure to improve Elisabeth's distress and anxieties, and rather than question his therapeutic advice, he maintained his basic concepts, writing a book on the passions (Lloyd 2008, pp. 170–177).

6.3 The Relevance of the Passions of the Soul

As discussed above, the seed for Descartes's theory of the passions is found in the epistolary exchange with Elizabeth. In the very important letter dated 6 October 1645 (AT 4:304) Descartes proposed the rudiments of a mechanism of the passions, which he later developed into Part One of *The Passions of the Soul.* Descartes suggests that impressions in the brain are formed by external or internal sensory stimuli, memory traces, "the agitation of the spirits coming from the heart",[16] or the agent's behaviour. Descartes defined "passion" as a thought produced by the agitation of the spirits in the soul.[17] Passions are not 'simple'

[16]The most comprehensive definition of "spirits" is provided in PS10: "For what I call 'spirits' here are only bodies, and their only properties are that they are very small and fast-moving…As a result they are never stationary, but while some are flowing into the cavities of the brain, others are simultaneously flowing out through the pores of the substance of that organ. Through the pores they are conveyed into the nerves, and thence into the muscles, by means of which process they move the body in all the various ways it can be moved".

[17]Hassing (2015, p. 6) suggests that Descartes used the term "thought" in both a narrow and a broad sense. In a narrow sense a thought is a clear and distinct cognition or volition, whereas in the wide sense, thoughts are "obscure and confused" objects such as sense-perceptions, internal (bodily) sensations (e.g. pain), appetites (e.g. thirst), memories, imaginations, judgments and passions.

sensations (i.e. thoughts produced by any external or internal stimuli), but are produced "by a particular agitation of the spirits." Descartes distinguished between passions "at random" from the passions produced in relation to a person's "temperament", which he illustrated with the example of inhabitants of a city who are told that the enemy is approaching. Descartes considered the "initial judgment about the evil that may befall them, as resulting from an action of their soul, not a passion." Suffering a passion (e.g. feeling fear), on the other hand, depends on habit, as not all people are "equally disturbed by it [the approaching enemy] emotionally." Furthermore, Descartes suggested that the production of passions is triggered by a judgment (e.g. the city will be destroyed), or by imagining the consequences of the event (e.g. producing brain "images" of slaughter and destruction).[18]

Descartes finished with a brief explanation of the mechanism of the bodily manifestations of fear: "spirits" flow from the nerves to the muscles and heart, producing the somatic changes of fear (e.g. paleness), whereas further agitation of the spirits produces images in the brain that result in the passion of fear in the soul. Elisabeth was impressed by this explanation but asked Descartes for clarifications on the manner in which the agitation of the spirits in the body produces passions in the soul (Letter 28 October 1645; AT 4:320). This was not explained in Descartes's response (Letter 3 November 1645; AT 4:330).

Several months later (Letter 25 April 1646; AT 4:403) Elisabeth, who by then had a copy of PS, insisted on a clearer explanation of the mechanism of the passions. Her main objection was about the mechanism by which the spirits produce "the five basic passions"[19] given that passions are rarely 'pure' (e.g. hatred may be accompanied by anger) and also depend on the person's temperament. Moreover, Elisabeth also wanted to know how passions can be distinguished from their physiological causes, and more importantly, given Descartes's mechanistic explanation

[18]In other words, judgment and imagination are sufficient to produce passions, but passions do not consist in judgments or imaginations.

[19]There are six basic passions listed in PS: wonder, hate, love, desire, joy and sadness. Interestingly, fear does not appear in this list.

of the passions, how remedies can be effective in the context of a life that is both contingent and unpredictable (Brown 2006, p. 23).

While answers to these relevant questions are not to be found in PS, this important work marks the beginning of psychophysical reductionism, that is, the explanation of psychological phenomena as being produced solely by specific physiological mechanisms. For a fully reductionist account passions are understood as nothing but physiological events. PS provides a step in this direction due to its novel method of understanding the passions as able to be analysed in terms of their putative biophysical components.[20] The humanistic treatment of fear is not only ignored by the new Cartesian philosophy, strongly rooted in the new science of Galileo and Harvey, but even treated with scorn. "I will treat the passions as a physicist" stated Descartes at the beginning of the treatise in order to separate his philosophy from the humanist and Aristotelian tradition. The break with Hellenistic philosophy is explicit in his remark that "there is nothing in which the shortcomings of the sciences we have inherited from the Ancients more clearly appear than in the writings on the passions" (PS 1).[21] I will now discuss the novelty of the Cartesian proposal for the mechanism of the passions.

6.4 Descartes's Philosophy of the Passions

Descartes was heavily influenced by the discovery of the system of the circulation of the blood by William Harvey in 1628 (less than 20 years before the publication of PS) (Harvey 1628). Descartes was impressed by Harvey's description of a circulatory system for nourishing the body, and he designed a mechanism for the passions that paralleled Harvey's. Thus, Descartes's system also has the heart as a central organ, providing 'nourishment' for the soul based on the circulation of "animal spirits".

[20] The reduction of psychological phenomena to physics is well rendered by Thomas Nagel (2012). Reductionism of emotions does not start with Descartes (Nagel 2012, p. 4), but his texts became extremely influential, and albeit with protestations (see Damasio, Chapter 7) still constitute the main framework for their analysis.

[21] Remarks are cited as originally numbered in PS.

But before examining Descartes's mechanism of the passions in more detail, several conceptual clarifications are in place.

6.4.1 Descartes's Definition of the Passions

As previously mentioned, in the letters to Princess Elizabeth Descartes defines 'passion' as a thought produced in the soul by the agitation of bodily spirits. He provides a more elaborated definition in PS, where he states that the passions of the soul are "perceptions, sensations, or emotions" caused, maintained and fortified by the movement of the spirits (PS 7). A 'passion-perception' is any thought that is not a volition (otherwise it would be an action rather than a passion), a 'passion-sensation' is a sensation "received in the soul", such as feeling hungry; and a 'passion-emotion' is a thought that most strongly agitates the soul (James 1999, p. 94). As already noted, Descartes postulated wonderment, love, hatred, desire, joy and sadness as the six fundamental human passions (PS 53–57). He considered wonderment as the principal passion, produced by being exposed to a novel object. The (secondary) passions of fear, hope, jealousy and complacency were grouped together, given that hope and fear are produced "by a desire that is more or less likely to occur" (PS 58).[22] Both jealousy and complacency were considered different types of fear. On the other hand, terror has an unclear position in Descartes's system of the passions. He considers terror as an excess of fear and astonishment, and not a true passion (PS 176). Nevertheless, he also considered terror to be an exception to his position that all the passions are beneficial, as it produces a paralysis of the body, which becomes "powerless to resist the evils it thinks are imminent" (PS 174–175). By this, Descartes implicitly admits terror as a type of passion.

Descartes famously stated that the soul "has its main seat in the little [pineal] gland", through which the soul "radiates" spirits, nerves and blood to the rest of the body (PS 34). He proposed that the sole function of the soul is to produce thoughts, which can be of two types:

[22]Descartes used the French *crainte* to design the initial affective apprehension of danger, whereas *peur* was used to denote a sudden urge to flee (Descartes 2015, p. 288).

actions which are always volitions[23]; or *passions*, which are "kinds of perception or knowledge" (PS 17) produced in the soul by representations of internal or external stimuli. Hassing (2015, p. 7) terms the basic principle of Cartesian dualism as "motion-thought," that is, motions in the pineal gland producing thoughts in the soul. This system replaces the Aristotelian hylomorphism, where form and matter are principles of a single substance not interacting with each other. The Cartesian "motion-thought" is an innate and relatively rigid system activated by stimuli producing a unique movement in the pineal gland, which causes a single passion in the soul. These constrained definitions and concepts require careful unpacking for a proper understanding of the Cartesian mechanism of the passions in general, and fear in particular, and this is provided below.

6.4.2 The Machinery of the Passions

Descartes begins PS by describing the elements that constitute the 'spiritual circulatory system'. The main components are the nerves ("little filaments or pipes" [PS 10]) coming from the brain which contain the "animal spirits", in turn a "highly subtle air" arising from the blood after being "rarefied" in the heart (PS 10). Like the blood in Harvey's circulatory system, the animal spirits are in constant motion, from the brain cavities to the rest of the body.[24] The core of the Cartesian system is the mechanism of perception, by which stimuli external (e.g. light) or internal (e.g. hunger) to the body push the spirits inside the nerves towards the brain. From this organ, the spirits move in two directions: towards the soul by moving the pineal gland,[25] or towards the muscles

[23]"Volition being the only or at least the principal action of the soul" (PS 13).

[24]Descartes used a rich metaphorical language, where the spirits are a "subtle air" coming from "rarefied" blood. The spirits are true matter, "very small and fast-moving" bodies (PS 10). Metaphors are frequently used in the PS to 'explain' physical phenomena linguistically in the absence of empirical information.

[25]Descartes decided on the pineal gland as the brain structure 'communicating' stimuli to the soul given that this is the only brain midline structure. The mechanism by which the pineal gland interacts with the soul remains unexplained, and this is one of the major objections that Elisabeth posed to Descartes's system of passions.

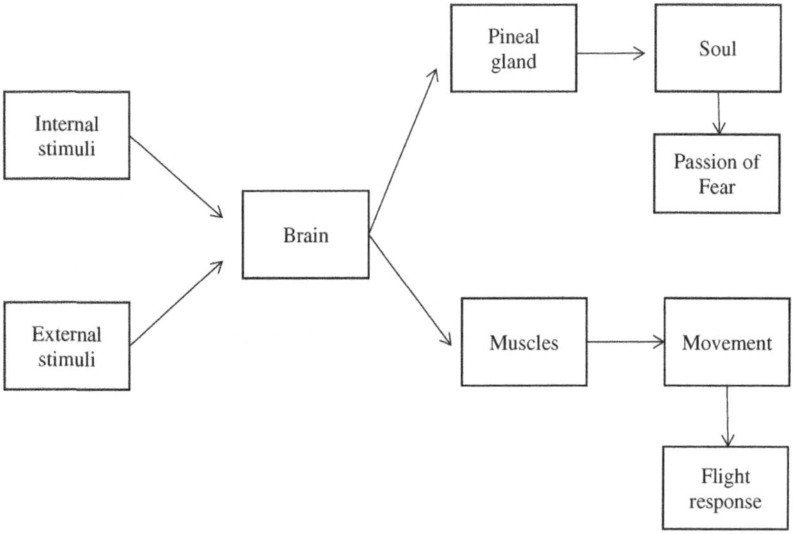

Fig. 6.1 Descartes's generic system of the passions (*Note* This diagram depicts Descartes's generic system for how the passion of fear arises in response to an external stimulus (e.g. a bear) or an internal stimulus (e.g. the idea of a future misfortune). The spirits transporting images produced in the brain by internal or external stimuli both move the pineal gland producing the passion of fear in the soul, and also flow to the muscles, generating a flight response)

of the limbs through efferent nerves. The soul 'perceives' through the movements of the pineal gland, and these movements are produced either by the nerves or by the outflow of spirits from the pores of the brain (see Fig. 6.1 for a schematic representation of this mechanism). The next question to be addressed is how this whole system works.

6.4.3 Descartes's Physiology of the Passions

Descartes suggests two mechanisms to produce the passions. The first, and simplest, is a 'reflex' mechanism in which a stimulus produces a motor response independent of the passion,[26] and the second, a

[26]Descartes considers sense-perception to be the most frequent stimulus producing passions. Other stimuli are thoughts produced by "bodily temperament" or by brain impressions (PS 51).

'complex' mechanism, in which the motor response results from a passion. Both mechanisms are described below, and the implications for Descartes's concept of fear will become clearer.

The 'reflex' mechanism is discussed in Article 38 of PS entitled "*An example of the movement of the body that accompany the passions and do not depend on the soul*". The system is activated by the sudden perception of an object (an animal in Descartes's example),[27] which imprints an image in the pineal gland. The perception of a frightful stimulus activates the legs for a flight response; and this motor act produces a movement of the spirits, and consequently of the pineal gland, "by means of which the soul feels and perceives this flight" (PS 38; see Fig. 6.2 for a schematic representation of the reflex model).[28] The example provided by Descartes is the response of closing our eyelids when a fist, even the fist of a friend, is suddenly aimed at our face. The soul is not involved in the motor response, as this reflex action cannot be inhibited by the will.

What requires clarification now is how the simple movements of the pineal gland are able to produce all the different passions, a query raised by Princess Elisabeth. The response to this question is provided, rather confusingly, in Article 51, where Descartes describes the "ultimate causes of the passions," which occur when the soul 'thinks' about a specific object (for instance, a frightening bear), as influenced by "bodily temperament"[29] (a typical innate way of responding with a specific passion), by "random impressions in the brain" such as feeling sad or happy for no apparent reason,[30] but primarily, by the attributes of the objects "moving the senses."[31]

[27]Passions are only produced by specific representations (e.g. seeing a piece of paper only produces a visual representation *simpliciter*), whereas reading what is written in that piece of paper (e.g. a love letter) produces both a perception and a passion.

[28]A more complex schematic representation of Descartes's machinery of the passions is presented by Hatfield (2007, pp. 23–25).

[29]This is a remnant in the Cartesian system of the passions of the Galenic humoral theory. Based on this theory, the individual's humours influence the type of passion that results from the movement of the pineal gland.

[30]In this case, it is the mood of the individual that influences the production of a passion. For instance, an individual with a fearful brain 'imprint' will tend to produce the passion of fear.

[31]This is a tautological statement, where a frightening image will produce the passion of fear in the soul. But the key question is: what makes the image 'frightening'? This relevant conceptual problem is discussed below.

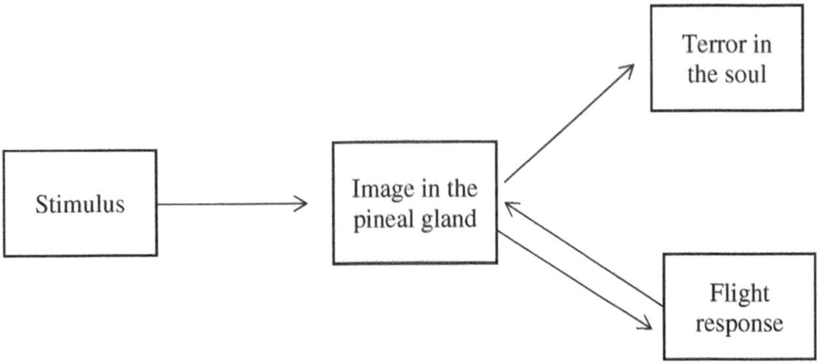

Fig. 6.2 Descartes's 'reflex' mechanism of the passions (*Note* This scheme depicts the mechanism by which a response to fear is enacted before feeling the passion of terror. In this schema, a given stimulus (usually external) prints an image of the fearful object in the pineal gland. This action moves the gland, and simultaneously a flux of spirits is generated towards the muscles for a flight response. In turn, these bodily movements generate a flux of spirits which move the pineal gland, generating the passion of terror in the soul)

6.4.4 The Purpose of the Passions

Descartes considered the principal function of the passions to be "to dispose the soul to will those things that…are [naturally] useful to us" (PS 52); in the same way, the animal spirits move the body towards a desired goal. An example may help to clarify this rather cryptic statement. The sense-perception of a bear may produce fear in the soul as the first passion. Depending on the individual's "physical temperament", "strength of mind," and previous outcomes in similar situations, the movement of the pineal gland may generate either of the two opposite passions: boldness or terror. For instance, an individual with a fearful temperament who has a history of bad outcomes develops a disposition to being fearful. In this case, the image of a dangerous object flows through a brain 'primed' by previous negative experiences, which innervates the muscles for a flight response. The heart is also stimulated to produce more animal spirits that flow to the brain to sustain and augment the passion of fear (this is the 'complex' mechanism illustrated in Fig. 6.3). To the question, why is it that some people feel boldness and others terror, Descartes simply responds that since "our brains are not all disposed in the same way" (PS 39), the same movement of the pineal gland produces different passions in different people. It is important to note that the passions are unable to directly produce or arrest bodily movements, but they are able to "incite and dispose" the soul "to will" the acts for which the body has been prepared by the spirits.

Thus, for instance, "the sensation of terror encourages it [i.e. the body] to flee" (PS 40). Once the soul "wills" an action, animal spirits move the pineal gland to enact the behaviour. Another indirect way of producing an action is to "consider the reasons, objects or examples" and "represent" the elements usually associated with the passion "we want to have" (PS 45). For instance, to switch from terror to boldness, it is not sufficient to will to do so, but we need to reason "and persuade [ourselves] that the danger is not all that great…that we can look forward to the glory and joy of victory" (PS 45).

6.5 Conflicts Between Soul and Body

Since they are ontologically independent, and both have the capacity to generate behaviours, soul and body can potentially generate opposite actions. In PS 47 Descartes depicts a scenario in which the soul by means of the will, and the body by means of the animal spirits, want to move the pineal gland in opposite directions. In Descartes's system, the animal spirits can only move the pineal gland in two directions. The first movement is produced by external sense-perceptions or by internal brain "impressions" which "exert no pressure in the will" and is therefore independent of the soul (PS 47). The second type of movement produces passions in the soul and exerts "some pressure" on the will (PS 47). Only the second type of movement can generate a conflict between passions and volitions. For instance, seeing a bear produces a movement of the pineal gland that generates fear in the soul and a flight response. To oppose this behaviour, a flux of spirits is generated by 'virtuous' volitions in the soul, which moves the pineal gland in the contrary direction and generates the passion of courage and a fight response (Fig. 6.3).

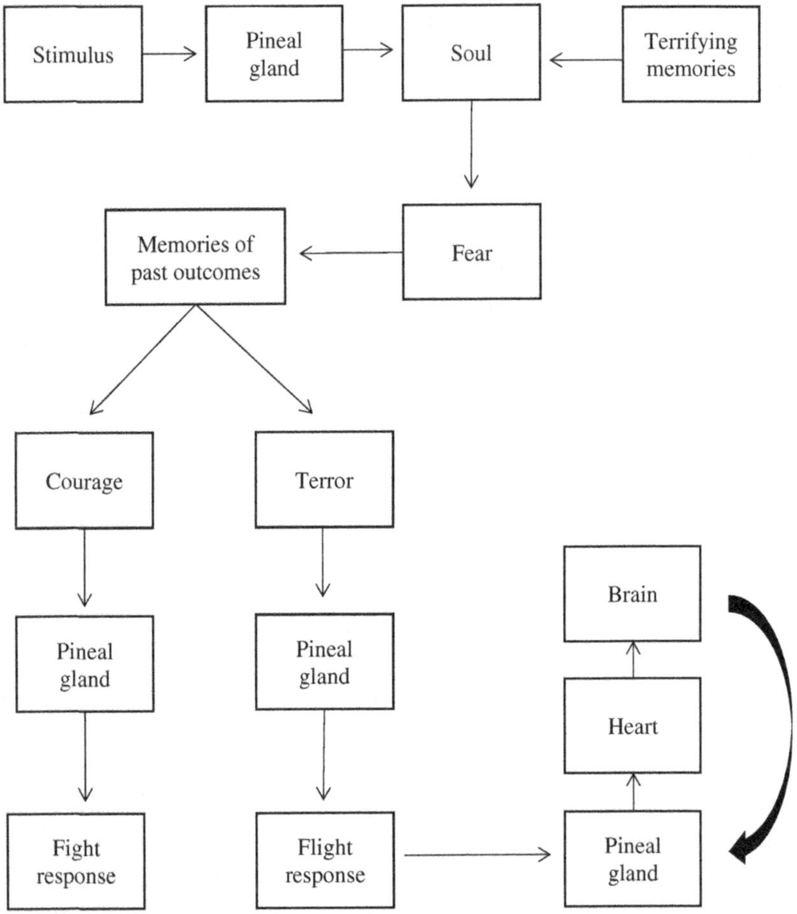

Fig. 6.3 Descartes's 'complex' mechanism of the passions (*Note* This scheme depicts Descartes's 'complex' mechanism of the passions. Fear is generated in the soul based on external stimuli or memories of fearful events. The passion of fear thus generated interacts with memories of past outcomes (good or bad), which, together with the individual's personality, result in the behaviours of courage (fight response) or terror (flight response). The behavioural response is sustained by a loop involving the heart, which sends additional spirits to the brain to that effect)

At this point it is important to remember that Descartes considered that volitions cannot act directly on the passions but only indirectly, by moving the pineal gland and generating antagonistic behaviours.

Thus, in the case of fear, this passion generated in the soul moves the pineal gland to generate a flight response, whereas the contrary movements produced by the will may move the pineal gland to produce a fight response. These series of pulls and pushes make the soul "almost simultaneously, to desire and not to desire one and the same thing" (PS 47).

A second type of conflict occurs, when for example, a dangerous object produces terror in the soul while simultaneously the animal spirits activate a flight response without "the contribution" of the soul. The soul, which first produced the passion of terror, on perceiving a bodily movement of flight may will the individual to act courageously, thus stopping the flight response (PS 47). In this conflict between the soul and the body those with the strongest soul will be the ablest to control their bodily passions. According to Descartes the strongest souls are furnished with "firm and definite judgments concerning the difference between good and evil" (PS 48), while the weakest souls are "swept away by the passions of the moment, which…reduce the soul to the most deplorable possible state" (PS 48). But having a strong soul is not sufficient to produce virtuous behaviour, since "knowledge of the truth" is required to guide behaviour (PS 49).

This is, in general terms, the rather convoluted and at times confusing Cartesian system of the passions. As stated by Hassing (2015, p. 55), "we begin to wonder if there is anything of our experience and behaviour for which Descartes could not make up a story in terms of pineal gland, animal spirits, thought-motion association, etc." Descartes' system of the passions seems to be infallible in being able to account for any contingency, but important conceptual knots in the system require specific discussion.

6.6 Conceptual Problems with Descartes's Mechanism of the Passions

Descartes's proposal of a physiological ('hydraulic') mechanism for the passions has historical interest only and is irrelevant to discussions of his philosophical concept of the passions. Dualism has been debated as a plausible explanation for the mechanism of emotions well into the twentieth century (Popper and Eccles 1977), and is still a subject of debate in philosophy of mind. However, again, this is of no central relevance to this chapter, whose main aim is to discuss the philosophical concepts of fear and the therapeutic suggestions gleaned from such concepts. Cartesian dualism is certainly alive in contemporary neuroscience as I shall discuss in the next chapters.

One of the main conceptual problems with Descartes's apparatus of the passions is present in both the 'reflex' and 'complex' mechanisms described above. Briefly, Descartes suggests that fear is produced by two mechanisms depending on whether the soul is involved. The 'reflex' mechanism starts with the image of the dangerous object being associated with memories of similar events in the brain cavities, followed by the animal spirits flowing to the lower limbs to activate a flight response. This seemingly simple explanation includes several unsupported assumptions. The first question is what makes a particular image (e.g. of a bear) "very strange and very terrifying" (PS 36). Descartes's simple answer is that fear is produced by the "close affinity" between the external image and memories of harmful events located in the brain cavities. Provided that images can be stored in the brain (a contentious topic discussed in the next chapter), we are still left with the problem of comparing images.

Assuming that there is a brain structure capable of bringing memory images to the fore, these have to be compared with the image produced by sense-perception which requires a 'comparator' capable of judging similarities between the images. Such a judgment has to be validated against definite criteria, which can only be provided by a comparator having its own memory system, thus falling into a regress. The second problem is that Descartes did not define the meaning of "affinity." If the meaning in the case of fear is the dangerousness of the object, the problem is how a value judgment is extracted from an image. In other words, what makes the image of a bear "dangerous"? Is the image of a bear always dangerous, even when it is printed in a picture book, or when the image is of a bear in a zoo? Brown (2006, p. 46) has suggested a mechanism where "the danger of the wolf" is "transmitted" to the soul in terms of its physical attributes (e.g. colour and shape) without the need of a special "apprehension" of danger. But this is different from Descartes's proposal, which combines the image with a value judgment based on a putative affinity with memory images. More importantly, it does not explain how fear is produced based on physical qualities alone.

Another significant problem stressed by Susan James (1999, p. 105) is the lack of consideration of contextual factors in Descartes's account. After all, the fearfulness of an object is not an intrinsic quality, but depends on several factors external to the object, such as the state of the agent (e.g. being sick or in good health), the place in which the encounter occurs, whether the agent is alone or in the company of individuals who can provide protection, and the experience of previous encounters.

Two further problems were brought up by Princess Elisabeth. Descartes's proposal is that fear in the soul is produced by a specific movement of the pineal gland but this interaction between the soul as *res cogitans* and the pineal gland as *res extensa* (the soul is affected by the body and produces somatic responses through the movements of the gland only) was incomprehensible to Elisabeth and one of her main criticisms of Descartes's system—an early version of the classic attack against his dualism. In addition to this infamous ontological problem, Elizabeth also drew attention to the fact that passions are complex constructs and commonly occur in combination. Thus, it may be difficult to discriminate envy from ambition, or apprehension from fear.[32]

The production of "volitions" is also an important conceptual knot requiring clarification. According to Descartes passions do not directly produce actions, but rather "incite and dispose the soul to will the acts…so that the sensation of terror encourages it [the soul] to wish to flee" (PS 40). Acts are produced by volitions of the soul, but how these volitions are generated is unclear. Descartes states that volitions are produced by the will, which is endowed with "its own weapons", basically the capacity to make value-judgements about what is good and what is evil (PS 48). The Cartesian (free) will also has several psychological

[32]PS 166 provides other examples: "when hope is…strong…it becomes complacency or confidence," and "when fear is so extreme that it leaves no room at all for hope…it is transformed in despair."

attributes such as being weak or strong, making good or bad decisions, being susceptible to being pulled or pushed by the passions, or on the contrary, being capable of resisting the "pressure" of some passions. But these attributes of the will rely simply upon metaphors that cover for a lack of a proper explanation about how the passions generate specific cognitions and actions. For example, the passion of fear 'produces' a given behaviour (for instance, a flight response), although the will may react to this response by 'producing' courageous behaviour instead (PS 47). Similar problems are found in current critical literature on PS. Thus Brown (2006, p. 22) suggests that the passions are able to bring specific sensations "to the foreground of the mind's attention," holding them in working memory for the soul to make a rational decision. Brown is proposing a 'Cartesian theatre' where the passions can somehow set up images to be attended to and worked out by the soul. This goes back to the Aristotelian model of the mind (the soul having a *vis estimativa*) which Descartes wished to reject with his proposal of a unitary soul, both sensitive and rational (PS 47, 68). However, images can be ambiguous: the image of a physician, for example, could equally represent a feared sickness or the person who will protect against an illness. It might well be asked whether a hypochondriac with the image of a physician, conjures up a representation of health or death?

Another conceptual problem is that behaviour and passion are not independent entities. Behaving in a fearful way is an essential part of the concept of fear and not just a post-effect of the passion. If someone says he is in terror but continues calmly playing cards with his partner, his statement will be understood as a joke or as irrational. If a child says he is scared but keeps playing in the sandpit, we would conclude he has not yet mastered the concept of being scared and is using the word incorrectly. On occasions, fear is manifested in a specific behaviour, without the agent being conscious of being afraid. This is the case when on my usual drive to work I avoid driving through dangerous neighbourhoods, or when I always use the train rather than planes due to my fear of flying. Moreover, to go back to the previous point, it is unclear which images could 'represent' the above types of fear-related behaviours. These difficulties lead to another conceptual problem which is rarely discussed, that is, that Descartes treats fear in the narrow sense of an individual being exposed to a dangerous object.[33] The examples of fear provided in PS (e.g. suddenly being exposed to an animal) relate to only a minor proportion of human fears. Fear should not be reduced to a feeling produced by sudden dangerous events, as people also fear life events that cannot be represented in a concrete way, such as the ominous impact of an economic recession on their jobs, discovering a lump in the body and worrying about having a fatal disease, and becoming concerned about the probable exposure of one's adolescent children to alcohol and drugs.

In the Cartesian model of passions, as already noted, memory plays an important role both in the production of passions and in the selection of behavioural responses. According to Descartes, remembering depends on the soul's "wishes to remember" (PS 42), which move the pineal gland to send animal spirits to "different places of the brain" until those wishes find traces left by the object "we wish to remember" (PS 42). This is facilitated by the fact that the object to be remembered has produced repeated movements of the spirits, making the pores of the brain more susceptible to being reopened upon successive presentations of the same object. This habit assists the flow of spirits towards the pineal gland, "which represents the same objects to the soul, so that it realises that this is the thing it wanted to remember" (PS 40). It is obvious that this system is riddled with conceptual difficulties. I will briefly address the most prominent of them. Descartes's system bestows the animal spirits with the capacity to remember, since they flow "through the different corners of the brain" (PS 42) in search of the memory image. Thus, the spirits already have a concept or an image of what they are looking for as well as the capacity to compare images, which implies they have their own memory system.[34]

The conceptual objections to the Cartesian system of passions outlined above would be of historical relevance only if the concepts had

---

[33]As we shall see in subsequent chapters, the same reductionist concept of fear affects its treatment in current philosophy of mind and cognitive neuroscience.

[34]A similar problem lies with Descartes's statement that a specific movement of the pineal gland "represents the same object to the soul, so that it realizes that this is the thing it wanted to remember" (PS 42).

been discarded together with the hydraulic mechanism. However, as I shall discuss in the next chapter, similar conceptual flaws resurface in the work of William James, one of the most prominent philosophers and psychologists of the nineteenth century, as well as in recent trends in analysing human emotions in the growing field of the neurosciences.

6.7 The Cartesian Concept of Fear

Fear is not only excluded from the six principal passions proposed by Descartes, but it is not even discussed as an individual passion, unlike others that may have less impact on life, such as disdain (PS 163) or derision (PS 178). Furthermore, the concept of fear is not cohesively rendered in PS. For instance, in PS 36 Descartes uses fear to illustrate the automatic mechanism of passions (see Fig. 6.1). Fear is described as a specific behavioural (flight) response after seeing a "frightful" object, but also defined as a passion instituted by nature to dispose the soul to produce volitions for the safety of the body. In the example, fear is already implied in providing value to the object, and the question again arises as to how the perception is qualified as frightful. The response is provided in PS 37, where Descartes states that the "terrifying" attribute of an object is based on shared similarities with memories of "harmful" objects. In PS 38 Descartes simply describes fear as a flight reaction, but a more elaborated definition of fear is provided in PS 165, where fear is described as "a disposition of the soul, which persuades it that the thing [in this case, what is desired] that will not come to pass". This definition is provided as a counterpart to hope without description of an intervening mechanism. Part Three introduces "indecision" as a type of fear (PS 170), defined as the situation in which the soul is unable to decide between different courses of action. This state of uncertainty may be increased by the fear of making a bad decision. Descartes also provides definitions for some other passions related to fear. Thus, he defined "faint-heartedness" as a "lethargy" preventing the performance of a given action (PS 174). This passion is transformed into "terror or horror" when mixed with the passions of astonishment and fear (PS 176). Given the limited attention that Descartes gives to the passion of fear, it should not be surprising that his therapy of the passions should provide limited options for fear and related passions, and this is the focus of the next section.

6.8 Descartes's Treatment of the Passions

I have already discussed Descartes's therapies in the practical context of his advice to Princess Elisabeth. His more formal discussion of treatments for the disruptions of the passions is mostly based on Neo-Stoic arguments and unrelated to the sophisticated mechanism proposed in the first two parts of PS. Most of Part Three deals with the proper management of the passions, and Descartes finishes the treatise with an article entitled "*A universal remedy for the passions*" (PS 211)[35] in which he voices his well-known conclusion that "it is the passions alone that make for all that is good or bad in this life." The "remedies" for the passions, claimed Descartes "would be sufficient if everyone took the trouble to apply them." Thus, not only had Descartes clarified once and for all the mechanism of the passions in Part One of the PS, but in Part three he explains the definitive therapy. Let us then discuss Descartes's remedies for the passions and their potential usefulness.

Against the Stoic tradition, Descartes considered the passions to be positive guides for human life, and in need of control but not extirpation (PS 170). During the seventeenth century, most thinkers considered the passions to be helpful when they were properly directed, thereby producing positive habits to strengthen the moral virtues (Hatfield 2007, p. 7). For instance, in the case of indecision, Descartes suggests developing the habit of forming "definite and determinate judgments about whatever things we are confronted with" (PS 170), and to accept that we are doing our best when judging the most adequate way to act, even when it may end up being wrong.

[35]This title illustrates important conceptual contradictions in PS, where passions are considered as always being good for the individual and yet some of them are in need of treatment due to becoming excessive (such as fear changing into terror) or inappropriate to the situation (such as a flight response triggered by fear when courage and a fight response would be more appropriate).

Perhaps the essential aspects of Descartes's therapy of the passions are conveyed in PS 156, an article entitled "*The properties of nobility of soul, and how it acts as a remedy for all the disorders of the passions*". In this article Descartes suggests that being virtuous is the best remedy for the passions. What is being virtuous for Descartes? It is being "most humble", and having a natural capacity for doing "great things" while at the same time knowing the true extent of one's capacities. Nobility of soul consists in having a "firm and constant resolution" to use one's free will to undertake those actions considered to be the best using the force of understanding (PS 153). The Cartesian virtuous person is in full control of their passions, and "always perfectly courteous, affable, and helpful towards one and all". Their desires are modest, since they do not esteem anything as having great value; they never hate since they "esteem all human beings"; and never have terror, being strengthened by the "confidence in their own virtue". Finally, the Cartesian person of virtue is never angry given that they will never be upset by events outside their control, such as what their "enemies" may plot against them.

In a letter to Princess Elisabeth (18 May 1645; AT 4:200) Descartes adds that the main difference between noble and vulgar souls is that the latter's happiness depends totally on the facts of life, whereas noble souls, in possession of a strong and powerful mind, are able to use reason to control all passions, thus achieving "perfect felicity," a heavenly happiness they can "enjoy already in this life." The Stoic sage may pale in comparison with the Cartesian noble, and Elisabeth may have felt that Cartesian sainthood was an impossible goal. In the case that her cure depends on achieving the Cartesian virtuosity she will never be healed.

Descartes also provided additional advice for treating excessive passions. A successful therapy of the passions requires self-examination to determine the "strength and weakness in a soul" (PS 48). For instance, some people are unable to make definite judgments about choosing virtuously and deciding on an appropriate course of action. Their souls are dominated by passions such as fear, reducing "the soul to the most deplorable possible state" of doubts, irresolution and inaction (PS 48). Regrettably, when a soul oscillates between fear and ambition it is condemned "to wretched slavery" (PS 48), and when under the passion of terror, the individual so affected will always have the desire to flee rather than honourably confront danger. The challenge for these weak souls is how to change the automatic movements of the pineal gland which produce fear and terror. To this end, Descartes recommends the technique of diversion, thus detaching the noxious movements of the gland created "by force of habit" and developing new healthier movements of the gland and spirits. He further considers this change may be achieved "by a single action", similarly to the way dogs can be easily trained not to run after hearing a shot (PS 50). Descartes is confident that if animals can so easily change their hydraulic machinery, humans who are endowed with reason should certainly be even more successful: "even those who have the weakest souls could acquire a very absolute command of all their passions, if one were to take the trouble to train them and guide them properly" (PS 50). I shall now describe Descartes's method for producing this change.

Descartes considered that passions cannot be controlled voluntarily given that they are independent from "acts of the will." Therefore, he suggested an indirect method consisting in thinking about the passions one wants to obtain, which is contrary to the passion to be suppressed. This requires several cognitive steps, such as, in the case of fear, examining the dangerousness of the object and considering reasons for 'willing' a specific response based on previous examples. Thus, one can convince oneself "that the danger is not at all great" and that by being courageous rather than fearful "we can look forward to the glory and joy of victory" rather than suffering the shame of fleeing (PS 45). Descartes further suggested that the activity of the soul can easily control "lesser passions" (PS 46) but not the most violent ones, given the great excitation with which they affect the heart and spirits. In this situation, his advice for overcoming the violent passions was to wait until after "the excitation of the blood and spirits had passed" (PS 46).

6.8.1 Descartes's Treatment of Fear

Following the Stoic tradition relating to fear, Descartes accepts the inevitability of 'first movements' (see Chapter 3), but refers to them as affecting those who have a "strong natural propensity" to fear (PS 211).

In such cases, a stimulus may produce a marked impact on the imagination and produce tremor as an expression of fear. While for Seneca first movements had no emotional value, Descartes considers them as useful, since "the blood stirred in this way" alerts a person to the fact that it is easy to be deceived by the imagination, and therefore, he recommends that it is better to wait before acting on the stimulus.

For the treatment of fear Descartes's advice is to aim at distracting oneself with other thoughts until time and tranquillity have altogether calmed the blood disturbance (PS 46). In the case of terror, Descartes suggests using the ancient remedy of premeditation. He considers that thinking about negative outcomes in advance will allow the person to prepare "for all events the fear of which might give rise to it" (PS 176). Descartes explains the technique of premeditation in terms of his dualistic physiology as the activity of "separating within oneself the movements of the blood and the spirits from the thoughts to which they are habitually attached" (PS 176). Descartes did not elaborate on this mechanism, although he was aware of the complexity in the implementation of his advice, stating that "there are few people who are sufficiently prepared" for such a feat.[36] When danger is imminent, and one is seized by fear, there is no time for deliberation. Thoughts should then be displaced from the danger towards nobler notions, for instance, focusing "on the reasons why it is always much safer and more honourable to stand and fight than to flee" (PS 211). Nevertheless, Descartes seems to accept that some kind of deliberation is in place since he concedes that "if the odds are heavily against one, it is better to retreat honourably…than to expose oneself blindly to certain death" (PS 211).

In conclusion, Descartes's "universal remedy for the passions" is no more than a mixture of ancient philosophical techniques (mainly premeditation and distraction), combined with the Aristotelian advice on pursuing a virtuous life as the main source of happiness. *The Passion of*

[36]"…the movements aroused in the blood by the objects of our passions follow so swiftly from mere impressions in the brain and the disposition of our organs, without any contribution from the soul, that there is no human wisdom capable of withstanding them if one is not sufficiently prepared" (PS 211).

the Soul ends by stating, rather circularly, that mastering the passions is a sign of great wisdom, and that for the virtuous person even the evils caused by the passions can be a source of joy (PS 212).

What was the impact of the treatise in real life? As for the therapeutic aspects of the text, little is known, and it was soon forgotten. Nevertheless, we have in Princess Elisabeth an intelligent patient who provided revealing feedback on Descartes's therapeutic technique. As discussed earlier in the chapter, Elisabeth told Descartes (Letter 10 June 1643; 3:683) about her limitations in meditating in accord with Cartesian rules, which basically consist of meditating on virtue by withdrawing oneself from sensory stimulation and all preconceptions.[37] Elisabeth's frustration is understandable as this advice is more relevant for philosophers investigating metaphysical matters whilst relieved from social duties than for a person hard-pressed by major life problems.[38] The second remedy was to remind Elisabeth time and again that virtuous people are not enslaved by fears and can master them by

[37]"Indeed, I shall go so far as to say that I seek to be read by none, except those who will be able and willing to meditate seriously alongside me, and to withdraw their minds from the senses, and at the same time from all their preconceptions. Of these I well know already that there are very few" (Descartes 1991; Introduction, p. 15).

[38]As already mentioned, Genevieve Lloyd (2008) elaborated extensively on the therapeutic relationship between Descartes and Elisabeth. Since the Princess suffered from sadness, distress and anxiety, Lloyd's comments on Descartes's therapy should be at least briefly mentioned. Like Nye (1999), she stresses the "asymmetry" (p. 172) between the philosopher and his 'patient' and suggests that the notion of 'providence' underlies Descartes's selection of Stoic remedies. By "asymmetry," Lloyd means the gender hierarchy, as expressed in Descartes's and Elisabeth's different life-styles, social relations and daily problems, as well as their different approaches to self-knowledge. For instance, Elisabeth is unable to practice the meditation towards self-knowledge that Descartes recommends, but this is not due to any intrinsic limitations, but to gender differences in their opportunities and social roles. Descartes is unable to understand the reason why Elisabeth is not improved by his remedies, which are based on right reason and ultimately depend on God's providence. The Princess writes to Descartes that she is enslaved by the physical weakness of her sex, although the implications of this statement, perhaps ironic, go beyond bodily differences and refer to a different embodiment in daily life practices (while the philosopher was able to practice the *vita contemplativa*, the Princess had to deal with actual misfortunes). In the end (Letter 18 May 1645; AT 4:200) Descartes recommends the Princess to seek advice from true doctors.

the use of reason.[39] This again proved to be of no benefit to Elisabeth who had "real reasons to be distressed" (Letter May or June 1645; AT 4:218). Descartes's counsel was to use the Epicurean method of distraction[40]: the distressing event had to be completely ignored and attention should be focused on cheerful subjects. Unfortunately, this strategy, as well as the use of premeditation and reading Stoic philosophers all failed. Elisabeth's main problem was the impossibility of controlling her constant distress and worries about real life misfortunes even when considered irrational by Cartesian standards. Descartes believed that by rational thinking disturbing passions would be subdued, but this ignores the fact that a person in a state of distress and worry may be unable to think about lofty matters.[41]

In contrast, Descartes's conceptual approach to the passions, based on mind-body dualism had a very different fate. While his ideas were heavily criticised by renowned philosophers of his time, they survived in the "mechanical" school of medicine, which emerged in the seventeenth century with the aim of explaining medical phenomena in physiological terms. Descartes provided a basis for medicine to reduce mental phenomena to physiological changes.[42] Ontologically and functionally,

[39]"...the difference there is between the greatest souls and those that are base and vulgar consists mainly in this, that vulgar souls give way to their passions, and are happy or unhappy only in so far as the things that happen to them are pleasant or unpleasant; whereas those of the other kind can reason so powerfully and convincingly that, although they too have passions, which are often indeed more vehement than those of common souls, their reason nonetheless remains in command, and ensures that even afflictions are of use to them, and contribute to the perfect happiness they enjoy even in this life" (Letter 18 May 1645; AT 4:200).

[40]"...if a person with any number of real reasons to be distressed applied himself so thoroughly to turning his imagination aside from them that he never thought of them, except when compelled by practical necessity, and devoted the rest of his time to thinking only about what could bring him contentment and joy, not only would this greatly help him to judge more wisely about matters of concern to him, because he would consider these without passion, I am certain that this alone would be capable of restoring him to health" (Letter May or June 1645; AT 4:218).

[41]Descartes himself could not help worrying about the risk of being condemned by the Calvinists in Leyden, and this fear was one of the main reasons he left the Low Countries for Sweden.

[42]Gaukroger (2002, p. 394) and other authors suggest caution when labelling the Cartesian system of the passion as 'reductionist'. Part Three of PS, as already noted, is mostly about how to manage the passions using psychological tools, and Descartes's approach to the passions is more

dualism could not be satisfactorily explained. Medicine eventually took over the treatment of fear from philosophers and the clergy, and the humanist tradition was lost. Descartes's reduction of fear to the product of a hydraulic mechanism was perhaps unfortunate, as it re-oriented the understanding of this emotion away from philosophy, while still basing its treatment on a dry account of ancient techniques.

6.9 Humanism Versus Cartesianism[43]

At this stage I should take stock and discuss some of the conclusions presented in this and the previous chapter. I have presented a rather benign picture of Hellenistic and Roman philosophy of fear, and also a positive analysis of Montaigne's approach. Hobbes's concept of fear has been considered as illuminating the use of this passion to cement human social organization, although the proposal of using fear as a tool for social control can only result in chronic anxiety. With Descartes, the overall conclusion regarding his conceptualization of fear appears to be negative, suggesting a conflict between humanism and Descartes's concept and therapy of fear. It was Descartes himself who criticized the "Ancients" and in PS his aim was to treat the passions as a physiologist rather than a philosopher.

holistic in this section of his work. But the aim here is not to blame Descartes for the problems of reductionism; I merely want to note the tremendous influence of dualism and reductionism that is present in current medicine, neurobiology, and even some trends in philosophy. This is discussed in the next chapters.

[43]The term 'humanism' derives from the Latin *humanitas* as used by Cicero, but it was only in the nineteenth century that it became a noun standing for, among other things, a deep interest in the humane values in the literature and philosophy of ancient Greece and Rome (Kraye 2010, p. 2). Renaissance humanism extended from the mid-fourteenth century to the seventeenth century, and it is Descartes who develops a new philosophy that marks the end of humanism. Descartes's advice on using ancient remedies in Part Three of PS could be considered as a return to humanist values, but as Lloyd remarks (2008), Descartes main therapeutic concepts were drawn from ancient Stoicism and were based on ascetic detachment, reliance on 'right reason,' and faith in a providential god (p. 183). Descartes's rigid Stoicism is very close to the one rejected by Montaigne and far removed from the nuanced Stoicism of Seneca.

My assessment of Descartes's approach as being more negative than Montaigne's is based on his less appealing and perhaps less fruitful approach to the therapy of fear. Montaigne teaches different types of fear, taking place in different times and contexts, and uses himself as a paragon of fear. In Seneca, we have a Stoic philosopher, but as I described in Chapter 3, his approach to the treatment of fear is extremely eclectic, keeping his 'affiliation' with Stoicism but using any remedy he considers adequate. Descartes's concept and mechanism of the passions is very innovative, but in the end, incoherent. He applied the Galenic mechanical tradition to the field of the passions and opened a new way of looking into their physiology. He placed understanding of the passions on a scientific path, which offered the possibility of providing a better solution for the ravages of fear.[44] But on the other hand, the therapy suggested by Descartes is not novel, and is mainly based on strict Stoic remedies. For Descartes, all passions have to be under rational control, and to this end, it is necessary to acquire a 'nobility of soul' manifested in virtuous actions. The Cartesian noble lives in perfect virtue, detached from the "vulgar," and related to Divine providence. But most importantly, Descartes's therapy does not follow from the mechanism of the passions that he attempted to describe with clockwork precision.

On the other hand, Montaigne seems to only offer confusion. He was certainly not a systematic thinker, and yet reading the *Essays* is strongly therapeutic. Fear is prominent in his text, whilst it remains hidden in PS. Montaigne describes fear in himself, and teaches by example. He is able to adapt to the different circumstances in life, and mortality also becomes better accepted. In contrast, the Cartesian rules accept no bending, requiring clear and distinct ideas in the context of life events that are far from clear and distinct. They are fixed and enduring. Montaigne appreciated and valued human diversity, which stimulated the learning, understanding and acceptance of different life experiences, emotions, and ways of life, whereas Descartes saw diversity as

[44]Discussing the transition of studying and treating passions from the philosophical to the scientific-medical domain will be the focus of the next chapters.

an obstacle to his strategy of explaining the passions in terms of bodily machinery (De Marzio 2010, p. 309).

A few years before his death, Descartes wrote to a friend (Chanut, 15 June 1646 (AT IV, 442) that he felt satisfied with his achievements in medicine "on which I have spent much more time" than on other scientific endeavours. Yet he acknowledged that "instead of finding ways to preserve life, I have found another, much easier and surer way, which is not to fear death." Montaigne would have happily agreed with this conclusion, but he may have asked Descartes about the method he used for arriving at such a peaceful state.

References

Boros, G. (2006). Seventeenth-century theories of emotion and their contemporary relevance. *European Journal of Analytic Philosophy, 2*(1), 125–142.

Brown, D. J. (2006). *Descartes and the passionate mind.* Cambridge: Cambridge University Press.

De Marzio, D. M. (2010). Dealing with diversity: On the uses of common sense in Descartes and Montaigne. *Studies in Philosophical Education, 29*, 301–313.

Descartes, R. (1984). *The philosophical writings of Descartes* (J. Cottingham, R. Stoothoff, & D. Murdoch, Trans., Vol. II). Cambridge: Cambridge University Press.

Descartes, R. (1991). *The philosophical writings of Descartes* (J. Cottingham, R. Stoothoff, D. Murdoch, & A. Kenny, Trans., Vol. III—The Correspondence). Cambridge: Cambridge University Press.

Descartes, R. (2015). *The passions of the soul and other late philosophical writings* (M. Moriarty, Trans.). Oxford: Oxford University Press.

Dixon, T. (2003). *From passions to emotions.* Cambridge: Cambridge University Press.

Gaukroger, S. (2002). *Descartes' system of natural philosophy.* Cambridge: Cambridge University Press.

Gross, D. M. (2007). *The secret history of emotion.* Chicago: The University of Chicago Press.

Harvey, W. (1628). *Excitatio Anatomica De Motu Cordis et Sanguini in Animalibus.* Frankfort: The Warnock Library.

Hassing, R. F. (2015). *Cartesian psychophysics and the whole nature of man*. London: Lexington Books.

Hatfield, G. (2007). The *Passions of the Soul* and Descartes's machine psychology. *Studies in History and Philosophy of Science, 38*, 1–35.

James, S. (1999). *Passion and action: The emotions in seventeenth-century philosophy*. Oxford: Clarendon Press.

Kraye, J. (2010). *The Cambridge companion to renaissance humanism*. Cambridge: Cambridge University Press.

Lloyd, G. (2008). *Providence lost*. London: Harvard University Press.

Nagel, T. (2012). *Mind & cosmos*. Oxford: Oxford University Press.

Nye, A. (1999). *The princess and the philosopher*. Oxford: Rowman & Littlefield Publishers.

Popper, K., & Eccles, J. C. (1977). *The self and its brain: An argument for interactionism*. London: Routledge.

Shapiro, L. (2011). Princess Elizabeth and Descartes: The union of soul and body and the practice of philosophy. *British Journal of the History of Philosophy, 7*(3), 503–520.

7

James's Fears and Wittgenstein's Therapy

> Common-sense says...we meet a bear, are frightened and run...The hypothesis here to be defended says that this order of sequence is incorrect... [rather] we feel... afraid because we tremble.
>
> William James, *What is an Emotion?* 1884, pp. 247–248

7.1 Introduction

The last chapter examined the dawning of a new era in the concept of emotions brought by Descartes's proposal of a mechanism for the passions couched in biological terms. From the perspective of the history this work traces, the Cartesian revolution relates not so much to the separation of soul and body, but to the advancement of a system for the emotions based on specific interactions between brain regions and motor effectors to produce behavioural responses. Descartes's mechanistic tradition was mostly continued by physicians, such as the renowned Thomas Willis (1621–1675) (Willis 1672), who ignored dualism but created a model of "human hydraulus" (Kassler 1998), and physicians such as Franz Joseph Gall (Wickens 2014, p. 134) who developed the

S. Starkstein, *A Conceptual and Therapeutic Analysis of Fear*,
https://doi.org/10.1007/978-3-319-78349-9_7

theory of phrenology, where different mental functions have a precise localization in the brain cortex.

Many other theories of mind-brain interaction were advanced in the seventeenth and eighteenth centuries (James 1999), but it was only by the end of the nineteenth century that the study of the mechanism of emotions was radically reformulated by the American philosopher, physician and psychologist William James (1842–1910) (Wassmann 2014). James's theory of emotions "became a landmark that physiologists, neuroscientists and historians alike refer to today" (Wassmann 2014, p. 166), and it has also been highly influential in the fields of psychology and philosophy up to the present (Ellsworth 1994; Reisenzein and Achim 2014). One of the main reasons for a revival in the study of emotions in the nineteenth century was that the care of people with emotional problems progressed from being of interest to non-specialized medical practitioners in lunatic asylums, to become the specialty of psychiatry.

During the nineteenth century there also was a growing interest in the study of brain functions and their relation to emotional and cognitive disturbances (Wassmann 2014). By the end of the nineteenth century psychiatry became divided into a psychodynamic branch, led by Sigmund Freud in Vienna (see next chapter), and a biological branch lead by Emil Kraepelin in Munich (Berrios 1996). Kraepelin pioneered the detailed examination of the brain to unravel the mechanism of emotional disorders, a tradition that is still current in the work of cognitive neuroscientists such as Antonio Damasio (Bechara and Damasio 2005; Damasio and Carvalho 2013). In parallel, during the first half of the twentieth century, the Austrian philosopher Ludwig Wittgenstein initiated one of the most significant philosophical movements of the century, with a strong interest in conceptual analysis which included profound reflections on the philosophy of emotions (Monk 1991). In part Wittgenstein's work responded to the way in which increasingly, especially during the nineteenth century, science made significant inroads into providing all-encompassing explanations of human psychology, a tendency known as 'scientism' (Williams and Robinson 2014). Wittgenstein considered scientism as "a disease of the intellect" (Hacker 2001, p. 272) to be extirpated by his new method of conceptual analysis. He was especially critical of James's theory of emotions, with its tendency towards reducing and explaining psychological phenomena in physical terms. Despite Wittgenstein's criticism, however, it was James's concept of emotions that succeeded in influencing the novel and fast-growing field of cognitive neurosciences, with a branch of philosophy actively collaborating in these endeavours.[1]

In this chapter I shall firstly discuss James's influential theory of emotions, showing its origin in Descartes's work on the passions and its further development by the so-called 'Neo-Jamesians', a group of prominent philosophers and neuroscientists such as Damasio, who developed James's theory of emotions in different directions but shared the concept of reductionism and increasing physicalism. Second, I shall discuss the important criticism provided by Wittgenstein to James's theory, and how Wittgenstein's conceptual analysis of emotions is still relevant to contemporary neurosciences.

7.2 William James's Theory of Emotions

Why was James so significant to the psychology and philosophy of emotions? A brief answer, according to Wassman, is that together with the German psychologist Wilhelm Wundt (2014), James stressed the importance of neurophysiology in the mechanism of emotions at a time when emotions were considered spiritual phenomena unrelated to bodily mechanisms (2014). The second half of the nineteenth century was an exciting period for the young specialty of neurology, with the discovery of language centres in the brain and areas specialised in motor and sensory functions. It is in this context of the increasing relevance

[1]Among neuroscientists the most active in this field are Antonio Damasio (1994, 1999, 2003, 2010) (who considers James to be a referent for his synthesis of neuroscience with philosophy), Joseph LeDoux (Debiec and LeDoux 2004; LeDoux 2000, 2013; Schiller et al. 2008), a pioneer in studying the fear mechanism in rodents, and Jap Panksepp (2004), a renowned neuroscientist interested in adopting a 'non-reductionist' approach to the study of emotions in humans and primates. Among philosophers perhaps most influential has been the work of Patricia Churchland (1989) to combine philosophy with the burgeoning field of cognitive neurosciences to form a new philosophical sub discipline termed 'neurophilosophy.'

of neurophysiology that James's theory of emotions developed. James's best known text on emotions is *What is an Emotion?*, published in 1884 (James 1888), followed by a chapter (Chapter 25) in his *Principles of Psychology* (1890) (James 1890), and *The Physical Basis of Emotion*, James's last work on this theme (1894) (James 1994).

7.2.1 What Is an Emotion?

What is an Emotion? is the most often quoted text by James dealing with emotions. The main objective of the work was to propose a novel mechanism for the emotions by stressing the relevance of specific "processes" occurring in motor and sensory brain regions (James 1888, p. 189). James's theory is not based on empirical studies but, similar to Descartes in his *Meditations*, James's idea "grew out of fragmentary introspective observations" (James 1888, p. 189). Surprisingly, James opened *What is an Emotion?* with an empirical proposition: emotions are either "affected" (that is, related) to specific brain centres, or they are related to sensory-motor processes in a generic way (James 1888, p. 188). Thus, James couched the concept of emotions, much like Descartes, in neurophysiological terms. He further considered that emotions should be studied by experimental psychologists and neurophysiologists, no longer being the realm of the antiquated conceptual tools of philosophers.

In James's theory of emotions, bodily or somatic changes, consisting of muscular, sensory and visceral activity, have a *necessary* role in the production of emotions. This important concept notwithstanding, his most puzzling proposal is the reversal of the so-called common-sense theory of emotions. According to James, 'common sense' suggests that emotions start with a perception, for instance and most famously, the sight of a bear, triggering the emotion of fear *after* the appraisal that there is risk at hand, and finishing with a behavioural response, such as running away from danger. James's perplexing proposal inverts the common-sense process, so that the perception of an object first produces bodily changes, and the emotion is limited to the perception of the bodily changes. In James's own words:

> Common sense says...we meet a bear, are frightened and run...The hypothesis here to be defended says that this order of sequence is incorrect, that our mental state is not immediately induced by the other, that the bodily manifestations must first be interposed between, and that the most rational statement is that we feel...afraid because we tremble, and not that we...tremble, because we are...fearful. (James 1888, p. 190)

In *Principles of Psychology* James further clarified this novel concept of emotions remarking that:

> "...bodily changes follow directly the perception of the exciting fact, and..... our feeling of the same changes as they occur IS the emotion... the one mental state is not immediately induced by the other, that the bodily manifestation must first be interposed between, and that the more rational statement is that we feel...afraid because we tremble". (James 1890, vol. 2, pp. 449–450)

James's definition of emotions in *What is an Emotion?* and in *Principles of Psychology* looks misleadingly simple, and requires detailed examination. First, what James is proposing is that emotions are produced by a reflex mechanism that excludes appraisals. Thus, the psychological scheme of the common-sense theory is converted into a neurophysiological one. In other words, James's novel mechanism consists of an "exciting" stimulus which automatically produces a bodily response, independent of conscious awareness (James 1888, p. 190).[2] The challenge for James was how to explain a behavioural response occurring automatically in the absence of any appraisal. His reflex circuit (perception → behaviour) may work for innate responses such as a startle reaction to a loud noise or a similar sudden threat, but it is unclear how such a reflex system could produce a fear response to more complex "objects", such as the fear of a financial crisis. James responded to this objection by referring to Darwinian evolutionary theory, where

[2]"My thesis on the contrary is that *the bodily changes follow directly the* PERCEPTION *of the exciting fact, and that our feeling of the same changes as they occur* IS *the emotion*" (James 1888, pp. 189–190) (italic and upper-case in the original).

a system that is adequate to manage basic threats may adapt to manage novel and more sophisticated ones. James further suggested that the reflex system works as a neural "lock" which can only be started by predetermined stimuli, with no need for appraisals.

According to James, somatic responses could range in intensity from very subtle, such as states of "inward tension" to states of gross behavioural turmoil. James concluded that no emotion is "without a [unique] bodily reverberation" and a particular "mental mood," and suggested a one-to-one correspondence between stimulus and somatic change (James 1888, p. 191). In the case of fear, James speculated that this emotion corresponds to "the feelings…of quickened heart-beats… shallow breathing…trembling lips…goose flesh [and]…visceral stirrings…" (James 1888, pp. 193–194). Somatic changes are therefore the end point of James's behavioural/neural reflex circuit, and are both sufficient and necessary to produce an emotion.[3]

What are these somatic changes and how are they generated? James's emotional reflex includes the perception of an object by a given cortical region, or the stimulation of this cortex produces an "idea" of the object. "Quick as a flash" (James 1888, p. 203) the brain stimulates the skin, muscle and viscera through specific neural channels. The effects of this stimulation are perceived in somatosensory regions of the brain, and when combined with the perception of the object "in consciousness", the perception is transformed from "an object-simply-apprehended" into an "object-emotionally-felt". In other words, the first perception is emotionally neutral, thus I see the bear but feel nothing, whereas the somatic perception of our legs moving or our viscera stirring, when combined with the image of the object, produces the emotion. It is after this second perception that the object is emotionally-laden. James adds that the number of potential somatic changes is "indefinitely numerous" as the whole organism works as a "sounding board" to produce feelings (James 1890, vol. 2, p. 308).

James was adamant that his theory included no additional components "beyond…ordinary reflex circuits," rejecting any process of

[3]James will later claim that visceral changes are *necessary* but not sufficient (see below).

"appraisal" taking place as part of the mechanism of emotions (James 1890, vol. 2, p. 324). Nevertheless, James was ambiguous about the role of contextual factors, implying appraisal in the production of emotions. For instance, he stated that "the most important part of the environment is my fellow-man", who has the capacity to "unlock" our fears (James 1888, p. 195). James also stated that fear may arise when one feels observed by another person, and has its extreme expression in "stage-fright" (James 1888, p. 195). Given the sophistication of human emotions and the myriad of novel stimuli in modern society as compared to tribal ones, James had the challenge of explaining how a simple neural reflex is activated by complex social events. His answer was that this phylogenetically primitive mechanism works as well for the "civilised man" as for the "member of a tribe" (James 1888, p. 196). In other words, James suggested that the brain mechanisms he had described as part of the reflex system of emotions are flexible and adaptable enough to accommodate any stimuli, from simple events affecting human ancestors as well as the more complex and elaborated stimuli affecting contemporary humans.

Finally, to support his theory, James advanced his famous thought-experiment ("a vital point of this theory" (James 1888, p. 193)), which consisted in imagining the subtraction from consciousness of all the feelings produced by the somatic changes associated with any particular emotion. According to James, this subtraction leaves no "mind-stuff" to create the emotion, and the person is left with a mere "cold and neutral" cognitive perception (James 1888, p. 193).

7.2.2 The Conceptual Position of Fear in James's System of Emotions

James used fear as a paradigmatic emotion and, like Descartes before him, the well-known example of running away from the perennial bear. In a state of fear, a person either runs or remains "semi-paralysed." According to James, 'instinct-like' fear is a rather uncommon event in modern life due to the great progress of civilization and he adds the astonishing comment that some people may have never felt fear in their lives (James 1890, vol. 2, p. 285). This comment exemplifies the way that James narrowed the emotion of fear to an instinctual and extremely intense somatic reaction, a reductive approach that will find fertile soil a century later in the field of cognitive neuroscience. Nevertheless, in the *Principles of Psychology* the ontological status of fear became unclear, since James stated that fear is not only the feeling of somatic changes but also a "psychical state…consisting of mental representations" (James 1890, vol. 2, p. 327). This is certainly not a minor correction of his original hypothesis, and the rationale for this change unfortunately remained unexplained.

While the ontological status of fear started to drift from the original proposal, James provided interesting but conceptually unclear descriptions of the phenomenology and nosology of this emotion. He refers to "pathological cases", those instances when fear occurs in the absence of a triggering object, or when a fearful reaction is out of proportion to the danger posed by the object (for instance, the case of intense fear of insects). He suggests that "unmotivated fear" (James 1890, vol. 2, p. 313) results from a high sensitivity of the "nervous machinery" in responding to somatic and visceral changes. Thus, if a person is unable to breathe deeply, has a flutter in the heart, and epigastric discomfort while sitting in a crouching attitude in the absence of a cause, the feeling of these somatic changes "*is* the emotion of dread" (italics in the original), a state James termed "morbid fear." In these cases of severe fear, James stated that the individual "is not afraid of anything; he is simply afraid", thus stressing that morbid fear has no object (James 1890, vol. 2, p. 314). James provided a clinical example demonstrating the interface between these clinical descriptions and his theory of emotions. He described the case of a friend who was affected with episodes of shortness of breath, palpitations, and epigastric pressure. The best treatment for his friend's morbid fear, James claimed, was to breathe deeply and assume a supine position, and "the dread, ipso facto, seems to depart" (James 1890, vol. 2, p. 314). This clinical anecdote illustrates the application of James's theory of emotions to real life therapy, and reinforces his thesis that somatic changes are the cause of emotions.

Although James reduced fear to a somatic response to a sudden threat,[4] he could not ignore the evidence that in many cases fear occurs as the expectation of a bad outcome, with no somatic changes necessarily involved. For instance, this is the case in the anxious expectation of a potentially dreadful event, such as awaiting the results of a biopsy to determine whether one has cancer. James considered these fears as "ideal emotions" (James 1888, p. 197), that is, an emotion that originates "internally," from a "representation" of somatic changes, but without being actual bodily changes. Regrettably, James did not comment on whether "ideal emotions" are exceptions to his rule that all emotions are feelings of somatic changes. James's theory is further complicated by his suggestion that even when fearful ideation seems to produce an "immediate…emotional feeling", further analysis suggests that "pure cerebral emotions" do not produce 'true' feelings unless these are related to "a bodily reverberation of some kind," a mechanism revealed by "careful introspection" only (James 1890, vol. 2, p. 322). Unfortunately, James never described how 'true' feelings may be recognised by using introspection (see below).

James's discussion of the therapy of fear was in line with this theory. In *The Physical Basis of Emotion* (1894) (James 1994) he recommended that individuals with a "frightful disposition" should persistently practice those behaviours that are "contrary" to the undesirable behaviour produced by their emotions. Thus, in the case of fear, he surmises that the affected person should lift their head and look straight at the object of fear, walking resolutely towards it with a stern facial expression to get rid of this emotion.[5]

---

[4]For an in-depth discussion of the reductionism of James's theory of emotions see Dixon (2012).

[5]Whether such a strategy may be useful is an empirical question, although as stated by Wittgenstein (2001) forcing oneself to smile while feeling sad may even increase rather than ameliorate the feeling of sadness. In any case, James's therapeutic suggestion is of limited applicability, given that for common daily fears there are no somatic changes to be countered. For instance, the fear of becoming unemployed, of having a serious illness, or that the person we are anxiously expecting may not come, may not be associated with typical bodily changes.

7.2.3 Challenges and Further Clarifications

Soon after being introduced, James's theory of emotions was strongly challenged by his contemporaries (Canon 1927). The first objection listed in the *Principles of Psychology* is the lack of evidence that stimuli produce somatic changes prior to becoming conscious. James answered this objection by referring to the startle response: he suggested that watching a dark object moving in the woods produces tachycardia and fast breathing before any conscious idea of danger emerges (James 1890, vol. 2, p. 288).

The second objection was that for James's theory to be correct, somatic changes should always produce an emotion. The objection was illustrated by the fact that actors can mimic emotional expressions such as crying, without feeling sad. James responded that his hypothesis cannot be empirically tested by voluntarily mimicking emotions, given that not all somatic changes can be voluntarily reproduced, such as visceral stirrings (James 1890, vol. 2, p. 316). Eventually, James's theory of emotions continued to drift away from his original hypothesis, and in *The Physical Basis of Emotion* he accepted that in some instances somatic changes are not sufficient to produce emotions, given the inability of these changes to fully reproduce the feelings of a putative "emotional wave." By switching the bodily response from muscular to visceral changes James placed his theory of emotions safely beyond empirical refutation.

The third objection was that the same emotions can be produced by different somatic changes. For instance, fear can result from running away or from freezing in a posture. This objection was dismissed by James with the unclear statement that the somatic changes that produce emotions occur "within limits" and that symptoms of fear can "still preserve enough functional resemblance" among different individuals, thereby allowing the use of "identical names" (James 1994, p. 520).

Still, the main objection to James's theory was the failure to include any cognitive appraisal of stimuli in the production of emotions.[6]

[6]The unnamed critic had stated that we run from the bear because we may otherwise be eaten,

In *The Physical Basis of Emotion*, the final and definitive version of his theory of emotions, James addressed the objection that the idea of danger has to precede the motor response by suggesting that emotional objects produce a somatic change in the context of a "total situation" (James 1994, p. 520), and added the critical remark that the emotion ensues "as soon as an object becomes …familiar and suggestive…" (James 1994, p. 518).

This is a major departure from his original theory and James can be seen to be conceding defeat, since by "total situation" he can only be taken to mean appraisal of the stimuli and context before the behavioural response. James even stated that the object "suggests" a total situation "on any theory of emotion." In other words, we no longer automatically run after the appearance of the bear, since in the amended theory the object triggers a fight or flight reaction based on an "overpowering idea" (i.e. an appraisal) of what the best course of action should be. To repeat, James's implicit admission that there is appraisal before the behavioural response is of critical importance since it shatters the heart of his theory.[7]

These major shifts in James's theory of emotions were partially accepted by some "Neo-Jamesians" such as Ellsworth, who suggests that in *The Physical Basis of Emotions* James introduced a *second* theory of emotions where contextual appraisal *does* occur before the behavioural response (Ellsworth 1994, p. 225). This second theory, according to Ellsworth, includes, as already mentioned, the proposal that visceral movements are critical to the mechanism of emotions, and stresses the relevance of discriminating between severities within the same emotion, implying that only the stronger feelings should be considered true emotions. In other words, to become an emotion, a feeling has to include "a very minimum of properly emotional excitement" (James 1994,

---

but "…according to Professor James the reason we dislike to be eaten is because we run away" (James 1994, p. 518).

[7]In other words, James conceded that the emotional response is no longer a reflex act consisting of object → somatic change; but now, object → appraisal of the "total situation" → behavioural response.

p. 519). According to James, if the intensity of the somatic changes is below this threshold, we no longer feel "*fear*" (italics in the original) but only an "unpleasant sensation" (James 1994, p. 519). The true emotion of fear is "a general seizure of excitement" accompanied by subtler sensations "often hard to describe" (James 1994, p. 523).

While this work deals primarily with conceptual rather than empirical issues in relation to fear, I have dwelt at length on the empirical conundrums of James's theory of emotions because these are the bases on which he builds his conceptual framework. Furthermore, we shall see similar problems with the interpretation of empirical studies as well as major conceptual quandaries resurfacing in the contemporary neurosciences of fear. James's theory of emotions[8] is still extant in contemporary cognitive neuroscience, but the conceptual problems are not so easily dismissed. Therefore, before moving on to contemporary elaborations of the Jamesian schema, I shall first introduce Wittgenstein's illuminating criticism of James's theory.

7.2.4 Conceptual Problems with James's Theory of Emotions

> The best thing I can say…is that in writing it, I have almost persuaded myself it may be true.
>
> William James, *What is an Emotion?* (James 1888, p. 205).

To support the theory that emotions are feelings of somatic changes, James states that actors who play "with their heart" report that the emotion of the role they play "masters them whenever they play it well" (James 1890, p. 317). In relation to this statement, Wittgenstein asks, rhetorically:

---

[8]This theory is known as the 'James-Lange theory' as it was independently developed by James and the Danish physician Carl Lange. Like James, Lange considered that all emotions are caused by physiological phenomena (Dagleish 2004).

> ...What is it that is so frightful about fear? The trembling, the quick breathing, the feeling in the facial muscles? – When you say: "This fear, this uncertainty, is frightful!" – must you go on "If only I did not have this feeling in my stomach"? (Wittgenstein 1980b; 728)[9]

Thus, following Wittgenstein's remark, should we treat our stomach whenever we feel anxious? This *reductio ad absurdum* should be sufficient to dismiss James's theory without the need for empirical refutation. In *Zettel*, Wittgenstein posited that the descriptor "a horrible fear" does not mean that the feeling is horrible (Wittgenstein 1967; 492, 496). Similarly, awareness of the somatic concomitants of some fears (e.g. the fast breathing and the tension in the face) is not that these responses are themselves "frightful" feelings (Wittgenstein 1967; 499). In response to James's hypothesis that somatic and visceral changes cause emotions, Wittgenstein argues that the *cause* of fear is not in our body, but in the danger we are facing. Thus, when asked why we are scared "...we wouldn't point to the stomach...rather, perhaps, at what gives us our fear" (Wittgenstein 1980a; 729). Moreover, what is frightful is the *object* of fear (e.g. losing my job), and not the tension in my chest. This is not to dismiss the fact that somatic changes are typical concomitants of some emotions, but the relation between the emotion and somatic changes is contingent and not causal. One of James's conceptual errors lies in this failure to distinguish between the cause of an emotion and its contingent concomitants (Ter Hark 2001, p. 215).[10]

An important distinction should be made between the *object* and the *cause* of an emotion. Most often what constitutes an object of emotion, that is, what the emotion is about is clear. The nature of the object may vary, from a tangible thing (e.g. James's bear), to a specific natural or social context (e.g. the experience of imagination of height or giving public talks), or a future event (e.g. the possibility of a divorce). In rare circumstances, there is no immediately identifiable object of fear, and emotions are considered as 'objectless fear,' or 'free-floating anxiety.'

---

[9]The numeral stands for the number of the remark in the text.

[10]As Wittgenstein puts it: "...Possibly one could be sad because he is crying, but of course one is not sad *that* he is crying..." (Wittgenstein 1980b; 323).

What is the relevance of these different objects for James's theory of emotions? As discussed earlier, James's example of fear is the unexpected appearance of a bear, and running away from the animal is an obvious response. But it is unlikely that the fear of a financial crisis, for example, is accompanied by a behavioural change. I have already discussed that, for James, only emotions occurring in the presence of a major behavioural upheaval should be considered true fear. But the fear of being late to an appointment with my boss, worrying about my children being sick, how I will go in an examination and many other such examples are the most common fears in our daily lives. With or without a "minimum of excitement", they are certainly much more relevant than the unlikely chance of meeting a bear in the street.

What constitutes a *cause* of an emotion also deserves discussion given the different events that may fall into this category. For James, the cause of an emotion was the somatic change; but it seems clear that he was wrong, as, at least in contemporary colloquial usage, the cause of an emotion is its motive or reason. In other words, the cause of my fear is in the answer to the question: *Why* are you afraid? Thus, whereas the object of fear is my car making a strange noise, the cause of my fear is the possibility that the engine may fail. It may be argued that fear is caused by brain mechanisms which are necessary to produce emotions; but brain mechanisms are not sufficient to produce fear unless there is also a reason and an appropriate context. Episodes of sudden fear in the absence of a motive or reason are considered to be an expression of pathology, such as the fear produced by some types of seizures. Kenny suggests that in some instances the object and the cause of an emotion coincide (Kenny 2003, p. 25). For instance, a sick man's frailty may be both the cause and the object of his fear. Nevertheless, it may be argued that the cause of fear in this example is not (only) being frail, but a host of other factors relating to the meaning of frailty, such as fear of death, fear of leaving a widow, etc.

To conclude, James's theory results in a double reduction of emotions, one conceptual and the other empirical. Empirically, James reduces the concept of fear to a rare and violent emotion, a limitation that makes the emotion more amenable to empirical examination, but at the same time, drastically reducing its human relevance. The second reduction occurs when fear is explained conceptually in neurophysiological terms. The upshot is that, using relatively simple concepts, James is able to divorce fear and other emotions from philosophical analysis, and establish them as objects of physiological experimentation.

7.2.5 Neo-Jamesians to the Rescue

James's theory of emotions is still defended fully or in part, by a number of neuroscientists, philosophers and psychologists. Thus Laird contends that "creating facial expressions increases emotional feelings, and preventing expressions reduces feelings" (Laird and Lacasse 2014, p. 29). Some Neo-Jamesians admit a step of stimulus appraisal as part of James's theory. For example, Laird (Laird and Lacasse 2014) again, while regarding James's reflex theory as correct, also accepts that appraisal of the social context is *necessary* for the production of emotions. Similarly, Barbalet (1999, p. 288) states that the object of an emotion "will *necessarily* vary with social experience" (my italics). Ellsworth (1994, p. 222) suggests that whereas somatic changes are necessary for the production of emotions, emotions are not limited to the feeling of those changes. Quite strikingly, Ellsworth admits that the restriction of emotion in James's theory to the perception of somatic changes "seriously impeded the study of emotions" (Ellsworth 1994, p. 223). In her view, it is the somatic change *in combination* with the appraisal that produces the emotion. Ellsworth states that ever since James's theory of object→ somatic/visceral change→ feeling, psychologists have tried to rearrange these elements as these would be 'real' entities rather than psychological constructs. These concepts have been used "like billiard balls" (Ellsworth 1994, p. 227) one pushing the other in sequence, when in fact these events do not occur in a time-locked manner (see also Dixon's criticism (Dixon 2012) [11]).

[11]Dixon considers that James's last version of his theory in *The Physical Basis of Emotion* "included so many concessions and qualifications as to amount virtually to a retraction of his own theory" (Dixon 2012, p. 342).

The current field of the neuroscience of emotions goes beyond James's use of introspection to access bodily changes by using, instead, sophisticated machinery to study brain activity. Thus, James's "bodily-sounding board" has been turned into brain circuits able to register every somatic change. Where James suggested that the human cortex has specific centres activated by changes in sensory terminals, which form a "representation" of emotional processes, many years later Damasio has resurrected the theory in the form of neural representation of somatic changes to explain the mechanism of both emotions and feelings (see below). The current cultural *zeitgeist* that affirms science as the most authoritative source of truth, adds strength to this move that largely restricts understandings of fear as well as the best methods to manage it to the scientific field of the cognitive neurosciences. Further consolidating this form of explanation and therapy, conceptually, the field of 'neurophilosophy' has emerged mostly among Anglo-American philosophers (Churchland 1989; Northoff 2016) with the aim of collaborating with neuroscientists in their research endeavours. It is against this context, and considering his major influence on the neurosciences and neurophilosophy, that the next section discusses the work of Damasio on emotion.

7.3 The Neuroscience of Fear: Damasio

By the mid-twentieth century, and with the advent of sophisticated tools to image the brain, there was a renewed interest in studying mental functions (Wickens 2014). Initial research focused on language and memory, and investigations into the neural mechanism of emotions did not begin in earnest until the last decades of the twentieth century. Damasio has been at the forefront of both empirical studies and conceptual work in the neurosciences of emotion. His research program has mostly focused on the neural systems underlying emotions, since "neurological disease provides a unique entry into the fortified citadel of the human brain and mind" (Damasio 2003, p. 5). I will discuss the conceptual continuity between James and Damasio, the increasing role of neurosciences in providing explanations for emotions that go far beyond what empirical findings suggest, and the relevance of philosophical discussion in the context of the massive influence of neuroscience on the epistemology of emotions.

7.3.1 "The Strange Case of William James"

The heading above is the title of one of the sections in Damasio's *The Feeling of What Happens* (Damasio 1999). Damasio considers that the relevance of James's reversal of the common-sense concept of emotion "cannot be overemphasised... [and] ...modern research entirely supports it" (Damasio 2010, p. 123). Nevertheless, Damasio points to major problems with James's theory of emotions. First, against James's (ambiguous) rejection of appraisals in the mechanism of emotions, Damasio explicitly accepts this cognitive step (Damasio 2010, p. 123). Above all, the critical break with James is Damasio's rejection of James's dictum that emotions are feelings of bodily changes, proposing instead, and even more reductively, that emotions *are* bodily changes and not feelings, thus separating emotions from feelings and creating the new concept of the "feeling of emotion", which I discuss below.

Damasio separated emotions from feelings since, he believes, they have different "essences" (Damasio 2010, p. 117). Accordingly, emotions are automated programs of bodily actions, either "external" such as changes in facial expression, or "internal" such as visceral and hormonal changes, which are triggered by an "emotional competent object". According to Damasio, the emotional programs are unlearned, automated and predictable, and originate in genetics and in Darwinian natural selection (Damasio 2010, p. 131).

In *Descartes' Error* and *Looking for Spinoza* Damasio defines "feelings of emotions" as the mental process of mapping a particular bodily state (Damasio 2003, p. 88), expressed as "mental images" (Damasio 1994, p. 186). Thus, feelings of emotions are "always hidden" (Damasio 2003, p. 5).[12] A more succinct definition is provided in *The Feeling of What*

[12]Damasio claims that emotions are "public" and "play in the theatre of the body" (Damasio 2003, p. 6) although emotions also include visceral and hormonal changes. On the other hand,

Happens, where feelings of emotions are defined as mental images produced by neural representations (Damasio 1999, p. 282). As hinted by these definitions, Damasio's major claims are metaphysical rather than empirical, and therefore in need of philosophical clarification.

7.3.2 Damasio's Mechanism of Emotions

Given the philosophical complexity of the terms "representation" and "image" which Damasio frequently uses in the definition of emotions and feelings, these concepts require brief discussion. For Damasio a "representation" is synonymous with a "mental image". The perception of an object generates a neural pattern, and Damasio's concept of representation also includes the specific processes in the different brain regions involved in generating mental images (Damasio 1999, p. 320).[13] In other words, the perception of an object generates a mental image which also works as a representation of the neural processes involved in its creation. In *Descartes' Error* Damasio claims that mental images derive from ("are based on") neural representations that are topographically organised in sensory cortices (Damasio 1994, p. 98). Interestingly, he acknowledges that there is a "mystery" regarding how images emerge from neural patterns, but optimistically suggests this dilemma will be clarified with more empirical research.[14] Damasio argues that the "essence" of an emotion is constituted by a number of

feelings are "private" and "play in the theatre of the mind" (Damasio 2003, p. 6). Damasio's texts are replete with these metaphors which in this case demonstrate a clear Cartesian divide.

[13]Damasio owes us an explanation about how a physiological process generates images in non-extended matter.

[14]"How a neural pattern becomes an image is a problem that neurobiology has not yet resolved. When I say that images arise from neural patterns I am not slipping into inadvertent dualism. There is a gap between our knowledge of neural events and the mental image…I maintain two levels of description, one of the mind and one for the brain. This separation is a simple matter of intellectual hygiene and… not the result of dualism" (Damasio 1999, p. 323). Reference to this Cartesian gap is also made in (Damasio 2003, p. 198) where Damasio says, in agreement with James, that currently we can go as far as describing "neural maps with the help of neurophysiology, and we can describe images with the tools of introspection" (Damasio 2003, p. 198). Unfortunately, all his protestations against dualism are in vain, as I discuss below.

somatic changes controlled by specialised brain centres responding to specific stimuli. Following James, he states that emotional behaviours are "wired in" at birth in a "preorganized fashion" (Damasio 1994, p. 131). Emotions are elicited by the critical detection of an "emotional competent stimulus" (Damasio 2003, p. 3). This process of "detection" is unclearly conveyed as an "appraisal-evaluation phase" (Damasio 2003, p. 53). Damasio defines appraisal as "the process leading to emotion rather than emotion itself", and considers appraisal to be "partly accessible to introspection", but he offers no further information about this strategic step in the mechanism of emotion.

Whatever the mechanism, the emotional competent stimulus may be an external event, a memory, or a product of the imagination which may be detected even before conscious attention (Damasio 2003, p. 60). The perception of this stimulus produces "images" and "signals" that are available to specialised brain centres, such as the amygdala in the case of fear. The interaction between the emotional competent stimulus and brain physiology is described as an automated process in the fashion of a key opening a lock (Damasio 2003, p. 57).[15] For instance, the activation of the amygdala produces a fear cascade, with typical somatic changes such as increases in heart ratio, blood pressure, and respiratory frequency. This also results in a motor response (e.g. freezing or fleeing) influenced by contextual cues as well as education and culture.

Another crucial element for the mechanism of fear is Damasio's hypothesis of the "somatic marker" (Bechara and Damasio 2005). According to Damasio, dangerous events produce specific bodily changes which are "marked" as a neural imprint (a "marker"). These neural markers act as an "automated alarm signal," guiding the selection of actions that may prevent the agent from falling into dangerous situations.[16] This marking is carried out by conscious bodily changes

---

[15]This creates a problem for the appraisal process, which drops from consideration whenever the emotional competent stimulus works 'automatically' on the brain. In *Looking for Spinoza* (p. 53) Damasio states that the process that produces emotion "begins with an appraisal-evaluation phase, starting with the detection of emotional competent stimuli," suggesting that the emotional competent stimulus is selected first, but this very important step is not further discussed.

[16]"When a negative somatic marker is juxtaposed to a particular future outcome the combination functions as an alarm bell" (Damasio 1994, p. 173).

or by subconscious mechanisms.[17] The somatic markers do not make decisions, but "assist the deliberation by highlighting some options" (Damasio 1994, p. 174). Finally, Damasio states that most somatic markers are influenced by education and social cues which become associated with specific somatic states under the control of an "internal preference system" (Damasio 1994, p. 179).

Damasio's hypothesis of a "somatic marker" is riddled with conceptual problems. For a start, it is unclear how the marker system can 'sense' that a given event is potentially dangerous without falling into an infinite regress. The somatic marker is considered to be an "automated alarm signal" but it is doubtful how this automaticity works in a world with complex events. For instance, if I laugh in the midst of a fearful situation, is this event marked as 'positive' based on my behaviour, or as negative, based on the fearful context? Damasio states that previously "marked" mental images of danger are "mapped" with new images of potential danger, but the mechanism for such a comparison is not described. In other words, it is not stated which instance makes the comparisons, and on what basis, or how a 'good fit' is established. Damasio explicitly rejected the idea of a homunculus and proposed instead a "proto-self" which "participates in the process of knowledge without starting it" (Damasio 1999, p. 79). But exchanging a homunculus for a proto-self is no more than switching metaphors and does not explain how appraisal works.

Another contentious subject is that, according to Damasio, an individual who is automatically "well adapted" to social life requires "that both brain and culture be normal" (Damasio 1994, p. 177). Damasio does not clarify what he means by a "normal" brain, but he provides examples of "sick cultures." It seems that these biological and contextual factors have greater importance for decision-making than the innate mechanisms described for the primary emotions, as Damasio explains that "the automated somatic marker device of most of us *lucky enough to have been reared in a relatively healthy culture* has been accommodated

[17]This marking is achieved "quite overtly, as in a gut feeling", or "covertly, via signals occurring below the radar of our awareness…" (Damasio 1994, p. xii).

by education to the standards of rationality of that culture" (emphasis added) (Damasio 1994, p. 200).[18] Thus, having 'rational' fears is in all probability limited to a small portion of the western world with cultures that correspond to a specific type of socio-economic system with high educational and ethical standards.

7.3.3 The Concept and Mechanism of "Feelings of Emotions"

According to Damasio, feelings are perceptions of bodily and mental changes that happen while humans engage in "emoting" (Damasio 2010, p. 116).[19] More specifically, feelings are a "composite perception" of emotions and ideas with changes in the visceral and musculoskeletal state (Damasio 2010, p. 116). This perception is mediated via a "body loop" which uses humoral and neural signals to map bodily changes in specific brain regions, resulting in "*feeling of emotion maps*" (italics in original) (Damasio 2010, p. 116). Feelings of emotion may also result from changes in a putative "as-if body loop," which occurs whenever an emotion originates in the brain. This "as-if" loop creates a representation of body-related changes in "body mapping regions" of the brain to

[18]Damasio further adds that assuming "the brain is normal and the culture in which it develops is healthy, the device has been made rational relative to social convention and ethics" (Damasio 1994, p. 200). Unfortunately, Damasio does not elaborate on how contextual factors may change pre-programmed brain systems.

[19]Damasio also defines the feeling of emotions as having mental images arising from neural processes representing bodily and brain changes which "make up an emotion" (Damasio 1999, p. 282). In Damasio's neuroscientific terms feelings are "a composite perception of (1) a particular state of the body during actual or simulated emotion, and (2) a state of altered cognitive resources and a deployment of certain mental scripts" (Damasio 1999, p. 118). More specifically (but confusingly) Damasio states that "a feeling depends on the juxtaposition of an image of the body proper to an image of something else such as the visual image of a face or the auditory image of a somebody" (Damasio 1994, p. 145). Even if we manage to understand the concepts of images of the "body proper" and images of "a somebody", we are still left with the problem of how these mental entities are "juxtaposed." Damasio explains this process, stating that as the two images remain physiologically separated there is a "combination" rather than a "blending". Nevertheless, Damasio concludes that "it might be appropriate to use the term *superposition* for what seems to happen to the images of body proper and 'something else' in our integrated experience" (italics in the original) (Damasio 1994, p. 145).

reproduce the changes of actual emotions, albeit the feeling is "fainter" than the actual ones (Bechara and Damasio 2005).

The ontological position of feelings is more comprehensively elaborated in *Looking for Spinoza* (2003), but in a similarly confusing way. Damasio states that feelings result from activity in "body-sensing brain regions", emerging when "the sheer accumulation of mapped details reach a certain stage" (Damasio 2003, p. 86). In full metaphysical vein, he says that feelings of emotions "are the idea of the body being in a certain way" combined with "the perception of thoughts with themes consonant with the emotion" (Damasio 2003, p. 86). Feelings result from constructing "metarepresentations" of mental processes, in which "a part of the mind represents another part of the mind" (Damasio 2003, p. 85). Whereas the content of feelings is for Damasio the representation of the body being in a specific state, the "essence" of feelings consists of "thoughts that represent the body involved in a reactive process." According to Damasio, if this essence is removed, "the notion of feeling vanishes" (Damasio 2003, p. 67). Finally, Damasio considers feelings to be "always hidden, like all mental images necessarily are, unseen to everyone rather than their rightful owner" (Damasio 2003, p. 28). I will try to clarify some of these conceptual knots in the discussion below.

According to Damasio fear is a useful emotion, shaped by natural selection, and which works automatically, that is, in a reflex way in line with James's (original) theory.[20] Thus, if while walking home at midnight I believe I am being followed, the brain automatically triggers a cascade of biochemical and neural reactions to elicit fear (Damasio 1994, p. 226). Damasio accepts that appraisal is part of the mechanism of fear (Damasio 2003, p. 138) and that the context has an important role in the production of fear. In the case of "false alarms induced by a culture gone awry" fear may be harmful (Damasio 2010, p. 121), and fear may also become an agent of stress which may "destroy life" (Damasio 2010, p. 121). Unfortunately, he does not further explore

[20] "the emotional action program we call fear can get most human beings out of danger…*with little or no help from reason*" (Damasio 1994, p. xi) (my italics).

these important concepts, with their implications of cognitive functions beyond what can be described in terms of putative brain mechanisms alone.

In this connection Damasio also makes several strong statements concerning the signal role of science in being able to reveal the definitive mechanism of emotions and reconcile humanism with neurosciences. Supporting this view, he often cites philosophers to show that they were either conceptually wrong (e.g. Cartesian dualism) or that his own empirical studies have confirmed and even surpassed propositions from other philosophers (e.g. James and Spinoza). I have already examined major problems with Damasio's mechanism of emotions, and shall now address the main problems with Damasio's concept of emotions, with a focus on fear.

7.3.4 Problems with Damasio's Concept of Emotions

Some of the problems with Damasio's hypotheses on emotions arise from his philosophical position and are amenable to meaningful discussion, whereas others arise from his use of obscure metaphorical descriptions or his hints towards concepts and arguments that he never develops in a formal way. Perhaps the main criticism, which extends to current cognitive neuroscience, is the tendency to reduce the concept of emotions, and especially fear, to its biological underpinnings, without being able to avoid incorporating non-biological factors. Biological and scientific understanding may be relevant for the fear-conditioning that can be easily elicited in rodents in experimental conditions, but it is not clear that it is exclusively relevant for the rich, multi-layered and complex terrain of human fear, which is mostly related to psychological attributes such as emotional dispositions, beliefs and desires. Fear responses depend on the context in which they occur, the psychological attributes of the agent of the emotion, and the personal relevance of the object of fear, which may change with time and contextual events. In their tendency to extrapolate from limited empirical findings, neuroscientists of emotion, of whom Damasio is one of the most prominent, attempt to provide an encompassing epistemology of emotions like fear, drifting, often unwittingly, from their empirical world into metaphysics.[21]

Damasio commits a specific type of reduction, which Bennet and Hacker term the "mereological fallacy" (Bennett and Hacker 2003, pp. 68–70). This consists in taking a part for the whole. For Damasio, it is the brain rather than the person that feels and makes decisions; it is the brain rather than the whole person who is afraid and evaluates the best way of facing danger. The brain is obviously necessary to feel fear, but it is not sufficient, as fear also depends, as Damasio agrees, on contextual and psychological factors. Damasio reifies brain processes to the detriment of other factors such as historically changing beliefs (for example, fear of witches and the devil existed in pandemic proportions in the Middle Ages, but are much less frequent nowadays), education (for example, people educated in some religious faiths fear God, whereas this fear is absent in non-believers), and contextual events (for example, being afraid of losing one's job in the context of financial recession). Damasio makes the reductionism of his theory explicit by separating emotions from feelings based on a "research intention" without discussing the conceptual problems implicit in this artificial separation. It is striking that social communication has no role in Damasio's system of emotions. Since humans have the capacity to use language and are able to communicate their emotions and feelings, it is incorrect to say that emotions are no more than bodily changes, and that feelings are always hidden. Emotions cannot be identified in abstraction from their context, or as Wittgenstein puts it, not "what *one* man is doing *now*, but the whole hurly-burly, is the background against which we see an action, and it determines our judgements, our concepts, and our reactions" (Wittgenstein 1967) (567). Wittgenstein's philosophy of emotions provides a useful framework against which Damasio's conceptual system may be compared, and this will be addressed below.

---

[21]See Bennett and Hacker for a thorough review and discussion (Bennett and Hacker 2003).

7.3.5 Neo-Jamesians or Neo-Cartesians?

Damasio's model of emotions appears to be more sophisticated than James's, but in fact is little more than a capitulation to Cartesian dualism. For example, as discussed already, Damasio posited that emotions begin with an emotionally competent stimulus activating specific brain regions, a proposal that raises two main problems. First there is the issue of what provides the stimulus with the attribute of being "emotionally competent". James, himself, had to face the criticism that his bear would produce fear in the forest but not in the zoo. As we shall see in the next section Wittgenstein argues far more plausibly that a stimulus is made 'emotionally competent' when occurring in a pattern of life. But neither James nor Damasio have any way of incorporating this evaluative educative process into their mechanistic explanations.

The second issue is the perennial Cartesian problem of a mental entity 'resulting' from extended (brain) matter, since according to Damasio, brain activation results in a "flow of mental processes" which somehow trigger somatic changes (Damasio 2003, p. 67).[22] Damasio has frequent recourse to the language and conceptual notion of images, and the notion of brain representations permeates all of his texts. As pointed out by Bennett and Hacker, these ideas bring back all the limitations of eighteenth century empirical philosophy. Several examples suffice to illustrate this point. Damasio posits that the processing of "mental images" activates brain regions that 'contain' knowledge of emotional processes in the shape of "acquired representations" (Damasio 1994, p. 133). And later, these representations are mental images or neural patterns which render an object "with some degree of fidelity" (Damasio 1999, p. 12). These statements illustrate the confusing interweaving of mental phenomena and somatic/neural patterning that is common throughout Damasio's work.

[22]We may add statements such as "To say that the mind *comes* from the brain is indisputable" (my italics) (Damasio 1994, p. 251), and paraphrasing Descartes, "When I started musing about how the brain managed to create the mind..." (Damasio 2003, p. 4).

To be fair, and as already noted, Damasio cautions "that emergence of mental images from neuronal patterns is not a fully understood process" (Damasio 2003, p. 88), and acknowledges that "there is a major gap in our current understanding of how neural patterns become mental images" (Damasio 2003, p. 198). However, the problem is not a gap in empirical understanding, but the conceptual error of Cartesian mind/body dualism, nowadays transformed into mind/brain dualism. Damasio's dualism is even more evident in statements such as his claim that whereas neural patterns are studied with the tools of neurophysiology, mental images are described with the tools of introspection (Damasio 2003, p. 198). While Damasio seems to reject dualism stating that "neural patterns *are* simultaneously mental images" (italics in the original), he also postulates a "self" who becomes aware of mental images (Damasio 2010, p. 16). But Damasio seems to be confused by his own language. First, the 'emergence' of ethereal (mental) images from brain matter is a metaphor and therefore should not be reified to explain psychological phenomena; second, there is no gap in understanding mental events but straightforward conceptual confusion as a result of dualistic thinking; and third, 'introspection' is an expression used to refer to the act of reflecting (for example, about how we feel) but not the searching and inspecting of images in the mind. In *Descartes' Error* (Damasio 1994), Damasio explicitly rejects dualism, embracing instead a kind of neutral monism (i.e. mental and neural processes are understood as two aspects of the same entity). However, most of Damasio's accounts of mind/brain interaction are clear instances of Cartesian dualism, with mental images *arising* from neural patterns (Damasio 1999, p. 282), neural patterns *resulting* from bodily changes, and feelings that "emerge…provided neural patterns *become* mental images" (italics added) (Damasio 1999, pp. 79–80). As already noted, in *Looking for Spinoza* Damasio also acknowledges that his theory of emotions implies a separation of mind and brain, but rather than addressing the major implications of his philosophical statement, he makes the astonishing remark that "maintaining this mind/brain gap is a matter of intellectual hygiene" (Damasio 2003, p. 198).

What Damasio refuses to accept is that explaining emotions is not simply a scientific problem, but goes to what is fully human, meaning drenched and philosophically significant phenomena. It might be said that there is a need for some philosophical therapy for Damasio's conceptual confusions. In what follows I shall use the work of Wittgenstein to provide it.

7.4 Wittgenstein's Concept of Fear

James approached emotions in a scientific way, proposing, initially at least, a reflex model that reduced emotions to a concept amenable to empirical refutation. He was a philosopher and scientist who hoped that science would eventually solve the riddle of human psychological phenomena. It is not surprising, then, that cognitive neuroscience, as exemplified by Damasio's work, adopts James's reductionism with some adaptations. As might be gleaned from his criticisms of James, Wittgenstein's concept of emotions, and fear in particular, could not be more different, as, unlike Descartes, James and Damasio, with their bear paradigm, he expanded the semantic field of fear by showing how this concept is used in multiple different ways in everyday life. Wittgenstein coined the term 'language game' to refer to the different connotations of words, like 'fear', when in common use. I will therefore explain the meaning of 'language game' using a pivotal example of fear in Wittgenstein's *Philosophical Investigations* (PI; II. ix, 160e):

> Are the words "I am afraid" a description of a state of mind?
> I say "I am afraid": someone else asks me: "What was that? A cry of fear, or do you want to tell me how you feel; or is it a reflection on your present state?"—Could I always give him a clear answer? Could I never give him one?
> We can imagine all sorts of things here, for example:
> "No, no! I am afraid!"
> "I am afraid, I am sorry to have to confess it."
> "I am still a bit afraid, but no longer so much as before."
> "At bottom I am still afraid, though I won't confess it to myself."
> "I torment myself with all sorts of fears."
> "Now, just when I should be fearless, I am afraid!"

> To each of these sentences a special tone of voice is appropriate, and a different context.
> It would be possible to imagine people who as it were thought much more definitely than we, and used different words when we use only one.
> We ask: "What does 'I am frightened' really mean, what I am referring to when I say it?" And of course we find no answer, or one that is inadequate. The question is: "In what sort of context does it occur?"

And following on from this (PI, II, ix 161e):

> What is fear? What does "being afraid" mean? If I wanted to define it at a *single* shewing – I should *play-act* fear.

Wittgenstein illustrates in the above examples that fear is a broad-ranging construct which can be used in a variety of ways. Canfield (2009) suggests that the question "what is fear?", as raised by Wittgenstein above, has no generic answer but requires a detailed investigation of the 'language game' for the term 'fear', as described below.

7.4.1 The Semantic Field of 'Fear' and Its 'Language Games'

Wittgenstein's term 'language game' refers to his understanding that words have no single connotation, but may be used in different ways to provide different meanings (Glock 1996). The meaning of a word is its use in the stream of life and as a consequence, "it is part of an activity, a form of life" (Wittgenstein 2001) (23) as reflected in the overall practice of a linguistic community.[23] There is no unique meaning of 'being afraid', and understanding its sense requires a description of the context in which fear arises, awareness of danger, and spontaneous reactions.

[23]"A language game [consists] of language and the actions in which it is woven" (Wittgenstein 2001) (PI 7); and the concept is used "to bring into prominence the fact that the speaking of language is part of an activity, or a form of life" (Wittgenstein 2001; 23).

The remarks in *Philosophical Investigations* 160e, quoted above, illustrate how fear can be manifested in multiple ways, from a simple cry to complex verbal expressions. A cry of fear, itself, has multiple connotations, such as being an instinctive response to a fearful object, for example, or a request for protection, a call of alert about a danger; or an expression of a mental state that can no longer be endured. A cry may be produced by a relatively simple brain mechanism, and yet its meaning is a constitutive manifestation of fear which can only be understood against a backdrop of life events including the crier's beliefs, desires and characteristic emotional disposition. As Wittgenstein remarks, "the background is the bustle of life. And our concept points to something within this bustle" (Wittgenstein 1980b; 625).

What about the *verbal* remarks provided in PI 160e? Shouting "I am afraid!" may just be the oral manifestation of a primitive cry or a way to communicate how I feel. Sometimes after honest reflection, I may admit to myself that my behaviour was motivated by fear, and I may feel relieved after confessing this emotion to others. The semantic complexity of fear is further illustrated in PI 160e with some additional examples. I may insist my interlocutors that, against their opinion, I *do* feel fear, or that perhaps they have to insist that, even though I don't want to recognise it, I *do* feel fear. In this language game the beliefs of agent and interlocutor as well as their interaction are of the essence.

The remark "I am still a bit afraid, but no longer so much as before" provides an example of the importance of context and personal history as fear changes in intensity. The agent feels relieved as fear lessens; she/he may even feel happy about this change, an example that emotions do not occur in isolation but blend with one another, as discussed before. In this example, the agent is very aware about her/his fear, whereas in the next example (i.e. "At bottom I am still afraid, though I won't confess it to myself") the opposite is the case, as the agent discovers she/he wants to hide this emotion from herself/himself. Perhaps the agent suffered great fears in the past, and is now afraid of a relapse. This is not to say that fear was until now 'non-conscious,' but just to acknowledge that the person is fighting an emotion which can no longer be covered up.

The next example (i.e. "I torment myself with all sorts of fears") is of an individual whose fears may be considered 'pathological' if by this term we mean a persistently negative feeling that is not under voluntary control. This raises the interesting question of the threshold at which we consider that fear becomes pathological, which, in turn, opens a new language game relating to what determines whether an emotion is considered abnormal and how this determination is accomplished (see Chapter 9).[24] To this end, we may need more information, such as the duration of the tormenting fears and the context in which they arise.[25] The characteristics of fear become less relevant, as what is now important is the personality of the agent, and her/his tendency to be tormented and even incapacitated by feelings. In any case, the agent has been suffering with fears, unlike the next example (i.e. "Now, just when I should be fearless, I am afraid!"), where the agent is surprised to notice that fears are still present. This awareness may go with disappointment, sadness or even angry feelings, another example of how differing emotions become enmeshed.

By use of these examples Wittgenstein shows how complex the meanings of fear are, given the many different language games in which the term is used. Wittgenstein is interested in the praxis of fear, which gets its meaning when used in the "hurly-burly" of human life. This is a far cry from Damasio's "key opening a lock" system, where the key is both the object and the cause of fear. In Damasio's universe where the focus is on accounting for the physiology of emotions, beliefs and emotional dispositions play only a minor role as the substrate of fear and the meanings of specific fears in a person's life are not taken to be central to the mechanism, and perhaps to their therapy. Further, fear is not always experienced in a prototypical way, amenable to be reduced to feelings in restricted contexts; rather, as Wittgenstein shows, it is a nuanced emotion with a diversity of meanings. Therefore, it is not surprising that

[24]Wittgenstein (1980b; 614): "Sufficient evidence passes over into insufficient without a borderline."

[25]Wittgenstein (1980b; 624): "We judge an actor according to its (sic) background within human life, and this background is not monochrome, but we might picture it as a very complicated filigree pattern…"

Wittgenstein is unable to verbalise *the* meaning of fear and would rather "play-act" this emotion in the variety of contexts in which it arises. For instance, he may use the facial expression and the bodily demeanour of somebody who is in a state of terror (Wittgenstein 2001; 161e). But this is just a caricature of fear, whereas the 'true' experience of fear is the one that happens in life.

Fear is a dynamic emotion, changing in quality and intensity. Fear may explain our behaviour even when we explicitly deny acting under its influence (an illustration that, on occasions, behaviours may be more reliable than words). We may suffer from a disposition to feel fear (as in having an anxious personality) in which case the object of fear is of minor relevance. We may find that fear does not always have the expected duration as occurs when we get used to an object of fear, or we may drag our fear along with us even after its object has dissipated. Fear may not only explain how we feel, but may also explain our past behaviours, our current actions, and our future plans. For each of these variegated situations the language game of fear is engaged and Damasio's focus on explaining fear mostly based on describing brain processes, rather than recognising its meaning and meaningful implications in our lives, is quite inadequate to the task of understanding the import of the emotion and searching for useful therapies.

7.4.2 Family Resemblance

Wittgenstein rejects the idea of 'essentialism', which is the view that objects falling under a particular category, for example the category of fear, share necessary and sufficient conditions to belong to the category (Odeberg 2007, p. 18). Rather, he argues that the objects to which any particular word refers do not share a common essence but instead exhibit a "family resemblance," whereby objects designated by a particular term or concept are not united by a single defining feature but by "a complex network of overlapping and criss-crossing similarities" (Glock 1996, p. 121).

The concept of fear includes an extensive net of 'objects' or experiences as we can see in the list of examples quoted above. In addition, it is possible to see why it is impossible to categorically distinguish fear from other terms such as terror, fright, horror, alarm, panic, agitation, trepidation, dread, consternation, dismay, distress, anxiety, worry, angst, unease, apprehension, nervousness, timidity, disquietude, unrest, foreboding, doubt, and suspicion, since the emotions that fall under each of these categories are not united by a single defining feature, either. Each may share in part some features in common with the family resemblance characteristics that unite the variety of emotions commonly termed fear. An interesting example is the word 'anxiety', which Wittgenstein, like Kierkegaard (see Chapter 9), considers to indicate undirected fear (that is, fear with no discernible object) "in so far as its manifestations resemble or are the same as those of fear" (Wittgenstein 1980b; 724). For instance, anxiety may be manifest in a bodily demeanour similar to fear. But if the anxiety is about soon starting my holidays, this use of the term 'anxiety' is quite different from the use of 'fear' in the directed way Wittgenstein refers above, as this anxiety no longer has the negative connotation of fear, but indicates a positive expectation. This explains why Wittgenstein suggests "comparing fear and anxiety with care", since fear always seems to have a negative connotation, whereas anxiety, may have either a positive or a negative one (Wittgenstein 1980b; 731).

7.4.3 Fear Is Not Hidden

Wittgenstein considered that words acquire meaning when shared in public use (Sluga 2006). If he is right, Damasio's suggestion that feelings are "always hidden" is incorrect, because hidden feelings cannot provide a shared basis for understanding the meaning of the concept. Wittgenstein reveals another problem with "hidden feelings" relating to the epistemological question as to how emotional words are learnt. This issue is illustrated by Wittgenstein's famous remark concerning the "beetle in the box" (Wittgenstein 2001; 293).[26]

[26]The 'beetle in the box' example provides a conceptual argument against the validity of introspection for the identification of emotions. Language is a public practice, and the expression of

> If I say of myself that it is only from my own case that I know what the word "pain" means—must I not say the same of other people too? And how can I generalize the *one* case so irresponsibly?
>
> Now someone tells me that *he* knows what pain is only from his own case!—Suppose everyone had a box with something in it: we call it a "beetle". No one can look into anyone else's box, and everyone says he knows what a beetle is only by looking at *his* beetle. —Here it would be quite possible for everyone to have something different in his box. One might even imagine such a thing constantly changing. —But suppose the word "beetle" had a use in these people's language? —If so it would not be used as the name of a thing. The thing in the box has no place in the language-game at all; not even as a *something:* for the box might even be empty. —No, one can 'divide through' by the thing in the box; it cancels out, whatever it is.
>
> That is to say: if we construe the grammar of the expression of sensation on the model of 'object and designation' the object drops out of consideration as irrelevant.

In this example, the name 'beetle' is given to an object (whatever it is) in each person's box. If the object in every box is different no one could know it, since the world beetle that I use to denote whatever is in my box is dissociated from the public concept of the term 'beetle' (Hacker 1990, p. 111). Therefore, if a feeling is treated like a private object (e.g. the beetle in my box), nobody would understand it, as each person would have their own idiosyncratic concept of the term. We learn the names of feelings and emotions through public language and not through introspection of private objects.[27]

According to Wittgenstein, there is no feeling of fear which is independent of its 'external' expression, since this expression is 'constitutive' of fear. Fear is constituted by both 'inner' feelings and 'outer' behaviours.

emotions such as fear creates the rule for using the word 'fear' in public communication (Hacker 1990, p. 111).

[27]If the grammar of feeling and emotion is construed as an internal object which is given a name, then "the object drops out of consideration as irrelevant" (Wittgenstein 2001; 293), that is, whatever word I decide to use, is only valid to me.

Damasio's hypothesis that 'hidden feelings' may be examined by using introspection is a misconception with roots in the Cartesian concept of a body which is amenable to public examination and a 'private' mind which only the agent can access. On the other hand, and based on this hypothesis, since feelings are by definition always hidden, an individual can only surmise what others feel based on their 'outer' behaviour, which may manifest those feelings. Wittgenstein's conceptual change was to invert the 'first person/third person' privacy argument. Since a person cannot be wrong about what she/he feels, he explains, that person cannot be right either. Hence, there is no sense to talking of knowledge in the case of first person feelings.[28] Access to one's feelings is direct and does not require inference. On the other hand, a person may fail in correctly identifying the feelings of others, as the others may just pretend to feel a given emotion. But the possibility of making mistakes assumes that our assumptions are correct most of the time.

Before finishing this section, an important caveat requires discussion. So far, I have quoted Wittgenstein using his tempting aphoristic remarks, which seem to imply that for the praxis of fear, public criteria may be sufficient for using this concept. However, the understanding of a given outward expression is not sufficient for the formation of the concept of fear, as can be observed in the cases of non-human animals and infants that may be subject to this emotion without having acquired the concept of fear. Concepts with a strong somatic component such as fear are not fully determined by culture and social conventions, since fear is also manifested by non-linguistic natural facts, such as instinctive feelings and behaviours. This was also recognised by Wittgenstein, who remarked that beliefs or concepts are "held fast by what lies around [them]" (Wittgenstein 1969) (144) and by our "interpretation of experience" (145). It is what lies around a concept as well as the way the object of experience is tied in nature to human behaviour what makes a given concept such as fear a non-arbitrary one, in other

[28] I may use the expression "I know I have fear!" just to appease my interlocutor in her insistence, but this use of the first person is not epistemological but social.

words, a concept not solely depending on language but also on natural facts such as non-linguistic feelings and instinctive manifestations (Dilman 2002; Racine and Slaney 2013).

In conclusion, when a person says, 'I am afraid' that person is expressing the emotion directly rather than describing an object of introspection (that is, an "inner" fear), and this can be neither correct nor incorrect. On the other hand, to identify the emotion in others we have to consider not only their behavioural expression, but the context and the history of their verbal and non-verbal exchanges as well.

7.5 Concluding Remarks

The previous chapter discussed how Descartes started a new tradition in the understanding of emotions, explaining them in mechanistic and dualistic terms. According to Descartes, fear is a behavioural response to a dangerous object produced by a flux of spirits to the brain and muscles, as well as an emotion in the soul produced by specific movements of the pineal gland. William James continued with the Cartesian tradition of explaining emotions as the result of physiological changes. In his view, fear is the feeling of somatic changes such as increased heart rate, shallow breathing, tremor, and visceral motions. The prominence of physiological changes as a relevant component of the mechanism of emotions in James's theory allowed the empirical examination of emotions in contemporary neuroscience. Damasio followed in the steps of James by proposing that emotions are neural representations of somatic changes which are structured in specific programs that activate external behaviour or internal (visceral and hormonal) changes. Whereas Descartes reduced fear to movements of the pineal gland and James to the perception of somatic changes, Damasio reduced fear to an emotional system, mediated by so-called 'somatic markers', which results in mental images of putative bodily states produced by neural representations. Once the amygdala is stimulated in this fashion, the behavioural 'cascade' of fear ensues.

While Cartesian dualism is strongly rejected, Damasio proposes that emotions consist in a mysterious mechanism by which feelings are produced through the transformation of neural patterns into mental images. The conceptual import of these kinds of statements is easily dismissed by Damasio when he (wrongly) insists that these (conceptual) 'hiccups' will be solved by further empirical study. Thus, what started as an understandable theory based on empirical studies, ends up in full, if implicit, metaphysical speculation. These criticisms, however, should not be construed as completely undermining the physiological study of fear, given that empirical discoveries may help in improving the situations of individuals struggling with severe fear and anxiety. Nevertheless, solid scientific work in the field of fear risks highly problematic overreach without clear concepts.

Conceptual clarifications were brought by Wittgenstein, who provided enlightening criticism to the Cartesian and Jamesian approach to the emotions that may be of use for current neuroscientists like Damasio. Rather than reducing fear to body-soul (or more simply even to internal brain) interactions, Wittgenstein stressed the many ways in which fear can be understood in our lives, as fear, like other emotions, has no essential or necessary features. Thus, the 'language game' of fear includes various mental states and behaviours ranging from simple cries to delicate confessions, with fear sometimes mixed with other emotions such as frustration and joy, and against a backdrop of specific contexts, personalities and biographies. Accordingly, fear is no longer reduced to a cybernetic mechanism, but becomes an important thread in the human 'forms of life', dynamically changing in quality and intensity, and a major determinant of behaviour.

In conclusion, since the end of the twentieth century, emotions, and especially fear, have been the subject of intense scientific research. This has resulted in increased knowledge of the brain systems engaged in very specific fear behaviours in non-human animals. However, when these findings are extrapolated to humans, without understanding the limitations of experimental conditions, or when experimental findings in humans are used to explain the concept of fear at large, important problems arise. This occurs when Damasio moves from explaining interesting research findings to reducing fear to putative visual images, somatic markers and metarepresentations. Wittgenstein, on the other hand, put the emotions back on the philosophical agenda as "it is…perfectly possible that certain psychological phenomena cannot be investigated physiologically, because physiologically nothing corresponds to them" (Wittgenstein 1980a) (904), or at least, physiology may explain only partially the conceptual network of fear. Furthermore, Wittgenstein advanced the method of conceptual analysis, a critical philosophical tool to dispel the conceptual confusions of empirical studies.

It can be seen that the conceptual problems brought about by dualism and reductionism are a major obstacle for the empirical study of emotions (Bennett and Hacker 2003). I have discussed in this chapter how the dualist strategy to account for the emotions, begun by Descartes and continued in more recent times by James and Damasio, has major *conceptual* problems that invalidate their model. On the other hand, the strong reductionist approach to the *empirical* study of fear in the field of current neurosciences ignores the richness and complexity of this emotion and its diffuse connections with, rather than definite demarcation from, other emotions with which it shares a 'family resemblance.' As I discuss in the next two chapters, this narrow approach has strongly influenced clinical practice for more than a century, with a potentially negative impact upon therapeutic progress.

Reductionism is manifest in another twist in the history of the thinking about the concept of fear during this time that is also worthy of attention. Between James's publication of *What is an Emotion* in 1884 and Wittgenstein's publication of the *Philosophical Investigations* in 1953, a major revolution occurred in medicine. Sigmund Freud, the father of psychoanalysis, published *Inhibitions, Symptoms and Anxiety* (1926), in which he presented a conceptualization of fear and anxiety based on psychodynamic theories. This work not only changed the philosophical concept of fear and anxiety but had a great impact on the medicalization and treatment of these emotions. This development will be the focus of the next chapter.

References

Barbalet, J. M. (1999). William James' theory of emotions: Filling in the picture. *Journal for the Theory of Social Behaviour, 29*(3), 251–266.

Bechara, A., & Damasio, A. R. (2005). The somatic marker hypothesis: A neural theory of economic decision. *Games and Economic Behavior, 52*, 336–372.

Bennett, M. R., & Hacker, P. M. S. (2003). *Philosophical foundations of neuroscience*. Malden MA: Blackwell.

Berrios, G. (1996). *The history of mental symptoms: Descriptive psychopathology since the nineteenth century*. Cambridge: Cambridge University Press.

Canfield, J. V. (2009). The self and the emotions. In Y. Gustafsson, C. Kronqvist, & M. McEachrane (Eds.), *Emotions and understanding: Wittgenstenian perspectives*. London: Palgrave Macmillan.

Canon, W. (1927). The James-Lange theory of emotions: A critical examination and an alternative theory. *The American Journal of Psychology, 39*, 106–124.

Churchland, P. (1989). *Neurophilosophy: Toward a unified science of the mind-brain*. Cambridge, MA: The MIT Press.

Dagleish, T. (2004). The emotional brain. *Nature Reviews Neuroscience, 5*(7), 583–589.

Damasio, A. R. (1994). *Descartes' error: Emotion, reason, and the human brain*. New York: Penguin.

Damasio, A. R. (1999). *The feelings of what happens: Body and emotion in the making of consciousness*. Orlando: Harcourt Inc.

Damasio, A. R. (2003). *Looking for Spinoza: Joy, sorrow, and the feeling brain*. Orlando: Harcourt Inc.

Damasio, A. R. (2010). *Self comes to mind*. Toronto: Random House.

Damasio, A. R., & Carvalho, G. B. (2013). The nature of feelings: Evolutionary and neurobiological origins. *Nature Reviews Neuroscience, 14*, 143–152.

Debiec, J., & LeDoux, J. (2004). Fear and the brain. *Social Research, 71*(4), 807–818.

Dilman, I. (2002). *Wittgenstein's copernican revolution: The question of linguistic idealism*. Hampshire, UK: Palgrave.

Dixon, T. (2012). "Emotion": The history of a keyword in crisis. *Emotion Review, 4*(4), 338–344.

Ellsworth, P. C. (1994). William James and emotion: Is a century of fame worth a centiry of misunderstanding? *Psychological Review, 10*(2), 222–229.

Glock, H. J. (1996). *A Wittgenstein dictionary*. Cambridge, MA: Blackwell Publishers.

Hacker, P. M. S. (1990). *Wittgenstein: Meaning and mind* (Vol. 3). Oxford: Blackwell Publishers.

Hacker, P. M. S. (2001). *Wittgenstein: Connections and controversies*. Oxford: Oxfor University Press.

James, S. (1999). *Passion and action: The emotions in seventeenth-century philosophy*. Oxford: Clarendon Press.

James, W. (1888). What is an emotion? *Mind, 9*(34), 188–205.

James, W. (1890). *The principles of psychology*. New York: H. Holt.

James, W. (1994). The physical basis of emotion. *Psychological Review, 101*(2), 205–210.

Kassler, J. C. (1998). Restraining the passions: Hydropneumatics and hierarchy in the philosophy of Thomas Willis. In S. Gaukroger (Ed.), *The soft underbelly of reason* (pp. 147–164). Oxford: Routledge.

Kenny, A. (2003). *Action, emotion and will.* New York: Routledge & Kegan Paul.

Laird, J. D., & Lacasse, K. (2014). Bodily influences on emotional feelings: Accumulating evidence and extensions of William James's theory of emotions. *Emotion Review, 6*(1), 27–34.

LeDoux, J. E. (2000). Emotion circuits in the brain. *Annual Review of Neurosciences, 23,* 155–184.

LeDoux, J. E. (2013). The slippery slope of fear. *Trends in Cognitice Sciences, 17*(4), 155–157.

Monk, R. (1991). *Ludwig Wittgenstein: The duty of genius*. London: Penguin.

Northoff, G. (2016). *Neuro-philosophy and the healthy mind.* New York: W.W. Norton and Company.

Odeberg, D. S. (2007). *Real essentialism*. New York: Routledge.

Panksepp, J. (2004). *Affective neuroscience: The foundation of human and animal emotions*. Oxford: Oxford University Press.

Racine, T. P., & Slaney, K. L. (2013). *A Wittgenstenian perspective on the use of conceptual analysis in psychology* (T. P. Racine & K. L. Slaney Eds.). Hampshire, UK: Palgrave Macmillan.

Reisenzein, R., & Achim, S. (2014). More on James and the physical basis of emotion. *Emotion Review, 6*(1), 35–46.

Schiller, D., Levy, I., Niv, Y., LeDoux, J. E., & Phelps, E. A. (2008). From fear to safety and back: Reversal of fear in the human brain. *The Journal of Neuroscience, 28*(45), 11517–11525.

Sluga, H. (2006). Family resemblance. *Gratzer Philosophische Studien, 71,* 1–21.

Ter Hark, M. (2001). *Beyond the inner and the outer: Wittgenstein's philosophy and psychology*. Dordrecht: Kluver Academic Publishers.

Wassmann, C. (2014). "Picturesque incisiveness": Explaining the celebrity of James's theory of emotion. *Journal of the History of the Behavioral Sciences, 50*(2), 166–188.

Wickens, A. P. (2014). *A history of the brain: From stone age surgery to modern neuroscience*. London: Taylor and Francis.
Williams, R. N., & Robinson, D. N. (2014). *Scientism: The new orthodoxy*. London: Bloomsbury Academic.
Willis, T. (1672). *De anima brutorum*. Oxford: Dates.
Wittgenstein, L. (1967). *Zettel* (G. E. M. Anscombe, Trans.). Oxford: Blackwell.
Wittgenstein, L. (1969). *On certainty* (G. E. M. Anscombe & G. H. Von Wright Eds.). New York: Harper Torchbooks.
Wittgenstein, L. (1980a). *Remarks on the philosophy of psychology* (G. E. M. Anscombe, Trans. Vol. 1). Oxford: Blackwell.
Wittgenstein, L. (1980b). *Remarks on the philosophy of psychology* (G. E. M. Anscombe, Trans. Vol. 2). Oxford: Blackwell.
Wittgenstein, L. (2001). *Philosophical investigations* (G. E. M. Anscombe, Trans.). Oxford: Blackwell.
Wundt, W. (2014). *An introduction to psychology* (R. Pintner, Trans.). USA: Blank Spots Publishing.

8

Sigmund Freud and the Psychoanalytical Concept of Fear and Anxiety

Anxiety is not so simple a matter.

Sigmund Freud, *Inhibition Symptom and Anxiety* (Freud 1953–1975a, p. 132)

The problem of fear is the meeting point of many important questions, an enigma whose complete solution would be as a flood of light upon psychic life.

Sigmund Freud, *Fear and Anxiety* (Freud 1953–1975d, p. 340)

8.1 Introduction

In the last chapter I discussed how the Cartesian model of fear, based on a hydrodynamic mechanism, was continued by William James and his hypothesis that fear is the result of a neurological reflex arc with no cognitive intervention. Even though James himself revised this model and despite the strong conceptual challenges proposed by Wittgenstein, the model of fear has continued to be developed in mostly biological terms by the current field of the cognitive neurosciences.

By the time William James was publishing his *Principles of Psychology* and Wittgenstein was beginning his philosophical writings, psychiatrists

S. Starkstein, *A Conceptual and Therapeutic Analysis of Fear*,
https://doi.org/10.1007/978-3-319-78349-9_8

and neurologists were dealing with psychosomatic complaints that were affecting increasing numbers of the upper classes in Europe and America. Physicians, specialized in 'nervousness' used a variety of treatments ranging from hypnosis to long admissions to specialized spas (Shorter 1992, p. 233). It is in this social and medical context that by the beginning of the twentieth century psychoanalysis had taken psychiatry by storm. Sigmund Freud (1856–1939) became one of the main referents for the field of mental disorders and their treatment, with his development of a revolutionary conceptual framework and a novel therapeutic technique.[1] Despite the influence of James, many psychiatrists ceased looking into the brain for responses to the riddle of emotional problems, and adopted the Freudian framework in which fear and anxiety play a central role. A whole new set of psychological concepts (Freud's "metapsychology") was created, not only to explain the phenomenon of anxiety, but to provide theoretical support for psychoanalysis as a therapeutic technique as well. The influence of psychoanalysis also extended beyond medicine to influence diverse areas of human knowledge including philosophy, sociology, the arts, and psychology (Leavy 2010). Consequently, analysis and discussion of Freudian texts is of great relevance for this investigation of the concept of fear.

This chapter will examine the principal Freudian concepts of fear and its pathology.[2] I do not pretend to provide an exhaustive analysis of

[1]Rollo May refers to Freud as "a giant who, like Marx and Einstein…set the tone for vast changes on our culture" (May 1996, p. 132). He further considered Freud as "the preeminent explorer of the psychology of anxiety…and provided understanding to both the mechanism and therapy" (p. 134).

[2]Freud, like Kierkegaard and Heidegger, defined anxiety (*Angst* in the original German) as objectless fear, but he used the terms fear (*Furcht* in the original German) and anxiety interchangeably in his discussion of clinical examples and in his theoretical discussions. For instance, he used the term "anxiety neurosis" in his early writings, switching to "neurotic fear" to denote similar concepts in later texts. In the Appendix to *On the Grounds* (Freud 1953–1975c, p. 116), James Strachey, the book's translator, noted the overlapping connotations of the German words *Angst*, *Furcht* and *Schreck*, and considered that Freud was unable to provide a convincing technical connotation for Angst as distinguished with related terms (Freud 1953–1975c, p. 116). Furthermore, Strachey considered that *Angst* could be translated into English as 'fear', 'fright', 'alarm' and other related terms, and regards as "unfortunate" the translation of *Angst* as anxiety, a noun he considered to have only a "remote connection" with the German *Angst*. *Angst* is usually translated as

Freud's texts on fear and related conditions such as anxiety and neurosis, but only to present his major hypotheses on their causes along with a critical discussion of them. I will also address, albeit briefly, Freud's suggestions on the therapy for 'anxiety neurosis', a term and therapy created for and employed on a variety of extreme fears.[3]

8.2 Freud, Fear and Anxiety

By the beginning of the twentieth century, studies on the emotions were being pursued by philosophers and practitioners in the young sciences of psychology and sociology. In parallel, a rather dramatic change was taking place in the practice of psychiatry and neurology in America and Northern Europe, with strong social repercussions (Gay 1988, p. 593). This change had started by the end of the nineteenth century, when the American neurologist George Miller Beard published influential articles and books on "neurasthenia", a term used to refer to a variety of psychosomatic symptoms such as fatigue, anxiety, weakness, dizziness, fainting, headaches, neuralgias and depressed mood (Beard 1881). Physicians in large cities of the western hemisphere were treating an increasing number of individuals whose main complaint was the presence of 'nervousness' impacting on their daily lives. Nervousness was manifest as somatic symptoms and various fears, such as fear of illness ('valetudinarianism' or 'hypochondriasis'), fear of unemployment, and fear of impending war, and as a result of these developments the terms

anguish in both Spanish (*angustia*) and French (*angoisse*), and this significant problem in translation has been addressed by German Berrios (1996, p. 265). In Freud's work, fear and anxiety are conceptually distinguished when, for instance, for some people being in a train produces fear, whereas thinking about travelling by train produces anxiety. However, as one commentator on Freud's work on anxiety states "at present, it can be said there is no consensus on the difference between fear and anxiety" (Nersessian 2013, p. 180).

[3]Interestingly, Freudian writings on anxiety have, to my knowledge, never been the subject of philosophical scrutiny from a conceptual point of view.

'anxiety', used in an inclusive sense incorporating a variety of fears, and 'neurosis' become of common use in the twentieth century (Berrios 1999). Both terms are combined by Freud into the novel syndrome of 'anxiety neurosis', a term with strong clinical implications but, as I shall argue, with major conceptual problems.

8.3 Freud's *Angstneurose*

The Freudian analysis of fear and anxiety is classically presented in two chronologically separated conceptual systems, the first published as *On the grounds for detaching a particular syndrome from neurasthenia under the description 'Anxiety Neurosis' [Angstneurose]* (*On the Grounds*) (Freud 1953–1975c) in 1895, and the second published as *Inhibition, Symptoms and Anxiety* in 1926. In his early work, Freud acknowledged the clinical relevance of Beard's concept of neurasthenia, a term he continued to use. *On the Grounds* had two principal aims. The first was to distinguish from Beard's broad description of neurasthenia a new syndrome with a specific phenomenology and aetiology that Freud termed "anxiety neurosis" (*Angstneurose*); and the second, to demonstrate the importance of sexual impulses on the mechanism of human fear and anxiety.

Freud was successful in advancing the clinical syndromes of anxiety and fear that are still found in main psychiatric nomenclatures, but he failed to demonstrate the influence of putative sexual forces underlying the pathology of fear. In the following analysis of *On the Grounds*, I shall argue that Freud did not open new ground with his theory of human fear, but instead followed the Cartesian concept of emotions on two accounts: first, he followed Descartes's hydraulic explanation of the mechanism of fear, although now replaced with a more modern 'pneumatic' system. Secondly, Freud fully abided by Cartesian dualism in his two theories on the mechanism of fear and anxiety. I shall also argue that Freud never justified his hypothesis of the sexual origin of anxiety, and that he also failed to suggest any conceptually sound therapeutic approach to this condition.

8.3.1 Phenomenology of Neurotic Anxiety

Freud was a shrewd observer and provided excellent clinical descriptions of a variety of symptoms which he subsumed under the umbrella syndrome, anxiety neurosis. The main symptoms are briefly presented, as they are relevant to the understanding to his first theory of anxiety neurosis:

1. *General irritability*: This is a generic symptom, seen in a variety of anxious states. Freud considered general irritability as being "invariably" present in neurotic anxiety, and, according to Freud, the theoretical relevance of this symptom is that it "points" to an accumulation of sexual excitation (Freud 1953–1975c, p. 92).
2. *Anxious expectation*: Rather than providing a working definition, Freud illustrated this symptom with clinical examples. Thus "...a woman...who suffers from anxious expectation will think of influenza pneumonia every time her husband coughs...and, in her mind's eye, will see his funeral go past" (Freud 1953–1975c, p. 92). Anxious expectation is present in "normal anxiety",[4] and in "hypochondria," mostly featuring vague somatic complains. Another expression of anxious expectation is "moral anxiety," described as "exaggerated scrupulousness and pedantry" (Freud 1953–1975c, p. 93). Freud considered anxious expectation as the main symptom of anxiety neurosis, and speculated that somatic energy freely available to engage with an object of potential worry is the main mechanism of this anxiety (Freud 1953–1975c, p. 93). This symptom is the precursor of his later description of 'free-floating anxiety.'
3. *Anxiety attacks*: These attacks may consist of either somatic symptoms (e.g. "spasms of the heart", "difficulty in breathing", "sweating"), or psychological symptoms such as the idea of imminent death, having an acute illness, or going crazy (Freud 1953–1975c, p. 93). These symptoms may also present in mixed patterns, as "rudimentary

[4]Freud describes "normal anxiety" as having the connotation of "anxiousness" or the "tendency to take a pessimistic view of things" (Freud 1953–1975c, p. 93).

anxiety attacks" or as "equivalents of anxiety attacks" (i.e. somatic symptoms only) with vertigo being "among the gravest symptom of neurosis" (Freud 1953–1975c, p. 96).[5]

Freud's phenomenological descriptions were not original (Berrios 1999), but consolidating the above symptoms into a single syndrome proved to have a strong influence in psychiatry, as several of these descriptions are still extant. For instance, irritability is a symptom of Generalized Anxiety Disorder; anxious expectation is the precursor of the current syndrome of anticipatory anxiety, and the same is true for Freud's "anxiety attacks" and the current condition of "panic attacks" (American Psychiatric Association 1994). Freud describes phobias as the presence of anxious expectation combined with anxiety attacks. He described two "types" of typical phobia: first, a fear of "general physiological dangers" related to anxious expectation; and second, "phobias of locomotion" during anxiety attacks (Freud 1953–1975c, p. 96). These attacks of fear increase the human natural aversion to real threats (e.g. "a thunderstorm in the open"). According to Freud, locomotion phobias (which include agoraphobia) are usually preceded by attacks of vertigo, especially when the individual is in an inducing context (e.g. walking along a narrow street).

In conclusion, it might be said that Freud followed the zeitgeist of his times as many practitioners were unhappy with the concept of neurasthenia given the lack of specificity of this construct (Berrios 1999). In *On the Grounds* we see a young Freud devoted to clarifying clinical issues, providing nosological descriptions based on clinical experience. From a conceptual perspective, the most interesting material is Freud's theory on the mechanism of the pathologies of fear.

[5]Freud was following a consolidated tradition in psychiatry of linking anxiety to somatic disorders (Berrios 1999). Freud's listing of anxiety attacks includes the forms of (1) disturbances of the heart, (2) disturbances of respiration, (3) attacks of sweating, (4) attacks of tremor and shivering, (5) attacks of ravenous hunger, (6) attacks of diarrhoea, (7) attacks of vertigo, (8) attacks of congestion (vasomotor neurasthenia), and (9) attacks of paraesthesias.

8.3.2 The Mechanism of Anxiety Neurosis

Freud's first model for anxiety deserves close examination given this is an example of the persistence, in the late nineteenth century, of Descartes's system of emotions, with the crucial addition in Freud's theory of sexual forces underlying *all* cases of anxiety. Another novelty is Freud's inclusion of a homeostatic system of biological forces based on Fechner's biological principle of constancy (Ellenberger 1956), the theory that humans are naturally "striving to maintain excitation at a comfortable level." Freud's theory in *On the Grounds* was labelled "economical" in the sense that the aim is keeping a balance between somatic and psychological forces. This is also based on Fechner's theory that experiences of pleasure and displeasure depend on the stability of psychophysical forces (Yahalom 2014, p. 407).

Freud's main 'discovery' in *On the Grounds* is that the somatic excitation, which is abnormally regulated and results in anxiety, is sexual in nature. The essence of the mechanism of anxiety neurosis is that the constant production of somatic sexual excitation has to be channelled towards the psyche for adequate processing, and anxiety neurosis results from "a deflection of somatic sexual excitation from the psychical sphere" and the "abnormal employment" of this excitation (Freud 1953–1975c, p. 108). Later in the text Freud states that somatic sexual excitation is produced continuously, resulting in increased pressure within the seminal vesicles. When pressure reaches a given threshold, it overrides the resistance of an afferent pathway to the cerebral cortex, where this somatic energy is turned into "psychical excitation" or libido. This libido charges with energy a set of "sexual ideas" stored in the psyche which produce a state of "libidinal tension" and an urge to reduce it to preserve homeostasis. Freud considers that the "psychical unloading" of this tension depends on the unloading of the pressure from the seminal vesicles via a complex spinal reflex by a "*specific* or *adequate* action" (italics in original) (Freud 1953–1975c, p. 109). Following this process, the somatic sexual excitation is removed, and the resistance of the afferent neural pathway is re-established. Anxiety arises whenever the libidinal tension is not "discharged" in (what Freud considers) a normal sexual act.

The question now arises as to why Freud selected a sexual cause as the main aetiology for anxiety over the common sources of anxiety and fear discussed in previous chapters, such as death, poverty and disease. Are these not legitimate causes of fear and anxiety? Freud was adamant that anxiety was caused by sexual factors, and all other potential causes have to accommodate to his discovery. Thus Freud considered that non-sexual factors such as those mentioned above (which he terms "stock noxae" (Freud 1953–1975c, p. 99)) are non-specific triggers of anxiety. In other words, these factors have, in Freud's opinion, only a "contributory" effect and thus are neither necessary nor sufficient for producing anxiety. The necessary factor for Freud's anxiety neurosis is the presence of a "specific noxa" which is the pathological deflection of sexual somatic excitation, and stock noxae can only increase the amount of excitation. Whenever a psychological shock of a non-sexual nature seems to produce anxiety neurosis, Freud is unbending in his view that "careful enquiry directed to that end reveals that a set of noxae and influences from *sexual life*… [are operative aetiological factors]" (italics in the original) (Freud 1953–1975c, p. 134).

To repeat, Freud's surprising discovery is that abnormal anxiety is always related to a dysfunctional sexual life, a fact he believes to be demonstrated with "overwhelming frequency" (p. 99). Freud also briefly refers to a 'normal' type of anxiety, which he considers to be the result of the incapacity to deal psychologically with external dangers (p. 121), but unfortunately, he does not elaborate on this important concept.[6]

At the end of the treatise Freud listed what he considers relevant factors in the aetiology of anxiety neurosis, which include: (1) a hereditary

[6]"Normal" anxiety is summarily explained in Addendum B of *Inhibition, Symptoms and Anxiety* (Freud 1953–1975a, pp. 164–168). In this important section, Freud begins by defining anxiety as "indefiniteness and lack of object," whereas fear (*Furcht*) always has an object. He remarks that "the problem" of conceptually separating "realistic" from "neurotic" anxiety "awaits a thorough examination" (p. 165). Freud defines realistic anxiety as produced by a known danger, whereas in neurotic anxiety the danger is unknown but probably instinctual. Once neurotic anxiety becomes conscious through psychoanalysis, it is not different from realistic anxiety. Nevertheless, a paragraph later Freud remarks that "in some cases the characteristics of realistic anxiety and neurotic anxiety are mingled" (p. 165). More specifically, Freud states that realistic anxiety converts into neurotic anxiety whenever the reaction to the danger is exaggerated.

disposition, which is the most frequent predisposing factor although it is neither necessary nor sufficient to produce anxiety neurosis (p. 137), (2) a specific cause (that is, deflection of somatic sexual excitation from "the psychical field") which is both necessary and sufficient to produce anxiety neurosis, and (3) an auxiliary cause ("stock noxa") such as physical exhaustion, which, like the hereditary disposition, is neither a necessary nor sufficient factor (p. 135).[7]

8.3.3 Empirical and Conceptual Problems with Freud's Sexual Model of Anxiety

Before addressing specific problems with Freud's mechanism of anxiety neurosis, it is important to stress the interesting commonalities with Descartes's mechanism of the passions. Freud's process of anxiety neurosis provided in *On the Grounds* follows Descartes's model of the passions as described in *The Passions of the Soul*, with some modifications. In both systems, there is a separation between *res extensa* (the body in Descartes, and "somatic sexual excitation" in Freud) and *res cogitans* (the soul in Descartes and the "psyche" in Freud). More specifically, Descartes's 'spirits' become Freud's 'somatic sexual excitation,' Descartes's 'soul' becomes Freud's 'psyche,' and Descartes's hydraulic interaction between spirits and soul becomes Freud's 'pneumatic' interaction between sexual somatic energy and its 'processing' in the psyche. An important difference is that in Descartes's system, fear and anxiety are produced by specific movements of the pineal gland, whereas Freud's neurotic anxiety is produced by a deflection of sexual somatic energy from the psyche into subcortical brain regions, which Freud considered a wasted or "abnormal employment of that excitation" (Freud 1953–1975c, p. 108).

[7]Lowenfeld (Freud 1953–1975c, p. 125), suggests against Freud's sexual aetiology of anxiety disorder, that a severe fright may be sufficient to cause anxiety. Freud denied what he considered a "post hoc ergo propter hoc", an astonishing remark given his later acknowledgment that his work lacked empirical confirmation (p. 128).

Unfortunately, Freud's model is riddled with conceptual problems and empirical questions. Firstly, there is his theory that anxiety results from a deflection of sexual somatic excitation from appropriate channels of "unloading" (p. 112). Such deflection occurs with any sexual behaviour that departs from what Freud describes as a "normal *vita sexualis*" (italics in the original) (p. 129), that is, a sexual act between a man and a woman culminating in mutual orgasm, and the cause of anxiety neurosis lies in these abnormal sexual practices. Individuals with a "normal *vita sexualis*" never develop anxiety neurosis, not even after receiving a "psychical shock" from a stock noxa as explained above. What about people with a normal sexual life who still develop anxiety neurosis? Freud's answer to this challenge is that these people have a hereditary disposition to deflect sexual tension from the psychical sphere. In other words, these people (all women in Freud's explanation) inherit the mechanism of an abnormal "*vita sexualis*."

Freud neither explains how 'abnormal' sexuality results in a deflection of sexual somatic excitation, nor what the putative deflection of this excitation consists in. These omissions relate to the main conceptual problem of this Freudian treatise, which amounts to a paraphrase of Descartes's system of emotions and its unavoidable dualism. Sexual tension is the main factor in Freud's theory, producing anxiety by being deflected from psychological processing. The miracle of this Cartesian jump from body to psyche is never addressed, but more worrisome is the lack of explanation of how sexual tension is being processed psychologically. We can only speculate about this putative mechanism, but even that is difficult. The question then arising is how and why this sexual tension is deflected. And what is this 'deflection' about? These are not empty questions given that we are discussing the crux of Freud's theory of anxiety.

A sexual factor underlying anxiety neurosis is Freud's main contribution, but the question still arises as to what the role of other traumatic factors may be. Freud easily dismisses their efficacy in producing anxiety by stating that "stock noxae" only reinforce the sexual noxa (Freud 1953–1975c, p. 103). But how this reinforcement occurs is never explained. It is at times exasperating reading statements regarding the mechanism of anxiety that are fully speculative but accepted without any self-criticism. There is no hypothesis being tested, and his biased observations are the only bases of his theory.

In conclusion, Freud's main proposal in *On the Grounds* is that the only necessary cause of anxiety neurosis is the accumulation of libidinal excitation, with all other relevant factors in life playing second fiddle. From the perspective of the ancients, Montaigne and Wittgenstein, and indeed common understandings today, such a conclusion seems wildly counter-intuitive, not only because the somatic factors relate to sexual expression only, but because of the unsupported reliance on sexuality to the detriment of other significant contextual factors. On the other hand, it is possible to trace continuities between this early Freudian account of anxiety and the kind of investigations into somatic brain processes that I discussed as the tradition of 'Descartes-James-Damasio', in terms of its mechanistic basis and body-psyche dualism. With Freud, fear and anxiety became the main expression of sexual pathology couched in pneumatic terms. Freud's argument that dysfunction in sexual mechanisms accounts for human anxiety, and that therefore anxiety is *always* pathological, signals the origin of the medicalization of anxiety.

A final question concerns the patients' well-being. As a physician specialising in 'nervous' disorders we would expect Freud's theoretical speculations to be orientated towards devising a better treatment for his patients. It is therefore disappointing that therapy is not specifically addressed in *On the Grounds*, except for a brief statement that the cure for anxiety lies in resuming a 'normal' sexual life. But no suggestion, let alone proof, for this assertion is provided. External factors (Freud's 'stock noxae') such as the death of a father or suffering a heart attack (as in one of Freud's examples), only play an accessory role, and the fear of death is not even considered.

8.4 Freud's Early Therapeutic Suggestions for Anxiety Neurosis

8.4.1 Lectures 24 and 25

Ten years after *On the Grounds* and before publishing *Inhibition, Symptom and Anxiety*, Freud delivered a series of lectures (1915–1917) (Freud 1953–1975b) to clarify conceptual issues about psychoanalysis, and several of these lectures were devoted to anxiety. The relevance of this material is that Freud clarified and modified some of his previous concepts of fear and anxiety, and also provided provocative advice regarding the treatment of anxiety.

In Lecture 24, entitled "Ordinary Nervousness" (pp. 328–339), Freud accepts that "nervous" people have a temperament characterized by incomprehensible reactions, irritability and uselessness. Freud here refers to his recent discovery of the unconscious and to the mechanism of repression of sexual instincts. A more clinically experienced Freud now proposes that neurosis is an incurable disorder, and yet of potential benefit to the patient, given that anxiety signals the resolution of an unconscious event.[8] Moreover, the role of the physician is not to interfere with neurosis: "the physician takes the part of the illness he is battling against" (p. 332). Freud asserts that there is "incurable suffering" in the world. Thus, a neurotic person finds refuge in illness, which, Freud believes, may be justifiable. When neurosis ensues, "the physician…will retire silently and tactfully" (p. 332). And now, in a wildly speculative manner, Freud expands on the putative advantage of suffering from neurosis: exploited and abused women may "adopt the evasion of the neurosis" to avoid being brutally treated by their husbands. This may occur whenever "…the woman is too cowardly or too virtuous to seek secret solace in the arms of another" (p. 332); or when the woman does not separate from the husband, because "… she has no prospect of maintaining herself or of finding a better husband…" (p. 332). Freud's misogynistic approach to the treatment of anxiety neurosis is compounded by his suggestion of sadomasochism in women, since a woman may elect to stay in a relationship "especially when her sexual emotions still bind her to this brutal man" (p. 332). The sadism is expressed by the woman's "misuse" of the neurosis "for purpose of vengeance… She forces her inconsiderate husband to spare her, to attend to her wishes, to permit her absence from the house and thus free her from the oppressions of her married life" (p. 332). In these cases, the neurosis is used

[8]"There are cases where even the physician must admit that the resolution of the conflict into neurosis is the most harmless outcome and one most easily tolerated by society" (Freud 1953–1975b, p. 332).

for self-protection. She "...can complain of her illness..." and the physician "...becomes her assistant..." (p. 332). Given the considerable gain that women obtain from being in a neurotic state, the efficacy of psychosomatic therapy is "very slight" (p. 333). By considering this an 'advantage' of the illness, Freud seems to suggest that neurosis is in some instances an act of pretending by shrewd women who cheat on their husbands to effect a 'cure.'

Freud also proposed an additional advantage of anxiety neurosis suggesting that after a long time of illness, the neurosis acquires an independent life; it attains a kind of *modus vivendi* between itself and other parts of the psychic life (p. 333). The secondary benefit of anxiety neurosis is that the patient no longer has to work, and "learns to exploit his injury by begging" (p. 334). The disadvantage is that "man renounces the use of his best and loftiest powers" (p. 334). Thus, Freud's concept of anxiety neurosis includes an implicit dimorphism, where women benefit from the illness indulging in vengeance or deception, and men are limited to begging and suffering curtailment of their powers.

The concept of the sexual origin of neurosis re-emerges in this Lecture mixed with personal references and anecdotes. Freud recounts that he made his crucial discovery of the sexual basis of neurosis after he realised that the examination of nervous patients rarely included questions about their sexual lives (p. 335): "At that time I sacrificed my popularity among my patients to my investigations." Freud "forced" patients to "confirm" his suppositions, but some patients would go to other physicians rather than disclose their sexual lives (p. 335). During this period, Freud did not consider sexual abnormalities as the single cause for neurosis, but insisted that the main cause for neurosis was the poor handling of increasing libido and the production of "sexual toxins" which could result from physical or psychological sources.

Lecture 25, entitled "General theory of the neuroses: fear and anxiety", makes explicit the divorce between psychoanalysis and biology for the understanding of these emotions: "...nothing [is] more indifferent...for the psychological comprehension of fear, than knowledge of nerves..." (p. 341). In this Lecture Freud makes the striking suggestion that fear is an unnecessary emotion for the guidance of rational behaviour. As opposed to neurotic fear, Freud states that real fear *appears to be* a rational response to an external danger, and the expression of the instinct of self-preservation, but this theory should be "thoroughly revised" (p. 341). He suggests in the most orthodox Stoic fashion that a rational response to an external danger should not be fear, but "the cool appraisal of one's own strength in comparison with…the danger" (p. 341). Based on this appraisal, the agent is then capable deciding on the best course of action, "flight, defence, or possibly even attack". In this context of Stoic virtuosity, Freud considers that fear has no positive role to play since it should not influence the appraisal and decision process.[9] What is of advantage is the expectation of danger which allows, says Freud, the activation of sensory and motor processes preparing the individual for a fast behavioural response to the threat. This expectancy produces "the condition of fear" as a mere epiphenomenon (p. 342).

Freud also makes the puzzling statement that all emotions consist of "the perception of motor activities that have already taken place" which strongly resonates with James's theory of emotions (see previous chapter), and yet Freud, the psychoanalyst, wants to break from the psychological tradition: "What psychology has to say about emotions—the James-Lange theory, for instance—is absolutely incomprehensible for us psychoanalysts, and cannot be discussed" (p. 343). Fear is the key to making psychoanalysis into an independent scientific undertaking, and Freud is now ready to propose more ambitious hypotheses as well as novel nosological descriptions. He proposes that the category of "neurotic fear" include the emotion of anxiety, which he now defines as being free-floating or expectant fear. Freud adds that neurotically fearful people always expect the worst outcome from any event, and should be distinguished from the "many" people who are not suffering neurotic anxiety but just show a "tendency to anticipate disaster" (p. 344).[10] He also describes phobias as a separate type of pathological fear, which he considers to be independent from neurotic fear.

---

[9]Fear may be actually counterproductive, since "if fear is too strong, it proves absolutely useless and paralyses every action, even flight" (Freud 1953–1975b, p. 341).

[10]Freud adds that "a striking amount of expectant fear" is characteristic of anxiety neurosis, which he now subsumes under the generic category of neuroses (Freud 1953–1975b, p. 344).

In terms of their mechanism, the more mature Freud proposes that fear and anxiety are a repetition of relevant past experiences,[11] primarily the trauma of birth and separation from the mother.[12] He also relates neurotic anxiety to the individual's sexual life, in line with his first hypothesis in *On the Grounds*. Neurotic anxiety occurs when sexual excitation "is not brought to a satisfactory conclusion" (p. 346), and anxiety is the clinical expression of unspent "libidinous excitement" (p. 347). The next step is to generalise this theory to all fears by demonstrating that this mechanism is not only valid for neurotic fear but for real fear, that is the typical reaction to danger (p. 350). Freud remarks that in children fear is common and it is difficult to know whether it is of the neurotic or the real type. He arrives at the conclusion that "the child (and later the adult) fears the power of his libido because he is anxious in the face of everything" (p. 351). In other words, children and adults have a neurotic disposition to respond with fear. Freud finds his explanation "simple and convincing," but the fact is that it is based on the mere speculation that all children have fear, that this fear is anxiety about their sexual instincts, and that those predisposed to be anxious will develop anxiety (p. 351).

In conclusion, while claiming simplicity, Freud provides in these Lectures a long and convoluted classification of fear and anxiety, which suggests two types: 'neurotic fear' due to "misused libido" and 'real fear' as the normal reaction to external danger (p. 352). Eventually, Freud wants to explain *all* fears, neurotic and real, as a libidinal problem, but

[11]As already discussed, we should not expect a consistent use of the terms 'anxiety' and 'fear,' since Freud prefers avoiding "entering upon a discussion as to whether our language means the same or distinct things by the words anxiety, fear or fright" (Freud 1953–1975b, p. 342).

[12]The rationale provided by Freud to substantiate his hypothesis is rather shocking. He writes: "Many years ago we were sitting around the dinner table—a number of young physicians—when an assistant in the obstetrical clinic told a jolly story of what had happened in the last examination for midwives. A candidate was asked what it implied if during delivery the faeces of the newborn was present in the discharge of waters, and she answered promptly 'the child is afraid.' She was laughed at and flunked. But I silently took her part and began to suspect that the poor woman of the people had, with sound perception, revealed an important connection" (Freud 1953–1975b, p. 344).

the stumbling block in his theory is that real fear is an expression of the instinct of self-preservation rather than a response to sexual dysfunction. Doing away with this conceptual limitation is the aim of Freud's major work on fear and anxiety, namely *Inhibition, Symptom and Anxiety.*

8.5 Inhibitions, Symptoms and Anxiety[13]

Freud's *Inhibitions, Symptoms and Anxiety*, published in 1926, presents his most elaborated theory on fear, anxiety and neurosis. Freud's main aim in writing this text was to better address "…what anxiety really is…" and to this end he proposed to bring together "all the facts we know about anxiety" (Freud 1953–1975a, p. 132). The reason behind this renewed interest in fear and anxiety is Freud's novel consideration that these emotions are the "essential" problems for psychoanalysis as a therapy.

Before analysing the concept of fear, it is important to clarify Freud's idiosyncratic use of the terms fear and anxiety in this text. In *Inhibition, Symptom and Anxiety* Freud rarely uses the term "fear", which he now considers a mere automatic reaction to danger in non-humans, using the terms "normal", "natural" or "real anxiety" instead. Furthermore, Freud replaces the construct of "anxiety neurosis" with the new one of "fear neurosis," and used the terms fear and anxiety as synonyms as I shall discuss below.

Another important clarification is that in *Inhibition, Symptom and Anxiety* Freud makes frequent reference to his "metapsychology", that is, his understanding of the mechanism of the psyche, introducing his own concept of the unconscious, the structure of mental process in terms of the "ego," the "id" and the "superego," his concept of "repression" of sexual (libidinal) stimuli, and the "Oedipus complex". I shall

[13]The period during which Freud wrote this text was severely distressing for him. His beloved Vienna was in steep decline after the First World War. But more importantly, Freud suffered the deaths of both one of his daughters and a niece, and he was diagnosed with cancer, suffered from crises of anxiety and was in poor general health. In the same period Freud also suffered the deaths of his mentor and of his best disciple (Foresti 2010, p. 211)

concentrate on discussing Freud's novel concept of fear and anxiety, making reference to his metapsychology only when necessary for conceptual understanding. This is certainly not a minor limitation of the chapter, but I believe it is possible to bring out the important points Freud makes on fear and anxiety, and their therapeutic value, without the need of a full explanation of his metapsychology.

The main departure in *Inhibition, Symptom and Anxiety* from Freud's previous writings is his new proposition that anxiety may be a useful signal of danger, and not only a symptom of pathology. This is not of minor importance, as I have discussed in the previous chapter that current neuroscientists also consider fear and anxiety as relevant in signalling danger. Moreover, I shall discuss in the next chapter that current writings on the sociology of fear also accept the Freudian concept of anxiety as a useful signal of danger. But what explains the radical change between Freud's initial hypothesis of anxiety as an abnormal symptom produced by deflected sexual energy and the new hypothesis of anxiety as a useful symptom? Answering this important question is the aim of this section, which will begin by addressing Freud's concept of 'inhibition' and 'symptom' for a better understanding of his new concept of anxiety.

Freud defines inhibition as "the expression of a restriction of an ego-function" (Freud 1953–1975a, p. 88), which may be clarified with a clinical example he provided. He presented the case of a person who developed a phobia (or extreme fear) about going on the street. Freud argued that this incapacity to leave home, which he describes as an 'inhibition', has the positive role of allowing the person to avoid the anxiety or fear of going on the street (Freud 1953–1975a, p. 101). Two problems arise with this concept of inhibition. The first pertains to the clinical role of inhibition, considered as a psychological event with preventive value. But this value would only work in the very short term, for in the long term the inhibition implies suffering for the individual who sees her/his life progressively limited by fear. The second problem is that the inhibition rather than protecting the individual against anxiety, already *includes* anxiety, as the 'inhibited' person is chronically fearful or anxious about leaving the house. It seems more likely that it is fear which inhibits the action, not that the inhibition is a protection from fear.

Therefore, inhibition would better be construed as a manifestation of fear or anxiety.

According to Freud, anxiety, the "symptom", is the result of inhibition. For instance, the fear felt by an agoraphobic when on the street is a symptom of the inhibition against leaving home. Thus, Freud considers that a symptom has the role of removing the person from danger. In the case of agoraphobia, the fear of being on the street will force the individual to return to the safety of home. Freud also defined symptoms in mechanistic terms, as manifestations that replace an instinct that is supressed. Understanding this concept of a symptom, requires some basic understanding of Freud's metapsychology. According to Freud, psychological defences against *internal* dangers are structured in a similar fashion to defences against *external* dangers. Freud considers that external dangers are faced by activating motor behaviours, whereas internal dangers are dealt with by the mechanism of "repression," which he considers to be an equivalent of the flight response (Freud 1953–1975a, p. 92). To this end, sexual energy is "disengaged" from the instinct to be repressed, and this energy is released as anxiety (Freud 1953–1975a, p. 109). Freud stresses that this anxiety does not result from an automatic conversion of repressed energy, since "the ego is the actual seat of anxiety" (Freud 1953–1975a, p. 93).[14] In other words, there is a psychological instance that 'decides' whether and how much of the sexual energy is converted into anxiety, and this depends on individual factors, such as the amount of sexual energy and the capacity of the ego for dealing with this energy. No support is provided for this

[14]Rollo May in his otherwise excellent rendition of Freud's theories of anxiety tends to 'straighten' Freud's account, in order, perhaps, to make it more accessible to the general public (May 1996). For instance, May states that the ego 'perceives' the danger which produces anxiety. Therefore, to avoid greater anxiety, the ego represses the impulses that would lead the person into danger. The ego is "inoculated" with a small quantum of anxiety in order "to escape its full strength" (Freud 1953–1975a, p. 162). But May's explanation is still muddled. May refers to an 'ego' preventing the person (to whom this ego belongs) from suffering anxiety, and the "homunculus fallacy" described in the previous chapter is unavoidable. May's proposal raises additional questions such as: how does the ego perceive danger? Does the ego, therefore, have a full repertoire of mental functions and organs of perception? What is the mechanism by which the ego manages to repress impulses? What inoculates the ego with a little anxiety?

speculation, except for Freud's remark that this is a metapsychological description (Freud 1953–1975a, p. 93).[15]

Going back to Freud's concept of a 'symptom,' Freud considered anxiety as a reaction to danger, whereas in the term "symptoms" he includes emotional manifestations such as phobias and obsessions, which are created to avoid a danger-situation signalled by the generation of anxiety, as explained above with the example of agoraphobia. In Freud's view, it is the symptom that expresses a repressed sexual "impulse" rather than anxiety, which is construed as a "signal of unpleasure" that forewarns of a danger (Freud 1953–1975a, p. 100). Whatever the validity of this explanation for anxiety, Freud offers in the same text a different option, where anxiety is created in accordance with a mnemonic image, since "biological necessity demands that a situation of danger has an affective symbol" (Freud 1953–1975a, pp. 93–94). These "affective symbols" are memory images of remote events, such as the "trauma of birth" (already hinted at in Lecture 25), but, as already discussed in the context of Damasio's account of fear in the previous chapter, it is unclear how these putative 'images' 'translate' into the psychological and somatic aspects of anxiety. I shall now explain Freud's account of this mechanism of anxiety in more detail.

8.5.1 "What We Clearly Want Is to Find Something that Will Tell Us What Anxiety Really Is" (Inhibition, Symptoms and Anxiety, p. 132)

Whereas the account above seems to have settled Freud's new theory of anxiety, a few pages later he argues that "anxiety is not a simple matter" (Freud 1953–1975a, p. 132). Freud then defines anxiety as an affective

[15] I am unable to do justice to Freud's complex metapsychology in a chapter focusing on his concept of fear and anxiety. It is necessary, here, to set aside judgement of Freud on the validity of his theory of Oedipal complex and concepts such as the "degradation of libido," "the super-ego [becoming] exceptionally severe and unkind," and an obedient ego providing behaviours of "conscientiousness, piety, and cleanliness" (Freud 1953–1975a, p. 115).

state characterized by "unpleasure" accompanied by somatic symptoms such as shortness of breath and palpitations, and the *perception* of these somatic changes (Freud 1953–1975a, p. 133). But the question still unanswered is the function of anxiety, and Freud's initial hypothesis is that "the obvious response is that anxiety is a reaction to a state of danger" (p. 133). Freud's hypothesis now is that after a traumatic experience affective states are "incorporated in the mind," and these affective states may resurface whenever the traumatic situation recurs as memory images (p. 133).

Freud considers the need for binding the somatic aspects of anxiety and its perception, and suggests this is produced by "historical factors" in the shape of memory images (p. 133). Initially he considers that the "trauma" of birth is such a factor, with anxiety becoming the "reproduction" of this putative trauma. Freud not only suggests that "the trauma of birth" constitutes a "necessary" condition to produce anxiety, but that anxiety symptoms are a reproduction of such trauma (p. 133). In other words, any situation of danger that produces anxiety does so by bringing forward images of this momentous biographical event. Freud argues that such anxiety is "inexpedient" given that the response is based on early behaviours, inadequate to master external danger. In support of his theory Freud states that many adults exhibit puerile behaviours when facing danger, being overcome by infantile fears (p. 148).

After further analysis, Freud decides to change the timing of the 'historical trauma' from birth to the first years of life, and suggests that anxiety is a consequence of the loss of a loved object during this period. He considers that in the absence of the mother, the child develops feelings of helplessness, which are the "*key to the understanding of anxiety*" (my italics) (p. 137). This *helplessness* can be either "material" (due to a real danger) or "psychological" (due to instinctual danger) (p. 138). In this system, anxiety becomes a signal triggered by the danger of helplessness, and has the positive role in assisting in activating psychological and behavioural mechanisms necessary to successfully confront danger (p. 138). Freud speculates that in early infancy the symptoms of anxiety play an important role, for instance, in bringing the mother's attention to the baby's needs, and later in life the symptoms of anxiety are expressed every time there is a state of danger.[16] Thus, Freud suggests it is more "expedient" that anxiety occurs early in the process of confronting danger, alerting the individual to the implications of this event and therefore allowing the preparation of appropriate responses (p. 134). Once this is achieved, anxiety is cancelled, and the agent may proceed to face danger using "suitable measures" (p. 135). This is Freud's concept of anxiety as a signal of danger, or in his words, anxiety as a "rescuing signal" (p. 138).

To conclude, in this new theory, anxiety is no longer an automatic harmful reaction triggered by deflected sexual energy, but it is now endowed with a positive value, with the "only function" of efficiently triggering defensive mechanisms (p. 138). Freud's proposal expands the concept of anxiety, which includes a negative emotion that is the product of discharging instinctual energy, as well as a novel positive mechanism forewarning the individual about incoming danger. Nevertheless, the conceptual difference between expedient and inexpedient anxiety remains unclear. Both types of anxiety imply the recognition of danger, the difference being in the timing of recognition. The question is whether 'early' anxiety is always better as Freud implies, and the answer is that it depends on contextual factors, which Freud frequently neglects. In fact, for Freud's mechanism of anxiety to be universal, contextual factors *must* play a negligible role since they add very little to a preformed mechanism. However, this is certainly not true in the case of anxiety. Anxiety may be helpful when it activates the individual to be better prepared for an adequate (or 'expedient') response to danger, but this is a matter of degree since excessive anxiety may paralyse the individual with the response becoming 'inexpedient.' The timing is not as crucial as Freud remarks. Moreover, in some cases an early state of anxiety may create an unnecessary burden. Finally, not every event in life generating anxiety can be acted upon in a preventative way. For instance, living in the context of a financial recession carries a high risk

---

[16]With this insight Freud claims that "we have the key to an understanding of anxiety" (Freud 1953–1975a, p. 137).

of losing one's job no matter how 'efficient' the response produced by anxiety may be. In these cases, being anxious could result in making mistakes at work and increasing the chance of being laid off. In the end, Freud's timing of inexpedient and expedient anxiety is merely based on the chronological factor that the former is related to the trauma of birth, whereas the latter is related to separation from the mother during the first few years of life.[17] It is unclear how this chronological difference makes one type of anxiety more "efficient" than the other, let alone why the moment of birth should leave an indelible mark of trauma. However, more important than this is the question as to how adult responses to danger are shaped by the early trauma of feeling abandoned and helpless. How is anxiety triggered as a signal of danger based on this early trauma? How do early traumas help in recognizing present dangers, especially when not every potentially dangerous event produces an anxiety response? How traumas 'produce' memory images, and how memory images produce anxiety, let alone efficient and inefficient ones, remains explicable only in Freud's metapsychological terms. Finally, fear of death is simply dismissed as fear of the 'super-ego' "projected on to the powers of destiny" (Freud 1953–1975a, p. 140).

Freud asks the important question about why is it that relatively few people develop anxiety neurosis given that external dangers are universal and common to all human beings. It is here that we should expect proper consideration of contextual factors, and yet, this is not only absent, but Freud's response to this challenge to his theory is answered in the most pedestrian way. His answer comes in the form of obscure reference to defective organic and mental apparatus. More specifically he identifies biological, phylogenetic, and psychological causes accounting for anxiety neurosis. The *biological factor* is based on "a defect of our mental apparatus" which in Freud's opinion results from a relatively short pregnancy period: [humans] "…are sent into the world in a less finished state." This may explain, according to Freud, the child's

[17]Freud includes the fear of castration (a result of the Oedipal complex) as another important cause of anxiety, but discussion of this factor is not relevant to the conceptual discussion of the mechanism of anxiety.

great dependence on the mother, the feelings of helplessness when she is away, and "the need to be loved" (p. 154). The *phylogenetic factor* is based on differences in sexual evolution between humans and non-human animals. According to Freud, somewhere along the path of human evolution sexual instincts become identified as dangerous, and consequently repressed, the mechanism of repression being "...the most direct aetiology of the neurosis" (p. 155). Finally, the *psychological factor* is also based on a human mental defect. The ego, says Freud, being unable to protect itself from instinctual dangers responds by transforming sexual instincts into neurotic symptoms such as phobias and obsessions (p. 155). On the first count, we may argue that though the duration of infant and juvenile dependency is longer than that of most other primates, it is unclear why this would produce more anxiety in humans. On the second and third, Freud's theory that sexual repression may produce neurosis has never been substantiated; and the same is true for the putative transformation of sexual instincts into anxiety symptoms.

The section devoted to the therapy of anxiety neurosis, relegated to the Addenda of the text, is brief and enmeshed in Freud's metaphysical system. Freud states that the treatment begins by overcoming the resistance of the ego in dealing with objects of anxiety, which have been repressed in the unconscious. Once these objects are brought to consciousness, the psychoanalyst argues against those ideas using logical arguments (Freud 1953–1975a, p. 159). The therapy has to be continued, given the power of compulsions to repeat the unconscious objects ("the resistance of the unconscious" (p. 159)). Freud concludes that the therapist has to confront several types of resistance which arise from the ego, the id and the superego. The ego's resistance is produced by the "benefit of the illness;" the resistance of the id is produced by unconscious compulsions; and the resistance of the superego is related to a "need for punishment" (p. 160) which antagonises the patient's own therapy.[18]

[18]Given the complexity of Freud's metaphysical system, a critical analysis of this therapeutic technique is beyond the scope of this work. I may point, as an example, to the controversial aspects of Freud's concept of the "unconscious," which is critically discussed by Bouveresse (1995, p. 75).

In conclusion, *Inhibition, Symptoms and Anxiety* is an impressive exercise in using different theoretical approaches to explain the phenomenon of anxiety. And yet, Freud's main proposal amounts to little more than changing the old pneumatic model of anxiety, as a manifestation of deflected sexual excitation, into a system of infantile traumas generating images that produce effective or ineffective anxiety. The innovation in this text is Freud's proposal that anxiety may be on occasions a successful signal of danger, but surprisingly, there is no consideration of the suffering produced by severe anxiety and fear. The specificities of the agent's context are almost completely ignored in order to support a rigid theory that should fit all. Even less is said regarding therapy for those with fear neurosis or anxiety neurosis. Freud is a precursor of the move that separates theory from the practice of helping people suffering from fear, a trend that, as we saw in the last chapter, is still extant. In *Inhibition, Symptoms and Anxiety* Freud's aim was "to find something that would tell us what anxiety really is" (p. 132), but in light of his confusing remarks it is clear that something important eluded him.

What eluded Freud was pointed out by Wittgenstein in his brief remarks. Wittgenstein considered that, although Freud's theory of anxiety as the repetition of an early trauma cannot be empirically substantiated, it is "an idea which has marked attraction" (Barrett 1967, p. 43). This is not the attraction of solid conceptual thinking or impressive empirical findings, but that of mythological explanations, that "all is a repetition of something that has happened before" (Barrett 1967, p. 43). Once such explanations are accepted, emotions such as anxiety may become clearer and easier for people to accept. What was also repugnant to Wittgenstein was Freud's reductionism; for instance, that all fears and anxieties have the same explanation and treatment. In a premonitory remark at a time when psychoanalysis was flourishing, Wittgenstein's perspicuous intuition was that "Freud's work died with him. No one today can do psychoanalysis in the way he did," implying that the construction of psychoanalysis was mainly based on a charismatic leader (Bouveresse 1995, p. 4).

8.6 Conclusion

Freud has been regarded as one of the most original thinkers of the twentieth century, and psychoanalysis, the therapy he developed, as one of the most influential treatments for neurosis, a concept which includes various manifestations of anxiety. Freud produced an original and innovative concept of anxiety, which he initially considered to originate in sexual dysfunction in the context of a 'canonical' approach to sexuality. As we have seen, Freud's first theory takes the process by which fear develops to be akin to a pneumatic system, in which an excess of sexual energy that is not elaborated properly by putative psychological systems is discharged as anxiety. This understanding left Freud with the problem of death, not a minor cause of fear and one without any sexual connotations. Difficulties with the sexual energy explanation led Freud to a second theory of anxiety, now embedded in an intricate metapsychology which proposed that anxiety remits to infantile traumas. This in turn developed into his proposal of an expedient anxiety which produces a signal of danger, useful in preparing an adequate response to that danger, and an inexpedient anxiety, which becomes a symptom of psychopathology. Fear of death, no longer a theoretical obstacle for an encompassing sexual theory of anxiety, has been removed from Freud's metapsychological system.

Without questioning its originality, the main problem with Freud's model of anxiety is that it has to be taken on his word without plausible argument or evidence. In other words, we have to accept the pneumatic system of deflected energy, and that this energy is always sexual. We also have to accept that birth is a trauma and that anxiety is the unconscious recollection of the fear of separation from the mother. We have to accept a model of humans who do not fear the (Epicurean) gods, death, poverty or sickness, but rather the memory images of an early trauma. Freud's interesting clinical descriptions of his patients are not used as valuable material to examine the varieties of fears and anxieties, such as Montaigne provided when describing his own fears, but are reduced to fit a pre-elaborated theory. In his relatively rigid, dogmatic and reductive approach, Freud's concept of fear has similar limitations to Descartes's and James's theories. And finally, we have to accept that there are no fears or anxieties that could be the expected consequence of living in a social environment, since according to Freud, all fears and anxieties are in the end pathological. With Freud, the medicalization of fear started in full earnest because his identification of anxiety neurosis laid the ground for a pathological understanding of fear that required a medical approach and a specific therapy, and how this has developed up to contemporary times will be the focus of the next chapter.

References

American Psychiatric Association. (1994). *Diagnostic and statistical manual of mental disorders (DSM-IV)* (4th ed.). Washington, DC: American Psychiatric Press.

Barrett, C. (1967). *Ludwig Wittgenstein: Lectures and conversations on aesthetics, psychology, and religious belief.* Oxford: Basil Blackwell.

Beard, G. M. (1881). *American nervousness, its causes and consequences.* New York: G. P. Putnam's Sons.

Berrios, G. (1996). *The history of mental symptoms: Descriptive psychopathology since the nineteenth century.* Cambridge: Cambridge University Press.

Berrios, G. (1999). Anxiety disorders: A conceptual history. *Journal of Affective Disorders, 56*(2–3), 83–94.

Bouveresse, J. (1995). *Wittgenstein reads Freud: The myth of the unconscious* (C. Cosman, Trans.). Princeton: Princeton University Press.

Ellenberger, H. F. (1956). Fechner and Freud. *Bulletin of the Menninger Clinic, 20*(4), 201–214.

Foresti, G. (2010). Freud's writing in the twenties: Theory construction-and clinical research in *inhibitions, symptoms and anxiety*. In S. Arbiser & J. Schneider (Eds.), *On Freud's "inhibitions, symptoms and anxiety"*. London: Karnac Books.

Freud, S. (1953–1975a). Inhibitions, symptoms, and anxiety (J. Strachey, Trans.). In J. Strachey (Ed.), *An autobiographical study; inhibitions, symptoms and anxiety; the question of lay analysis and other works* (Vol. 20, pp. 87–175). London: The Hogarth Press.

Freud, S. (1953–1975b). *Introductory lectures on psycho-analysis* (J. Strachey, Trans., J. Strachey Ed., Vols. 15–16). London: The Hogarth Press.

Freud, S. (1953–1975c). On the grounds for detaching a particular syndrome from neurasthenia under the description 'Anxiety Neurosis' (J. Strachey, Trans.). In J. Strachey (Ed.), *Early psycho-analytic publications* (Vol. 3, pp. 87–139). London: The Hogath Press.

Freud, S. (1953–1975d). Twenty-fifth lecture: General theory of the neuroses; fear and anxiety. In J. Strachey (Ed.), *Introductory lectures on psycho-analysis* (Vols. 15–16, pp. 340–355). London: The Hogarth Press.

Gay, P. (1988). *Freud: A life for our time*. New York: W. W. Norton.

Leavy, S. A. (2010). What happened to psychoanalysis? *American Imago, 67*(1), 73–87.

May, R. (1996). *The meaning of anxiety*. New York: W. W. Norton & Co.

Nersessian, E. (2013). Psychoanalytic theory of anxiety: Proposals for reconsideration. In G. Saragnano (Ed.), *On Freud's "inhibitions, symptoms and anxiety"*. London: Karnac Books.

Shorter, E. (1992). *From paralysis to fatigue: A history of psychosomatic illness in the modern era*. New York: The Free Press.

Yahalom, J. (2014). Freud and Epicurean philosophy: Revisiting drive theory. *Contemporary Psychoanalysis, 50*(3), 395–417.

9

The Medicalization and Social Construction of Fear in the Age of Anxiety

9.1 Introduction

In the last chapter, I discussed Freud's identification of a syndrome he termed "anxiety neurosis" within the nebulous world of the neuroses. This syndrome was used to diagnose individuals with either common or unusual fears, sometimes acute and severe, or sometimes evolving into a chronic state of nervousness. Freud also created the technique of psychoanalysis primarily as a treatment for anxiety neurosis. This "talking cure" was an original approach to the treatment of emotional disorders, aimed at relieving the individual's fears by uncovering the 'unconscious roots' of anxiety. Thus, the loose categories of 'neuroses' and 'neurasthenia', previously managed by neurologists, became by the 1930s the therapeutic territory of psychiatry and psychoanalysis. Psychoanalysts considered anxiety as "the central problem in psychotherapy" (May 1996, p. ix), given that, in their opinion, a healthy personality depends on successfully dealing with unconscious fears.

During the mid-twentieth century the concept of anxiety became bifurcated into two different streams: the first elaborated by dynamic

S. Starkstein, *A Conceptual and Therapeutic Analysis of Fear*,
https://doi.org/10.1007/978-3-319-78349-9_9

psychoanalysts,[1] philosophers and sociologists, who conceptualised anxiety as resulting from either major changes of libidinal or social forces affecting the individual; and a second stream, mostly consisting of the increasing trend of biological psychiatry, which considers emotional problems such as anxiety to be the consequence of brain dysfunction amenable to treatment with psychoactive drugs. Whatever its origin, by 2001 anxiety was recognised as the most common mental health problem in the United States, whereas in 2002 anxiety was found by the World Mental Health Survey to be the most prevalent mental health problem worldwide (Dowbiggin 2009).

The aim of this concluding chapter is to discuss the medicalization of fear and anxiety, from its origin in Freud's psychoanalysis to the current concept of anxiety as a psychiatric disorder due to brain dysfunction. Medicalization is usually conceptualised as the process of defining a problem in medical terms, such as an illness or disorder, or treating the problem using medical intervention (Conrad 2005). In a competing but, as we shall see, also something of a parallel vein, thinkers in the fields of philosophy and sociology have conceptualised anxiety as a "social construction," that is, as being the result of social practices which surround the development and use of specific terms such as anxiety.[2] This view of anxiety as the result of social and institutional practices, is connected with arguments in favour of managing anxiety by modifying the social context, and empowering the individual to deal more successfully with life pressures. I will discuss these contrasting views and conclude with a critical discussion of both the medicalization and the social construction of anxiety.

[1]Dynamic psychoanalysis or psychotherapy developed as a branch of orthodox psychoanalysis during the early twentieth century, and is based on interpreting events in the 'unconscious' (in accord with Freud's metapsychology, see previous chapter) as they manifest in therapeutic relationships, to alleviate psychic tensions (Shedler 2010).

[2]Rollo May, a prominent psychoanalyst and thinker of the twentieth century states in *The Meaning of Anxiety* that "If one penetrates below the surface of political, economic, business, professional or domestic crises to discover their psychological causes…one runs athwart the problem of anxiety at almost every turn. The ordinary stresses and strains of life in the changing world of today are such that few if any escape the need to confront anxiety and to deal with it in some manner" (May 1996, p. ix).

9.2 Psychoanalysis and the Medicalization of Anxiety

Between 1950 and 1970, psychoanalysis had a prominent role in the treatment of anxiety and extreme fears ('phobias' in the psychoanalytical nomenclature) (Mayes and Horwitz 2005). Initially developed for use by practitioners trained in the psychoanalytical technique, psychoanalysis soon pervaded many aspects of social life, and the term 'neurotic' became increasingly used to refer to individuals suffering from excessive worry and major stress (Mayes and Horwitz 2005).

In parallel with the growth of psychoanalysis, since the beginning of the twentieth century 'alienists'[3] were leaving their reclusive jobs in mental asylums to join the ranks of academic psychiatry, which was modelled upon medical specialties such as neurology. This trend in psychiatry was dramatically boosted (and psychoanalysis virtually demolished) by the discovery of drugs capable of reducing or eliminating anxiety in a matter of weeks, as compared to the years a 'neurotic' had to spend on psychoanalysis, with uncertain results. The new trend of somatic treatments in psychiatry required a new nosology of "mental disorders," which was based on a biological framework. I shall first discuss how the Freudian concept of neurosis became the kernel of the future medicalization of fear and anxiety, and then address the shift into biological psychiatry.[4]

When Freud distinguished within the overarching concept of the neuroses a specific cluster of symptoms that constituted what he termed "anxiety neurosis", he not only proposed a mechanism for this novel construct (see previous chapter), but, as already mentioned, also created the technique of psychoanalysis to treat this condition. The process of

---

[3]'Alienists' were those physicians that took care of individuals with mental illness living in "lunatic asylums". Alienists had a low reputation among physicians, as they were rarely seen outside mental institutions (Rollin 2003).

[4]While the term 'medicalization' has been extensively used with negative connotations, implying that non-medical conditions have been illegitimately conceptualised and managed as medical conditions, it may also be considered in its positive connotations of new medical discoveries that provide better quality of life to humans (Conrad 2005). Conrad considers that psychiatry has been at the forefront of medicalization where power shifted in three decades from psychoanalysis to

medicalization of anxiety got started with the classification of a cluster of symptoms as a specific psychological disorder with a specific therapy. The definitive move into medicalization took place in the 50s in the USA through the restriction of the practice of psychoanalysis to professionally qualified psychiatrists, and by the contemporary discovery of anti-anxiety medications.

To recapitulate, intrinsic to the concept of medicalization is, first, that habitual emotional responses are considered abnormal emotions or full-blown mental disorders based on their severity and the social inadequacy they bring about, and second, that a specific treatment should be available and delivered by medical specialists. Psychoanalysis became the main therapy for anxiety neurosis in cosmopolitan cities, and scores of individuals were regularly assisted in their 50-minute sessions for months or years. In the dialectic relationship between analyst and patient, the former was progressively invested with powerful attributes, and the 'oracular' therapy which consisted in 'interpreting the unconscious' frequently generated increasing dependency of the patient on the analyst to solve even minor conflicts of daily life. On the other hand, psychoanalysis provided a place where, beyond the technical shortcomings of the treatment, patients could regularly relate their fears and anxieties in a nonjudgmental environment, and where they were cared for by a compassionate professional. In parallel, another revolution, of a different sort, in the treatment of anxiety was silently brewing. In 1955 the American Food & Drug Administration approved the first 'minor tranquilizer', a step that would lead to a dramatic shift in the concepts of fear and anxiety, and the practice of psychiatry for decades to come (Tone 2009).

---

psychopharmacology, genetics and neuroscience (Conrad 2005). Erik Parens, a sociologist investigating the ethical and social implications of using psychoactive drugs makes the important point that to investigate the problem of medicalization the sociologist must be able to distinguish, a priori, medical diagnoses that are 'true' health problems from those that are not (Parens 2013). However, Parens considers this is a conceptually impossible task, as the 'essence' of what a medical condition is has not been defined (and, I would add that it may be impossible to define, that is, to come up with the necessary and sufficient factors for something to be called a 'mental disorder').

9.3 Anxiety in the Age of Biological Psychiatry: The *Diagnostic and Statistical Manual*

During the mid-twentieth century, when psychoanalysis was the most popular therapy for anxiety in the USA, the American Psychiatric Association (APA) began the compilation of a new nosology of "mental disorders" that would change the practice of psychiatry (Mayes and Horwitz 2005). The early efforts of the APA at defining and classifying mental disorders were triggered by the sudden need to manage frequent and complex emotional disorders afflicting members of the armed forces returning from World War II. The first edition of the *Diagnostic and Statistical Manual* (DSM-I) was compiled by the APA in 1952 mainly to provide "an accurate account of the emotional morbidity among the armed forces, as well as to provide a suitable diagnosis for every case seen by the psychiatrist, a situation not faced in civilian life" (American Psychiatric Association 1952, p. vi). Therefore, there was a need for a new classification of neuroses, and the first modern nosology of anxiety was developed to suit soldiers exposed to traumatic war experiences, rather than the daily fears and anxieties of civilians.

One of the principal categories in the DSM-I was "Psychoneurotic Disorders" which, following the Freudian tradition, were considered as disorders of "psychogenic origin" (American Psychiatric Association 1952, p. 6). This category included anxiety as the main symptom, as well as dissociation, conversion, phobias, depression and obsessive-compulsive reactions. The Freudian influence on the DSM-I concept of anxiety was evident in definitions that are almost literal copies from Freud's work *Inhibition, Symptom and Anxiety*, such as "anxiety…is a danger signal felt and perceived by the conscious personality…and produced by a threat from within the personality" (Freud 1953–1975, p. 167) (see also Chapter 7). The DSM-I defined anxiety as a "diffuse" reaction not related to specific situations and objects, and as a state of expectation associated with somatic symptoms such as insomnia, muscle tension, and fatigue. This section on anxiety concluded with the warning that an "anxiety state" should be differentiated from the "normal apprehensiveness of fear", although the manual nowhere provides a definition of anxiety or clarifies how a "pathological anxiety state" should be differentiated from daily life anxiousness or fear (American Psychiatric Association 1952, p. 32). As I shall discuss below, this critical demarcation is not an empirical but a major conceptual problem. Based on the DSM framework, the classification of anxiety as a disorder or an illness requires the setting of a threshold to distinguish 'pathological' from 'everyday' anxiety, but this strategy overlooks the 'grey areas' characteristic of anxious people who do not qualify for a definite diagnosis of psychoneurosis and yet suffer from the emotional condition of anxiousness, or the different trajectories of anxiety, sometimes a constant burden but many times fluctuating in time.

The second edition of the DSM was published in 1968, and while still under Freudian influence, its main aim was to "facilitate maximum communication within the profession" (American Psychiatric Association 1968, p. viii), while avoiding the use of terms that may relate a psychiatric condition to specific mechanisms. The reason behind this decision is that the creators of the DSM wanted this instrument to remain 'agnostic' regarding the cause (psychological or biological) of any specific psychiatric condition. The DSM-II included a section entitled "Neuroses" (p. 39), with anxiety as the main symptom. The Freudian category of "Anxiety Neurosis," characterised by worrying or "anxious over-concern" and frequent somatic symptoms, was preserved in full (p. 39). Another relevant category included in the 'Neuroses' section was "Phobic neurosis", used to indicate severe and specific fears.

The third edition of the DSM (American Psychiatric Association 1980), however, marked a definite departure from psychoanalysis and a strong alignment with biological psychiatry (Mayes and Horwitz 2005). This edition was compiled by psychiatrists who mostly believed in the biogenesis rather than the psychogenesis of mental disorders (Frances 2013). Following an "atheoretical" approach, the DSM-III provided descriptive diagnoses without discussing potential mechanisms. One of the major changes in this edition was that the Freudian category of "anxiety neurosis" was broken into several syndromes, each with their own specific diagnostic criteria.[5] Thus, the DSM-III illustrates another aspect of the process of medicalization, which is the fragmentation of a syndrome into several sub-entities. Such a strategy ends up increasing the number of individuals who meet the criteria for a "mental disorder", opening the door for 'specific' treatments for these newly created conditions.

The fourth edition of the DSM lamented, in the Introduction, the distinction between mental and physical disorders, considered as a "reductionist anachronism of mind/body dualism" (American Psychiatric Association 1994, p. xxi). The section on "Anxiety Disorders" eliminated the category of "anxiety states" and included several new syndromes.[6] An interesting consideration in the DSM-IV is the difference between pathological and "unpathological [sic] anxiety" (American Psychiatric Association 1994, p. 411). Pathological anxiety is described as being difficult to control and interfering with daily life activities, whereas "unpathological" anxiety is considered more controllable, less likely to be accompanied by physical symptoms, and "able to be put off until later" (American Psychiatric Association 1994, p. 411).

The latest edition of the DSM (American Psychiatric Association 2013) (i.e. the DSM-5), defines anxiety disorders rather tautologically as characterized by excessive fear and anxiety. Fear is considered an "emotional response to real or perceived imminent threat," and to be related to flight/fight responses, immediate danger, and escape behaviours. Anxiety is defined as the anticipation of future threats associated with muscle tension and cautious and avoidant behaviours. Whereas the text acknowledges major symptom overlap between fear and anxiety, it nevertheless states that on "close examination" fear and anxiety may be differentiated by "the types of situations that are feared or avoided and the content of the associated thoughts or beliefs" (American Psychiatric

---

[5]These syndromes include phobic disorders, agoraphobia, social phobia, simple phobia, and anxiety states (comprising panic disorder, generalized anxiety disorder, obsessive compulsive disorder, and post-traumatic stress disorder).

[6]These are the new categories of acute stress disorder, anxiety disorder due to a general medical condition, substance-induced anxiety disorder, and anxiety disorder not otherwise specified.

Association 2013, p. 189). It is unfortunate that these differences are not further elaborated in the text. Furthermore, the rationale for modifying the diagnostic criteria of a given anxiety disorder or including specific anxiety syndromes is also unclear.

It is intriguing that the concept and diagnostic criteria for an "anxiety disorder" remained unchanged in the DSM-5, after major changes had been considered for inclusion in the new manual. In the preparation stages for the DSM-5, the committee responsible for the entries included in anxiety disorders considered the following changes: (1) that any severity of worrying (not just those that are "difficult to control", as in the DSM-IV) should be considered for diagnosis; (2) to reduce the number of somatic and psychological symptoms necessary to meet diagnostic criteria, and (3) to reduce the duration of anxiety symptoms from 6 months to 3 months (Andrews et al. 2009).

Starcevic, Portman and Beck consider that these proposed changes had the aim of reducing the number of "false negatives", that is, failures to diagnose an anxiety disorder based on diagnostic criteria among individuals that have "true" anxiety.[7] Unfortunately, in contemporary psychiatry there is no definitive concept of what anxiety truly is, as it is circularly defined by using the DSM diagnostic criteria. This is certainly not a limitation only with the DSM, as anxiety is a permeable diagnostic category that shifts in different contexts. I have discussed how anxiety came to be used in the medical nomenclature as a bodily symptom, how Freud used fear and anxiety interchangeably, and how Wittgenstein expanded the concept of fear and anxiety, so that anxiety could indicate a rational state of mind or a pathological one.

In conclusion, the concept of anxiety suffered a second 'wave' of medicalization when psychiatrists left the psychoanalytical school to adopt a more biological approach, looking for the cause of mental disorders in brain dysfunction. The practice of psychiatry became more constricted due to time and budgetary limitations, as well as the need

---

[7]Starcevic et al. (2012) also suggest that the proposed changes in diagnostic criteria (even if informed by empirical data) have the danger of increasing the prevalence of anxiety to "epidemic levels" which "will further damage the credibility of psychiatry and undermine its scientific standing" (p. 665).

to come up with a definition of pathological anxiety that could receive readily made pharmacological treatment (as discussed in the next section) and that could be accepted for patients' reimbursement by medical insurances and state agencies (Mayes and Horwitz 2005). I have explained in this section the major difficulties in reaching a unitary concept of pathological anxiety and the changes in diagnostic criteria that have plagued the major medical nosologies until current times. This problem is at the heart of the medicalization approach and one of its central difficulties. It must rely on definitions and reification of concepts, which remains an impossible task. As Wittgenstein remarked: "The classification of philosophers and psychologists: they classify clouds by their shape" (Wittgenstein 1967) (462). The emotions and pathologies of fear, anxiety, distress, phobias and similar others are such clouds, and psychiatrists have the expected problem of placing them in neat nosological boxes. I shall now discuss the main conceptual limitations of the DSM approach to fear and anxiety.

9.3.1 A Critical Analysis of the Concepts of Fear and Anxiety in the DSM Tradition

There is a vast amount of critical literature on the DSM classification of 'mental disorders', but my interest in this chapter is to restrict the discussion to conceptual problems within the category of "anxiety disorders." The first of these problems is with the concept of "mental disorder," which the DSM-5 defines as "a syndrome characterised by clinically significant disturbance in an individual's cognition, emotion regulation, or behaviour that reflects a *dysfunction* in the psychological, biological, or developmental processes underlying mental *functioning*" (p. 20) (my italics). Unfortunately, this definition is circular since 'mental disorder' is defined as the dysfunction of mental functioning. But beyond this minor conceptual remark, the DSM-5 does not provide a definition of 'mental functioning;' it does not specify what is needed for a putative mental disorder to achieve "clinical significance;" it does not explain the meaning of metaphors such as "emotional regulation" and "dysfunction in psychological, biological or developmental processes" (let alone how this putative dysfunction is "reflected" in behaviour); and it does not explain the mechanisms by which the above processes "underlie" mental functioning. These questions may be all dismissed as mere pedantic remarks, but they all pertain to the crucial concept of what is considered a mental pathology in need of treatment, a concept that lies at the core of the medicalization of anxiety. In addition, the DSM-5 is misleading in its statement that it is "atheoretical" in the formulation of nosological categories. Such a stance is not possible given that the manual is compiled by professionals with definite opinions about the potential mechanism of mental disorders. There was nothing inherently wrong when the preparation of DSM-III was entrusted to biological psychiatrists, with a firm belief that a better understanding of the workings of the brain could unravel the pathogenesis of mental disorders. In fact, the narrative of both the DSM-III and the current DSM-5, with their standardised diagnostic categories and rigid clinical criteria, are most conducive to the empirical testing of biological correlations and treatments. What is incorrect, however, is to insist, that since 1980 and after three editions, the DSM is ideologically 'agnostic' when in fact the tendency in psychiatry is moving towards a radicalised biological approach.

In an effort to move beyond the conceptual limitations of the DSM tradition, Wakefield and First (2013) have analysed the problem as to when anxiety should be considered a mental disorder. They argue that anxiety, like other emotion, is a normal response to life events, and have suggested that there is a major overlap between the symptoms of anxiety due to life events and the symptoms of anxiety due a mental disorder, an overlap which may result in many "false" positive cases of mental disorder. In their opinion, the problem with diagnosing anxiety relates to this significant blurring of the 'boundaries' of normal and abnormal anxiety. Wakefield and First argue that their "harmful dysfunction approach" theory is helpful in setting the threshold to distinguish normal from pathological anxieties. Their approach to defining anxiety as a "disorder" requires two judgements: first, that there is an "internal dysfunction" which they define as "a failure of some psychological mechanism to perform its biologically designed function" (p. 601), and second, that this dysfunction causes "distress or impairment."

They conclude that anxiety disorders are "pathologies of biologically designed psychological systems," but acknowledge that the biological foundations of pathological anxiety remain poorly known (p. 604).[8]

First and Wakefield consider that the strategy to determine what constitutes a mental disorder involves looking for "pathosuggestive" (sic) symptoms (First and Wakefield 2013, p. 665). For instance, according to these authors, auditory hallucinations are highly pathosuggestive given that this symptom is rarely present in normal individuals. On the other hand, they consider fear and anxiety to have low "pathosuggestiveness" (p. 665) given the ubiquity of these emotions in ordinary life. First and Wakefield consider that the best strategy for increasing the accuracy of the 'normal-disordered boundary' is to increase the degree of pathosuggestiveness (p. 665). To this end, they propose several strategies. The first is the "duration and persistence" strategy (p. 666) which entails that a relatively long duration of anxiety is suggestive of dysfunction. They acknowledge that setting a threshold for duration requires the assumption that the anxiety should be out of proportion to the trigger. The second strategy involves consideration of the intensity and frequency of anxiety; and the third is considering its "disproportionality" (p. 666), that is, similarly to the case of the "duration and persistence" strategy, that the intensity of the symptom is out of proportion to the trigger. For instance, in the case of Generalised Anxiety Disorder, the DSM-5 requires excessive worry and anxiety. The problem is, again, how to determine when worrying and anxiety are excessive. The last strategy is the "pervasiveness" of anxiety, that is, that anxiety as a disorder should be manifest in a variety of contexts (p. 667).

First and Wakefield's efforts to distinguish 'normal' from 'pathological' anxiety is laudable, but fraught with conceptual limitations. Besides the problem of circularity, their 'strategies' are a euphemism for a more severe anxiety. In other words, they propose that anxieties that are of long duration, have a high frequency and intensity, are disproportionate

[8]Wakefield and First have failed to discuss the circularity in this reasoning, given that searching for the biological mechanism of anxiety as a disorder requires having a concept for the disorder to be empirically characterised.

to the stimulus, and pervasive across contexts are more suggestive of pathology (they have higher "pathosuggestiveness") that anxieties that are short, rare and of low intensity, adequate to the trigger, and present in a specific context. This is not an empirical formulation, but a pleonastic description of qualities that are internally related to the concept of pathological anxiety.

In conclusion, rather than chasing an evasive 'magical threshold' that indicates disorder, it may be more parsimonious to accept that fear and anxiety occur in life in various severities and frequencies, and that the need for treatment depends not only on a threshold, but on a host of contingent factors such as the personality and biographical attributes of individuals, contextual and cultural factors, hopes and desires, and some such, as well as the experience, knowledge and empathy of the therapist.

9.4 The Age of Anxiolytics

The concept of anxiety, understood from a psychiatric perspective, has been dramatically influenced by the irruption of medications with high efficacy to reduce anxiety states.[9] The advent of these 'anxiolytics', diluted the already porous division between the DSM classification of pathological and "unpathological" anxiety. In the USA, where the first anxiolytics such as Valium were discovered, these drugs were not only advertised for individuals meeting the DSM criteria for "Anxiety Disorder", but also marketed for the businessman after a tense day, as well as for the housewife stressed by minor problems at home. With the discovery of these medications the process of medicalization of fear and anxiety has increased exponentially. Valium was approved by the Food and Drug Administration in 1963 and became the most widely prescribed medication in the Western world between the 60s and 80s (Tone 2005). In *The Age of Anxiety* Tone wonders whether the rising

[9]The story of this development is well narrated by Andrea Tone in *The Age of Anxiety* (2009).

consumption of anxiolytics was related to a true increase in the prevalence of anxiety, or whether daily life anxieties were medicalized by the availability of such medications. She concludes that in the 50s and 60s the concept of "excessive" anxiety was mostly driven by the extraordinary consumption of anxiolytics rather than by the consensus of professional committees.[10] Furthermore, Tone raises the question as to whether the widespread use of anxiolytics in the 60s and 70s may have influenced the inclusion of the category of "Anxiety Disorders" as a separate syndrome in the DSM-III.

The use of anxiolytics is still strong in the twenty-first century. A large epidemiological study published in 2014 shows that 5% of adults in the USA filled a benzodiazepine prescription during the course of one year (Olfson et al. 2015). It has even been suggested by social scientists and sociologists that the use of anxiolytics is tantamount to a form of social control, since it is the unfavourable socio-economic conditions of most humans, rather than "inner" psychological issues, that is at the root of anxiety (Koumjian 1981). This control is exerted in a non-coercive fashion, because usually it is the anxious individual that decides in consultation with a physician for a medication to alleviate anxiety. Koumjian et al. blame the drug companies, whose interest is financial profit; the physicians, who have in the anxiolytics a simple treatment tool; and even anxious people themselves, who demand medication, whereas the structural social conflicts that produce anxiety are left unchanged (Koumjian 1981). These criticisms mainly originate among sociologists who believe that the origin of psychiatry is not explained by a biological deficit, but in social forces strongly working on the peace of mind of individuals. This social construction of anxiety will be examined next.

[10]Tone claims that the medicalization of anxiety was a 'patient-driven' phenomenon, congruent with "the American tendency to seek individual solutions" to conflicts that have a social origin (p. 6), a political and social phenomenon rather than a medical one (p. 8). I discuss the implications of these interesting remarks in the section on sociology below.

9.5 Existential Angst and Anxiety

Rollo May published in 1950 an influential work entitled *The Meaning of Anxiety*, in which he examined the phenomenon of anxiety from cultural, historical and psychological perspectives. In the Foreword to the revised edition of the work, published 27 years later, May admits that despite the "thousands" of studies and dissertations published since the first edition of his book, "our knowledge [about the causes of anxiety] has increased but we have not learned how to deal with anxiety" (p. xiii). He claims that a healthy mind bereft of anxiety reveals "a radical misperception of reality", given that some amount of anxiety is needed to fight boredom, to become more sensitive to life events, and to help in keeping oneself safe. May was among the first thinkers to discuss Kierkegaard's concept of anxiety and its relevance to understanding the complexities of this emotion. Kierkegaard's *The Concept of Anxiety* (Kierkegaard 1980) not only shaped the views of existentialist philosophers such as Sartre, Camus and Heidegger on the relevance of anxiety for human life, but also influenced social constructionism and the contemporary sociology of anxiety.[11] I will therefore make a brief excursus into this major philosophical work before moving on to discuss contemporary sociological perspectives.

9.6 Kierkegaard's *The Concept of Anxiety*

Kierkegaard's *The Concept of Anxiety*, first published in 1844 under the pseudonym, Vigilius Haufniensis, and originally translated into English in 1944 with the title *The Concept of Dread*, is a philosophical work

[11]The concept of fear and anxiety are of particular importance to existentialist philosophy, from Kierkegaard to Heidegger, Sartre and Camus. It is impossible here to do justice to this vast field. It is worth noting, however, the rich depiction of fear and anxiety in the fullest range of human behaviour, found in Camus's *The Plague*. This work has much to contribute to a descriptive account of fear. *Fear and Trembling* (1843), and Sickness unto Death (1849) are other relevant texts by Kierkegaard offering a theological view of fear and anxiety. I have decided to discuss *The Concept of Anxiety* given that this is the text where Kierkegaard presents his most elaborated conceptualisation of this emotion.

mostly dealing with the topic of 'original sin' and human guilt, but it is also a major study into the phenomenology of anxiety.[12] Already in its Introduction Kierkegaard emphasises the importance of making conceptual distinctions when discussing psychological concepts such as anxiety. He was pessimistic (like Wittgenstein a century later) about the success of teaching conceptual differences in an age in which psychological phenomena were being reduced to simple constructs amenable to scientific study.[13] Against the *zeitgeist*, Kierkegaard embarked on a major didactic work to explain different phenomenological attributes of anxiety. He traced a radical distinction between fear and anxiety, the former having a definite object, and the latter being not attached to any object or circumstance. This separation of fear from anxiety based on the presence of an object was accepted as veridical by many other thinkers from Freud to the editors of the DSMs, also including philosophers and sociologists.

9.6.1 A Religious Point of View: Anxiety as Fate or Faith

Kierkegaard considered anxiety to result from the human capacity to choose,[14] becoming "the possibility of possibility" (p. 41). Later in *The Concept of Anxiety* Kierkegaard identifies fate as another important aspect of anxiety, stating that anxiety has "nothing" for an object and that "fate…is the nothing of anxiety" (p. 97). In other words, the possibility of choosing creates anxiety, given that the outcomes of choices

---

[12]Kierkegaard certainly did not lack in personal anxiety. In his diary on 17 May 1839, he writes: "All existence makes me anxious, from the smallest fly to the mysteries of Incarnation…My distress is enormous, boundless; no one knows it except God in heaven…" (Kierkegaard 1996).

[13]"The age of making distinctions is past, it has been vanquished by the system. In our day, whoever loves to make distinctions is regarded as an eccentric whose soul clings to something that has long since vanished" (p. 4). During Kierkegaard's lifetime, there were major changes in the field of psychiatry (a term coined by Reil in 1808). This was the period when phrenology was the dominating medical influence on mental disorders. Phrenology proposed that by observing and feeling the skull, it was possible to determine an individual's psychological attributes. William James was born a few years before Kierkegaard's death, and Freud was born one year later.

[14]"Anxiety is not found in the beast" (Kierkegaard 1980, p. 41). All subsequent references to this work will be given by page number only.

are often unknown; while fate is the 'true' object of anxiety as it determines the outcome of choices. Thus, in a rather indirect way, unknown but all-knowing fate becomes a cause of anxiety and anxiety becomes central (existential) to what it is to be human. Kierkegaard's concept of anxiety is permeated by religious connotations. He argues that being anxious about one's fate is characteristic of non-believers, whereas having Christian faith is a protective factor against anxiety, as a person with faith is no longer at the mercy of fate. In this connection, Kierkegaard, despite his view that anxiety is objectless, also separates anxiety into a 'vulgar' type having for its object "something external," and an "inner" and more spiritual type, which is the product of faith (p. 155). Whereas vulgar anxiety lures humans to desire terrestrial objects, inner anxiety educates humans about the dangers of being deceived by those objects.

Although Kierkegaard articulates a distinction between anxiety and fear, the text does not offer a straightforward concept of anxiety that enables it to be readily distinguished from fear. He initially conceptualises what he terms "anxiety" in the Stoic fashion, that is, as an exercise in premeditation to prepare oneself for future mishaps (see Chapter 3). For Kierkegaard there are two ways to be anxious: one, consistent with following the wrong path in life, where anxiety is related to external factors only, and a second in which there is understanding that anxiety is produced by the fact that nothing can be demanded from life, and that anxiety lies solely with oneself, directing one towards faith (Marino 1998, p. 325). Anxiety works for Kierkegaard like a spiritual cathartic, an anxiety that "takes fate away" by bringing faith (p. 159). In this contrast between faith and fate, where faith brings joyful reconciliation with uncertainty and fate conjures the possibility of adverse uncertainty, we can appreciate Kierkegaard's dialectical approach to anxiety.[15]

According to Kierkegaard, anxiety has either positive or negative connotations depending on whether the person suffering anxiety has the gift of faith (that is, the second path described above), or is a prisoner

[15]The person who has learned to live in the anxiety of faith "will dance when the anxieties of finitude strike up the music", whereas the believers in fate will "lose their minds and courage" (p. 161).

of fate (that is, the first path, with anxiety related to externals). The person with faith will still suffer, but will be recompensed with peace of mind in the midst of the most serious troubles. On the other hand, those that rely on fate are condemned to perpetual anxiety. To conclude, Kierkegaard understands anxiety as an existential condition and places it within a religious context, as a useful tool for spiritual education, rather than being a mental disorder in need of medical treatment (Marino 1998, p. 308).

Kierkegaard considered that the state of anxiety is not fixed in time, but evolves as an intermediate step between the possibility of choosing freely and the "actuality" of expecting the outcome of the choice.[16] Anxiety ('vulgar' anxiety) may sometimes refer to past events, but only because a past misfortune may happen again (p. 91). Kierkegaard also claims that anxiety about a past deed results from the incapacity of staying in the present due to the lack of repentance regarding past faults (p. 91). Consequently, Kierkegaard's therapeutic advice is to repent of past errors and to carry on with life by staying in the present moment, thus avoiding the "dialectical" (p. 91), or in other words, the return of anxiety attached to a past fault. In this analysis sin and guilt have a crucial role in producing anxiety, as Kierkegaard relates anxiety to Adam's freedom to choose to sin. Therefore, acts of repentance should be understood against this religious framework. They are highly significant, being "in a dialectical relation to the offense" (p. 91). In other words, we may be caught between accepting punishment for a past fault and, if we do not repent, being condemned being constantly dragged along with the anxiety of the past deed. But it is important to note that Kierkegaard's advice applies to terrestrial life, since the act of repenting implies forgiving oneself, accepting the deed and its consequences, and acquiring the freedom to choose how to live.

[16]We may say that possibility is intrinsically related to choosing, or in Kierkegaard's own words "anxiety is the dizziness of freedom" (p. 60).

9.6.2 The Phenomenology of Kierkegaard's Concept of Anxiety

According to Kierkegaard, anxiety has a positive role in human life, helping to navigate the "adventure of life" as an expression of human freedom (p. 155). Anxiety is inherent in being alive, and learning how to manage anxiety may allow a person to walk the middle path between dying due to poor foresight and being crushed by paralysing fears. Kierkegaard broadens the field of anxiety by noting that this emotion can be "strange," "bashful" or even "pleasing" (p. 41). By using the derivative term "anxiousness", he stresses the temporal attributes of anxiety, ranging from acute anxiety to a pervasive state of anxiousness. Thus, "pleasing anxiousness" (p. 42) is a state of being in enthusiastic "eagerness" for a positive outcome. Kierkegaard considers this type of spirited anxiety to be common in children, especially when they are engaged in a task of discovery, and claims that what he describes as "childlike" anxiety is a culturally relevant phenomenon, whereas seeking for the "enigmatic" and "spiritual" produces the most profound and constructive anxiety. Owing to 'spiritual' anxiety, however, humans may discover "the monstrous" as well as the pleasure of deep knowledge (p. 42).[17] This knowledge is constituted in a dialectic opposition between anxiety as a vehicle of pleasure and as a depressing force, due to the realisation of the unavoidable fate of death.[18] Anxiety may also act as a motivator, allowing the possibility "to be able" to achieve one's goals once actualised by faith (p. 49). Kierkegaard's dialectical approach to anxiety is further illustrated by his view that anxiety emerges as a continuous dialogue between prohibitions and desires.[19]

---

[17]Anxiety is the key to self-knowledge, and "only a prosaic stupidity maintains that this is disorganization" (p. 42). Anxiety is a search with a clear aim, not a disorganized one or a mental disorder.

[18]"This terror is simply anxiety" (p. 45).

[19]Kierkegaard employs the term "prohibition" in the Biblical sense of a limit that awakens desire. The Biblical prohibition, says Kierkegaard, produced anxiety in Adam, "the anxious possibility of being able" (p. 44).

For Kierkegaard, the concept of anxiety will sound like "foolish talk" (p. 156) to those that have never experienced anxiety. On the other hand, those in the grip of anxiety should follow Kierkegaard's therapy of accepting the anguish produced by this emotion. Acceptance implies that anxiety educates an individual's understanding of "freedom's possibility" (p. 155), that is, the exhilarating possibility of choice. According to Kierkegaard, the only way of achieving the solace of this stage is by following a spiritual path. The person who is "educated" in faith does not escape from even the most terrifying anxiety (p. 158) but instead 'welcomes' it, being ready to suffer pain. Once the pain of anxiety is accepted, that pain will be erased.

In conclusion, Kierkegaard's *The Concept of Anxiety* demonstrates a variety of ways in which anxiety may be conceptualised. In contrast to the current reductionist approach in psychiatry, anxiety is for Kierkegaard a state with either negative or positive connotations, depending on the individual's beliefs and situations in life. Like Wittgenstein with his 'philosophical therapy', Kierkegaard provides a profound philosophical analysis of the attributes of anxiety in relation to different life situations and perspectives. Like Wittgenstein, Kierkegaard is teaching differences. Anxiety is created through the freedom to choose as well as being itself the result of choosing. Anxiety is the torture of the spiritually ignorant and the joy of the enlightened. In a word, excessive or not, anxiety is for Kierkegaard the sign of being human.

9.7 The Social Construction of Anxiety

Kierkegaard is frequently cited in the texts of dynamic psychologists who address the twentieth century as the "age of anxiety" and sociologists analysing the socioeconomic and cultural bases of anxiety (for example, May 1996; Wilkinson 2001). For the past forty years the so-called "social constructionist" model of disease has embraced the theory that pathology is produced by culturally specific processes (Conrad 2005), and more recently, an eclectic sociological approach to human fear has moved towards a synthesis between social construction, Freudian theories and, perhaps counter-intuitively in light of the previous discussion, Kierkegaard's concept of anxiety (Wilkinson 2001). An important caveat, here, is that the religious connotations in Kierkegaard's concept of anxiety have been translated into a social emphasis on safety (Mythen 2004), a step far removed from Kierkegaard's high spiritual and ethical standards. The eminent sociologists Ulrich Beck and Anthony Giddens have written extensively on the fact that the twentieth century witnessed the emergence of what is called the "age of risk," a harbinger of increasing anxiety (Beck 2009; Giddens 1990, 1991).[20] Far from Kierkegaard's understanding of the anxiety of being human (inner dread), though as part of a sociological movement that frequently references it, these authors conceptualise anxiety as being determined by powerful socioeconomic factors acting on the individual, an understanding commonly referred to under the more generic term, the 'social construction of emotions'.

Boiger and Mesquita define the "social construction of emotions" as the understanding that emotions are primarily constituted, shaped and defined by social contexts (Boiger and Mesquita 2012). They also suggest that the social construction of emotions depends on three primary situations. The first, termed "moment-to-moment interactions", refers to the fact that emotions are constructed at the time of social exchange, for instance, when I develop anxiety after a friend tells me about future job cuts in my work place. Accordingly, anxiety is shaped by present social exchanges and their future implications for the individual. The second kind of situation occurs when social interactions directly produce anxiety, and the emotion impacts, in a circular way, upon the social interaction. For instance, this occurs when my boss's actions and words make me feel continuously anxious, and my anxiety further shapes interactions with my boss. The third situation relates to specific socio-cultural contexts. Based on this perspective, social norms are the framework on which emotions are constructed and interpreted, and the defining characteristics of mental illness depend on cultural rules

[20]There is a vast literature on this subject, far beyond the scope of this work. However, for a different view, see Frank Furedi's works (2013).

concerning what is normal or abnormal (Averill 2012). For instance, anxiety may be more frequent in developing countries, where the job situation is more precarious than in developed countries. In conclusion, the social construction of emotions is considered as a dynamic process of social interaction in given socio-cultural contexts. Within this framework, the increasing use of anti-anxiety medications such as Valium is symptomatic of social construction and medicalization given that in the opinion of some sociologists this treatment only provides a temporary emotional relief without addressing the social forces that cause anxiety, such as work, family and social isolation (Koumjian 1981).

Ian Wilkinson's comprehensive sociological study of anxiety, *Anxiety in a Risk Society* (Wilkinson 2001), brings together the work of other sociologists into a thorough social constructionist approach that includes views from psychoanalysis and philosophy. Wilkinson proposes that modern societies produce feelings of insecurity about one's own identity and purpose in life, with anxiety becoming a symbol of this uncertainty. He remarks that, following Kierkegaard, anxiety results from the impossibility of escaping from the expected "course of our fate" (Wilkinson 2001, p. 17). In other words, individuals feel that they are at the mercy of whatever happens in their life, without the possibility of changing their situation. Wilkinson considers that one of the functions of anxiety is to alert humans of the fact that they are in danger. Following Freud, Wilkinson construes anxiety to be a consequence of the difficulty of knowing the cause of an "anticipated danger," and hence, the inability to effectively deal with potential dangers (Wilkinson 2001, p. 18).

Following Kierkegaard's distinction, Wilkinson conceives of fear as directed to a definite object, and anxiety as due to the unknown outcome of a feared situation. He accepts that it is difficult to separate the concepts of fear and anxiety, but in line with Freud's position, he suggests that action towards self-preservation depends on converting the uncertainty of anxiety into the certainty of fear. Thus, once the object of fear is known, anxiety is relieved.[21] In Wilkinson's view, the sociological

[21]"Where knowledge frees us from anxiety it may only bring us so far as to realise the proper identity of our fears" (Wilkinson 2001, p. 20).

causes of anxiety are frequent changes in the contexts in which humans live and in their changing social relationships, increased social pressure to decide about one's future, and the loss of communal social bonds and traditions, with the concomitant dissolution of support networks provided by traditional ways of community organization.

While the question as to whether life in pre-modern societies produced less anxiety than in contemporary western societies is anachronistic, given that feelings of insecurity have always accompanied human civilisation, nevertheless Wilkinson suggests that the increasing use of the term 'anxiety' in contemporary times denotes a new conception of this emotion, not present in earlier societies. On this basis, Wilkinson believes that there is more anxiety in contemporary society than in preceding times. He suggests that one of the main reasons for this phenomenon is that individuals in earlier societies were much more prone to display their emotions, whereas currently, emotions are more repressed, and, this repression (with a nod to Freud) results in increased anxiety. He further suggests that the impoverishment of community bonds and family relations, as well as the poor quality of social ties plays a major role in producing anxiety. Wilkinson considers the conditions of employment to be another important source of anxiety given that the stressful working conditions in contemporary societies, where, he believes, there is less opportunity to make choices about one's future, impose additional disruption on communal support. Finally, Wilkinson considers that the contemporary culture of "economic individualism" (Wilkinson 2001, p. 37), where people primarily consider their own interests, rather than those of others or of the community as a whole, is another source of anxiety. He notes, however, that this social framework is quite heterogeneous in its impacts as different socioeconomic groups have different social problems. For instance, the anxiety of the middle classes is mostly related to competition in the workplace, whereas anxiety in the working classes is associated to an increased risk of violence, poverty, and unemployment.

Based on empirical sociological studies Wilkinson concludes that high unemployment, decreased access to health care, increased job insecurity, and the increasing rate of divorce make people vulnerable to anxiety. He summarises by saying that anxiety is primarily a result of social conflicts and cultural factors, whereas problems at the individual level (such as personality traits) have a secondary role. In his opinion, anxiety construed as a psychiatric disorder only captures a fraction of those who are suffering from this emotion. Consequently, anxiety should not be conceptualised simply as an individual psychiatric condition given that this strategy is unable to encompass the social experience of distress. Arguing that social processes are critical in producing anxiety, Wilkinson suggests that the solution to anxiety does not lie in attending solely to individual personalities but in "questioning society" for appropriate socioeconomic solutions (Wilkinson 2001, p. 66). Thus, Wilkinson only accepts medical treatment of anxiety as a matter of "practical necessity" (p. 66), since the real causes of anxiety to be attended to are cultural and societal conflicts.

Wilkinson discusses empirical studies in the sociological literature showing that coping behaviours depend on an individual's socioeconomic status and type of social role. Accordingly, the capacity for coping is lowest in the lower classes and in women, who are subjected to worse quality of employment than men (Wilkinson 2001, p. 71). The significant association between economic deprivation and higher "psychosocial distress" (Wilkinson 2001, p. 71) suggests that interventions to alleviate anxiety should be aimed at changing socioeconomic policies. I shall now address the conceptual limitations of Wilkinson's approach to the social construct of fear and anxiety.

9.7.1 Conceptual Limitations of Sociological Models of Anxiety

Several of the arguments raised by Wilkinson to explain anxiety in contemporary times, such as socioeconomic inequalities, are conceptually sound and do not require critical discussion. There is no need for empirical studies to establish that limited access to health care, employment uncertainty and family crises are important causes of fear and anxiety. As previously proposed by Beck, Furedi and other sociologists, living in a society of increasing risks may also play a relevant role in causing anxiety. What is difficult to accept is his view that psychological attributes should be only of minor relevance. The correlation between anxiety and social factors is not absolute, and much of the 'noise' in this association may be explained by different 'thresholds' for developing anxiety depending on individual factors. Thus, Wilkinson is in danger of committing the same sort of error as that of the biological psychiatrists. While the latter reduce the cause of anxiety to biological mechanisms, Wilkinson largely reduces the cause of anxiety to social and cultural variables.

Radical postures on the social construction of anxiety have been criticised by other sociologists such as Williams (2000, 2003) and Francis (2007) who have warned against the extremes of the "organismic" approach of complete acceptance of the biomedical model of emotional disorders as well as the radical social construction of emotions which considers that the biomedical model of labelling moral emotions is used as a tool of social control. Francis has argued in favour of a model transcending current divisions of biological positivism versus social constructionism of emotions (Francis 2007, p. 594).

The challenge to Williams and Francis's otherwise sound proposal, however, is how this wider approach can be applied to real life. One main obstacle to this endeavour is the so-called continuous "redefinition" of anxiety (Koumjian 1981). The idea of "redefinition" is based on the fact that the concept of anxiety encompasses a range or states, from an emotion that the vast majority of people experience relatively frequently in their lives, to severe states of anxiety, in which this emotion has a profound negative impact upon individuals' lives. As already discussed, what becomes important is the vast territory lying between these extremes of anxiety and the consequent lack of a clear point of demarcation for the pathological state. "Redefinition" of anxiety occurs when people with anxieties related to daily life consult with doctors to access a pharmacological solution. Thus, day-to-day social problems are 'redefined' in terms of medical problems. As stated by Parens (2013), "It would be lovely if we could look to nature and discern the line between species-atypical and species-typical functioning, between the categories of disease and health" (p. 4). In this ideal scenario, we would "point to nature" to indicate the adequate timing for medical intervention.

Another limitation with Wilkinson's account, which extends to other sociologists such as Rollo May, is the apparently forced use of philosophical and psychoanalytical concepts on which his analysis is based. Wilkinson cites the works of Freud and Kierkegaard as providing the conceptual framework for the social construction of anxiety, but he provides no clear explanation as to how Freud's and Kierkegaard's very different frameworks 'blend' with his sociological conception of anxiety. In fact, Freud's concept of anxiety is ambiguous: he considers anxiety to be a protective factor while also medicalizing the emotion by describing anxiety neurosis as a frequent emotional disorder. Freud did not take up any social factors beyond the family circle for his account of anxiety neurosis. Kierkegaard's concept of anxiety, on the other hand, is framed within the religious concepts of sin, guilt and faith, and as discussed above, he mostly limits his analysis of anxiety to the personal existential level. Most striking is that, for Kierkegaard, it is acceptance and faith what redeems anxiety, and not ameliorative social factors.[22]

9.8 Conclusion

The main aim of this chapter was to describe the process of medicalization of fear and anxiety which took off in the early twentieth century and continues today. As a postscript to the previous chapter, I have discussed how Freud began medicalizing anxiety, with his description of a specific type of anxiety and the invention of a therapy for this condition. In the early 1950s the decision as to what counted as pathological fear and anxiety was taken over by committees of expert psychiatrists, and the age of the DSM was begun. Freud's notion of anxiety neurosis

[22]The philosopher Ian Hacking suggests a novel approach to social construction of psychiatric disorders which is not committed to either full social construction or full biological reductionism (Hacking 1999, p. 107). He advanced the concept of "interactive kinds," according to which human activity may change the context in which they are engaged, which in turn changes the way humans behave. This is contrasted with "natural kinds," a concept that includes homogeneous classes of inanimate objects. Thus, classifications in psychiatry may "change the way in which individuals experience themselves" (Hacking 1999, p. 104), which may itself change future psychiatric classifications.

was disassembled into a variety of sub-syndromes on weak conceptual and empirical bases. The reduction of conceptions of fear and anxiety to a new nosology consisting of a restricted set of criteria was accompanied by the design of biological models to explain their mechanism and treatment.

In parallel with the process of medicalization, sociologists and dynamic psychologists introduced more wide-ranging categories with their concepts of the "age of anxiety" and the "social construction of anxiety." But here again, extreme social construction falls into the same sort of mistake that is attributed to biological psychiatrists and neuroscientists, that is, the reduction of fear and anxiety to by-products of socio-cultural forces (as opposed to reduction to biological factors) while dismissing the role of personality attributes, the complex variability of contexts (internal and external), and idiosyncratic emotional responses. Sociologists have also minimised the potential of the psychopharmacological revolution, which is able to control mild to severe anxieties without the need to change social structures.

In conclusion, the radical biological approach to fear and anxiety promoted by contemporary psychiatry results in a fundamentalist approach to emotional disorders, which are all considered to be due to dysfunction of brain circuitry and genetic anomalies, with only lip service paid to contextual factors. A similar fundamentalism applies to extreme social constructionist approaches, which consider anxiety to be merely a result of socio-cultural factors, thereby ignoring personality issues. Thus, the so-called "age of risk" and "age of anxiety" give rise to therapeutic solutions that might be better characterised as part of 'the age of fundamental reductionism'.

References

American Psychiatric Association. (1952). *Diagnostic and statistical manual of mental disorders (DSM-I)* (1st ed.). Washington, DC: American Psychiatric Association Mental Hospital Service.

American Psychiatric Association. (1968). *Diagnostic and satistical manual of mental disorders (DSM-II)* (2nd ed.). Washington, DC: American Psychiatric Association.

American Psychiatric Association. (1980). *Diagnostic and statistical manual of mental disorders (DSM-III)* (3rd ed.). Washington, DC: American Psychiatric Association.

American Psychiatric Association. (1994). *Diagnostic and statistical manual of mental disorders (DSM-IV)* (4th ed.). Washington, DC: American Psychiatric Press.

American Psychiatric Association. (2013). *Diagnostic and statistical manual of mental disorders (DSM-V)* (5th ed.). Arlington, VA: American Psychiatric Association.

Andrews, G., Charney, D. S., Sirovatka, P. J., & Regier, D. A. (2009). *Stress-induced and fear circuitry disorders: Refining the research agenda for DSM-V*. Arlington: American Psychiatric Association.

Averill, J. R. (2012). The future of social constructionism: Introduction to a special section of emotion review. *Emotion Review, 4*(3), 215–220.

Beck, U. (2009). *World at risk* (C. Cronin, Trans.). Cambridge: Polity Press.

Boiger, M., & Mesquita, B. (2012). The construction of emotion in interactions, relationships and cultures. *Emotion Review, 4*(3), 221–229.

Conrad, P. (2005). The shifting engines of medicalization. *Journal of Health and Social Behavior, 46*(1), 3–14.

Dowbiggin, I. R. (2009). High anxieties: The social construction of anxiety disorders. *Canadian Journal of Psychiatry Revue Canadienne De Psychiatrie, 54*(7), 429–436.

First, M. B., & Wakefield, J. C. (2013). Diagnostic criteria as dysfunction indicators: Bridging the chasm between the definition of mental disorder and diagnostic criteria for specific disorders. *Canadian Journal of Psychiatry Revue Canadienne De Psychiatrie, 58*(12), 663–669.

Frances, A. (2013). *Saving normal*. New York: William Morrow.

Francis, L. E. (2007). Emotions and health. In J. H. Turner & J. E. Stets (Eds.), *Handbook of the sociology of emotions*. Boston: Springer.

Freud, S. (1953–1975). Inhibitions, symptoms, and anxiety (J. Strachey, Trans.). In J. Strachey (Ed.), *An autobiographical study; inhibitions, symptoms and anxiety; the question of lay analysis and other works* (Vol. 20, pp. 87–175). London: The Hogarth Press.

Furedi, F. (2013). *Authority: A sociological history*. Cambridge: Cambridge University Press.

Giddens, A. (1990). *The consequences of modernity*. Cambridge: Polity Press.

Giddens, A. (1991). *Modernity and self-identity: Self and society in the late modern age*. Cambridge: Polity Press.

Hacking, I. (1999). *The social construction of what?* Cambridge, MA: Harvard University Press.

Kierkegaard, S. (1980). *The concept of anxiety: A simple psychologically orienting deliberation on the dogmatic issue on hereditary sin* (R. Thomte & A. B. Anderson, Trans. Vol. VIII). Princeton: Princeton University Press.

Kierkegaard, S. (1996). *Papers and journals* (A. Hannay, Trans.). London: Penguin Books.

Koumjian, K. (1981). The use of Valium as a form of social control. *Social Science & Medicine. Part E: Medical Psychology, 15*(3), 245–249.

Marino, G. D. (1998). Anxiety in the concept of anxiety. In A. Hannay & G. D. Marino (Eds.), *The Cambridge companion to Kierkegaard* (pp. 308–328). Cambridge: Cambridge University Press.

May, R. (1996). *The meaning of anxiety*. New York: W. W. Norton & Co.

Mayes, R., & Horwitz, A. V. (2005). DSM-III and the revolution in the classification of mental illness. *Journal of the History of the Behavioral Sciences, 41*(3), 249–267.

Mythen, G. (2004). *Ulrich Beck: A critical introduction to the risk society*. London: Pluto Press.

Olfson, M., King, M., & Schoenbaum, M. (2015). Benzodiazepine use in the United States. *JAMA Psychiatry, 72*(2), 136–142. https://doi.org/10.1001/jamapsychiatry.2014.1763.

Parens, E. (2013). On good and bad forms of medicalization. *Bioethics, 27*(1), 28–35. https://doi.org/10.1111/j.1467-8519.2011.01885.x.

Rollin, H. R. (2003). Psychiatry in Britain one hundred years ago. *The British Journal of Psychiatry, 183*, 292–298.

Shedler, J. (2010). The efficacy of psychodynamic psychotherapy. *American Psychologist, 65*(2), 98–109. https://doi.org/10.1037/a0018378.

Starcevic, V., Portman, M. E., & Beck, A. T. (2012). Generalized anxiety disorder: Between neglect and an epidemic. *The Journal of Nervous and Mental Disease, 200*(8), 664–667. https://doi.org/10.1097/NMD.0b013e318263f947.

Tone, A. (2005). Listening to the past: History, psychiatry, and anxiety. *Canadian Journal of Psychiatry Revue Canadienne De Psychiatrie, 50*(7), 373–380.

Tone, A. (2009). *The age of anxiety: A history of America's turbulent affair with tranquilizers*. New York: Basic Books.

Wakefield, J. C., & First, M. B. (2013). Clarifying the boundary between normality and disorder: A fundamental conceptual challenge for psychiatry. *Canadian Journal of Psychiatry Revue Canadienne De Psychiatrie, 58*(11), 603–605.

Wilkinson, I. (2001). *Anxiety in a risk society*. London: Routledge.
Williams, S. J. (2000). Reason, emotion and embodiment: Is 'mental' health a contradiction in terms? *Sociology of Health & Illness, 22*(5), 559–581.
Williams, S. J. (2003). Marrying the social and the biological? A rejoinder to Newton. *The Sociological Review, 51*(4), 550–561.
Wittgenstein, L. (1967). *Zettel* (G. E. M. Anscombe, Trans.). Oxford: Blackwell.

10
Conclusions

I have examined understandings of fear through the work of western philosophers and thinkers selected based on their overall contributions to the concept and therapy of this emotion. I have discussed different perspectives, ranging from Greek Hellenistic philosophy to current neuroscience-informed biological psychiatry. The aim has not been to produce an historical review of fear, but to provide 'perspicuous presentations' from selected philosophers as well as from current psychology, the neurosciences, sociology and psychiatry. This strategy allows for fruitful comparisons of different conceptualisations of fear and how this rich variety of concepts translates into different therapeutic techniques.

A brief review of the highlights of this investigation will bring the range of different perspectives back into view.

For the hedonistic philosopher Epicurus, fear was one of the main obstacles to obtaining *ataraxia*. As we have seen the Epicurean treatment for fear requires living unnoticed, curbing human ambitions, understanding that death is the mere dissolution of atoms, and that living among friends is the best antidote against life misfortunes. Honest 'confession' of one's fears and worries to the philosopher-therapist, who will teach the techniques of concentrating on the present,

S. Starkstein, *A Conceptual and Therapeutic Analysis of Fear*,
https://doi.org/10.1007/978-3-319-78349-9_10

avoiding thinking about the future, and in times of suffering, finding refuge in sweet memories, is central to Epicurean therapy. It is delivered through simple aphorisms to memorise, rehearse, and repeat in times of hardship.

Fear and distress were also identified by Cicero as the most damaging and "bitter" of human passions. What is most important in Cicero's work is his systematic therapeutic approach to fear and distress. The philosopher becomes the physician of the soul, and both philosophy and rhetoric provide the proper remedies. Philosophy teaches that fear has deep roots, and for effecting a cure, all fears, one by one, must be turned over and investigated. Once the causes of fear are understood, rhetoric will furnish expertise in using words as potent drugs. Rhetoric will inform the philosopher which words to choose, how to best convey the message, and, most importantly, to select the proper time (*kairos*) to deliver the treatment. The final aim of the Ciceronian philosophical therapy is to empower individuals to become their own therapists in managing fear and distress.

A century later, Seneca borrows from both Epicurus and Cicero for his broad approach to fear. As a Stoic, Seneca promotes a virtuous lifestyle and self-examination as the main remedies against fear. The Stoic sage has no fear, only caution. But Seneca understands that the Stoic remedy is for the very few, and for most humans he recommends an eclectic and non-dogmatic selection of remedies, from the sheltered Epicurean life to the Cyrenaic dampening of fear by pre-rehearsing misfortunes. Even more important is the fact that Seneca's writings are already therapeutic in that the letters are directed to readers, who have the opportunity to identify their own fears with those discussed by Seneca, and thereby to benefit from his therapeutic advice. This technique of therapeutic writing and reading reached its pinnacle with Michel de Montaigne, who made himself and his many fears, the main object of study. Nothing is hidden in his *Essays*; all sorts of fears criss-cross the text, and Montaigne presents different therapies he has tried on others but especially on himself. Montaigne's fears were unmoved by even the best Ciceronian remedies, and after sampling remedies from different Hellenistic schools, Montaigne embarked in a dialectical exploration that allowed the design of his own therapy. This included understanding the limitations of the Stoic eradication of emotions to be practiced in life; the difficulty of suppressing the fear of death based on the Epicurean concept of death as dissolution into atoms; and assenting to the Sceptic stance that there may be no 'definite' therapy for fears. These understandings provided Montaigne with the necessary freedom to implement those remedies that suited him best, such as accepting that misfortunes of life are intrinsic to being human, understanding and accepting one's limitations to face fear, and enjoy what is at hand.

Montaigne's renaissance humanism is followed by the materialism of the seventeenth century, based on significant discoveries in human physiology and the need for political guidance to states at risk of social dissolution. It is in the context of social turmoil that Hobbes proposes a political system based on fear. Hobbes considers that enforcing social fear is the best 'therapy' to strengthen a sovereign. There is no better emotion than fear to subdue individuals under a powerful ruler. In parallel, Descartes developed a mechanism for the emotions that, after several iterations, would interest physicians and scientists during the latest two centuries. Common to both Hobbes and Descartes are reductive accounts of human fear: in the case of Hobbes, fear becomes a generic emotion amenable to political manipulation; for Descartes, it becomes a secondary emotion resulting from a dualist mechanism amenable to physiological experimentation.

The twentieth century witnessed major changes in the conceptualisation of fear. Reductive accounts were overwhelmingly accepted, undermining the complexity and depth of fear and related emotions, and understandings of their specificity in different contexts and individuals, to the detriment of their therapy. In line with Descartes's mechanistic approach to the emotions, William James argued that fear was a reflex response to the perception of visceral changes, thereby paving the way for the endeavours of the contemporary cognitive neuroscience focus on finding a brain circuitry mediating fear. Following James, fear became primarily reduced to a fight/flight response, identifiable in the brain, and this sort of understanding is later generalised to account for a generic type of human fear. Major conceptual problems with this strategy are overlooked, but this empirical approach continues to be the predominant paradigm in current psychiatric endeavours, which aim at treating fear by 'tuning' a malfunctioning 'fear brain circuit'.

A second reduction, influential the twentieth century, was Freud's conceptualisation of fear and anxiety as products of inadequately processed libidinal impulses, or later, from a return to primitive experiences of abandonment. Freud's psychoanalytical therapy consisted in a technique of bringing unconscious fears (about libidinal repression or infant memories) to consciousness for proper processing. As we have seen, Freud's theories of fear and anxiety are also marred by serious conceptual shortcomings. Further, the discovery of medications that could relieve fear and anxiety in a matter of days, and the predominance of biological psychiatry in current nosologies, signalled the demise of psychoanalysis. From a different angle, a third reductive development, according to which fear is understood as resulting from social forces acting on the individual emerged. The 'social construction' of emotions, mainly proposed by sociologists, is directly opposed to the biological reduction of psychiatry. Whereas social factors are certainly relevant, they cannot fully account for all fear-related behaviours and feelings because different people respond to social triggers in their own idiosyncratic ways, influenced by the myriad of factors that shape their personalities.

Against these relentless reductions of fear in the last few centuries, not only have the insights of the humanistic tradition been overlooked, but the more elaborated, comprehensive and didactic concepts of fear proposed by Kierkegaard and Wittgenstein have been given scant attention. Kierkegaard described anxiety as both oppressive and liberating. Oppressive fear arises from our attitudes to externals and vulnerability to fate, whereas liberating fear relates to faith, elevating the individual to a state that transcends earthly misfortunes. Wittgenstein provided a therapeutic "prelude" (Hutto 2009, p. 207) by clarifying conceptual knots in the understanding of fear, showing, against Freud that emotions are not purely inner hidden phenomena, but that fear is interwoven with human life, an emotion in constant flux, manifested in severities that range from almost inconspicuous states to paralysing terror. Wittgenstein teaches differences in the subtleties of motivations, contexts and personalities that shape fear, also stressing that fear relates to a variety of emotions connected by 'family resemblance' (Wittgenstein 1980). These efforts notwithstanding, the dominant contemporary concept of fear navigates between the Scylla of biological psychiatry and the Charybdis of social construction. It is paradoxical that after all the progress in the neurosciences and social sciences of fear in the last century, we are often seen to be living in a "risk society" in an "age of stress and anxiety" (Beck 2009; Dunant and Porter 1996; Jackson 2013), and that research on the brain mechanisms of fear and anxiety "have been disappointing as a source for novel treatments" (LeDoux and Pine 2016).

The oversight provided by these different understandings of fear and its therapies reflects my preference for a broad perspective on different aspects of fear and for empowering individuals in active participation in their own therapeutic process. This kind of understanding was variously argued for by the Hellenistic philosophers, Montaigne, Kierkegaard and Wittgenstein. However, I do not advocate for an anachronistic return to ancient remedies; that would contradict the insights relating to the careful consideration of changing differences, times and contexts that they championed. Rather, by setting out these different understandings it is possible to see how their concepts may be philosophically re-elaborated for delivering better therapies and further philosophical and empirical investigation.

References

Beck, U. (2009). *World at risk* (C. Cronin, Trans.). Cambridge: Polity Press.

Dunant, S., & Porter, R. (1996). *The age of anxiety*. London: Virago Press.

Hutto, D. D. (2009). Lessons from Wittgenstein: Elucidating folk psychology. *New Ideas in Psychology, 27*, 197–212.

Jackson, M. (2013). *The age of stress*. Oxford: Oxford University Press.

LeDoux, J. E., & Pine, D. S. (2016). Using neuroscience to help understand fear and anxiety: A two-system framework. *American Journal of Psychiatry, 173*(11), 1083–1093. https://doi.org/10.1176/appi.ajp.2016.16030353.

Wittgenstein, L. (1980). *Culture and value* (P. Finch, Trans.). Chicago: The University of Chicago Press.

References

Index

S. Starkstein, *A Conceptual and Therapeutic Analysis of Fear*,
https://doi.org/10.1007/978-3-319-78349-9

The manufacturer's authorised representative in the EU is Springer Nature Customer Service Centre GmbH, Europaplatz 3, 69115 Heidelberg, Germany. If you have any concerns regarding our products, please contact ProductSafety@springernature.com

Printed and bound by CPI Group (UK) Ltd, Croydon, CR0 4YY
30/09/2026
02225195-0005